ROGER STEVENSON
FEBRUARY, 1995

OVER 55

a handbook on health

Edited by Theodore G. Duncan, M.D.
Illustrations by Joyce Richman

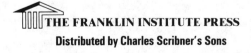THE FRANKLIN INSTITUTE PRESS

Distributed by Charles Scribner's Sons

Current printing (last digit):
5 4 3 2 1

Library of Congress Cataloging in Publication Data
Main entry under title:
    Over 55: A Handbook on Health.

Includes index.
1. Geriatrics. 2. Aging. 3. Gerontology. I. Duncan,
Theodore, G. [DNLM: 1. Aging—Handbooks. WT 104 096]
RC952.5.094 618.97 81-2134
ISBN 0-89168-031-4 AACR2

Printed in the United States of America

CONTENTS

PREFACE

Realizing the increasing needs of our population 55 years and over, the Director of The Franklin Institute Press asked that I gather together a group of experts to explain in an understandable manner some medical, social, emotional, financial and legal matters that concern this age group. It was impossible to record all the problems and solutions, but during discussions with Lynn Hubschman, Director of the Social Service Department, Pennsylvania Hospital, important topics were selected to enrich and support the portion of our population that has successfully completed the stages of childhood, adolescence and early adult life.

Never has there been gathered together in one volume so much information concerning these major issues of living. The selection of authors was relatively easy since an abundance of expert medical talent exists at the Pennsylvania Hospital, Philadelphia, our nation's first hospital. We are indebted to the contributing authors, all authorities in their specific areas of interest, for their cooperation, enthusiasm and patience. We hope that not only the person age 55 and over and those preparing for this age group will benefit, but also support groups of specialists, for example, social service workers, physicians, clergy, government health providers, will glean information about people entering the maturing years.

I specifically wish to acknowledge my gratitude and deep appreciation to the following: Joyce Richmond, artist, for her devoted interest and her ability to interpret doctors' ideas and record them in a pictorial form to convey specific ideas; to Margaret Bossard for precise and diligent work in keeping track of the authors, mailings, manuscripts, proofs, etc.; and to Christine Schwenk, our executive secretary, whose skill permitted us to take on the additional tasks of editing this book in conjunction with running an active medical practice.

I express my sincere appreciation to the staff of The Franklin Institute Press for their invaluable assistance in every area of this undertaking.

Theodore G. Duncan, M.D.

FOREWORD

Hugh Downs

It may not be obvious, but there is a dynamic change taking place in our population today. We are moving from a youth-dominated culture to one more oriented toward our maturing citizens. Right now in America there are 40 million people age 55 and over; beyond the year 2000, women over 65 years of age will be the largest segment of our population.

People over 55 don't necessarily decline at retirement age: Some are vigorous; many are skilled, intelligent and capable of starting new occupations, new businesses. More wisdom and freedom are available. These mature years often provide more security since the awkward stresses of adolescence, the hardships of getting ahead in business, and the growing pains of nurturing children through their problems have faded away. The mature years can be pleasant. There is time to savor talent and the joys of achievement and position. Age itself is an accomplishment; it is sign and proof of one's triumph over problems.

This expanding group of our population has somewhat different medical, emotional, financial, and social needs, from those it had earlier. The authors of this book, mostly physicians from Pennsylvania Hospital, Philadelphia, have presented in a clear, concise, and factual manner a review of the medical problems of patients over age 55. Specialists discuss signs, symptoms and methods of evaluation and treatment of the common maladies. They review information concerning other basic needs — for example, the social adjustment involved in living alone or living with someone new and the emotional crises one can encounter in life. The chapter about fraud points out how vulnerable one can be and how one can be protected. Other information includes financial planning, social security benefits, and insurance.

This volume will benefit not only those preparing for 55 over, but also those who deal professionally with this age group — including clergymen, social service workers, nurses, health administrators, and others.

Realize that terms such as "elderly," "senior citizens," "golden agers" are really destructive and undesirable, although they were euphemisms originally designed to offset the pejorative connotation of the word "old" by a thoughtless society. When we treat our elders (not "elderly") fairly, there will be no need of euphemisms. Arriving at an age that is "old" will become a matter of pride. We are not programmed for obsolescence and senility at age 65. It is better to realize that "old" is beautiful and that by remaining active, viable, and dynamic, the years after 55 can be the most rewarding of our entire life.

ARTHRITIS

Barry M. Schimmer, M.D.

Head, Rheumatology Section, Pennsylvania Hospital
Assistant Professor of Medicine, University of Pennsylvania
School of Medicine

Arthritis is the nation's leading crippling disease, second only to heart disease as a cause of prolonged disability. At present, 31.6 million Americans have arthritis. Approximately 16 million have osteoarthritis, caused by injury or a natural consequence of aging, 6.5 million have potentially deforming rheumatoid arthritis, 1.6 million have gout, and the rest have other forms of the disease. Estimates indicate at least one million new victims each year, and 7.3 million arthritics are now disabled. As the population ages, these figures can be expected to increase, since virtually everyone who lives to a ripe old age will develop arthritis in some form. Yet the majority of arthritics are under 65 years of age, including 250,000 children. For reasons not fully understood, arthritis strikes women twice as often as men.

The human cost of arthritis is even more staggering than the size of the afflicted population. These rheumatic diseases cause more suffering by more people for longer periods than any other group of related illnesses. They seldom kill, taking their toll in a more insidious fashion that can lead to crippling. Added to disability are the countless days of pain, limitation of activity, and the incalculable effect on the social and economic aspects of life. It has been remarked that rheumatic diseases do not impose a death sentence, but imprison a patient for life. Capabilities usually taken for granted are diminished as movements become painfully difficult and slow.

While arthritis is the leading chronic illness, it should be emphasized that the overwhelming majority of arthritics do well with their handicaps, leading normal lives, holding down jobs, and enjoying leisure activities. Much like hypertension and diabetes, for which there are also no rapid cures, arthritis is treated by control and management. In addition, many rheumatic diseases are subject to spontaneous remissions and exacerbations that are wholly unpredictable. Therefore, patients are guided through periods of active disease in anticipation of natural abatement.

As the economic burden of arthritis continues to grow, much attention has focused on medical costs, especially hospital expense. But the financial strains are not restricted entirely to the direct costs of hospitalization, physicians' fees, drugs, and X rays. There are also the indirect costs of lost income and non-financial deprivation due to disability and death. Although the money figures provide a basis for estimating the impact of illness on the economy, they offer little insight into the true cost to the individual.

Based upon recent government surveys, direct annual costs of arthritis include $1.6 billion in hospitalization and $860 million for physician office visits. Advances in pharmacology have sent the costs of prescription drugs soaring to over $1.25 billion. Especially alarming, however, is the nearly $1 billion spent on quackery in the treatment of arthritis. Long-term sufferers of diseases for which there is no immediate cure are understandably attracted by claims of new miracle remedies. To combat such quackery, the Arthritis Foundation allocates a significant portion of its annual budget to investigate innumerable questionable treatments. None of the claims of success for medicaments, herbs, vitamins, diet, pendants—or even acupuncture—has withstood the rigorous test of controlled study. With "evidence" largely attributable to the placebo effect (which can sometimes bring real relief to those who expect it strongly enough) and to the inherent variability of the symptoms of most forms of arthritis, benefit has been claimed for remedies ranging from bee venom to sarsaparilla tea.

The indirect costs of medical care now assume greater importance in a society struggling with endless inflation. It is estimated that more than $4.5 billion per year is lost in wages and over $1 billion in homemakers' services. One billion dollars is expended for disability insurance payments. A recent study of chronic disease costs showed that direct medical expenses to the patients of rheumatoid arthritis were three times the national average, and only 58 percent of this was covered by insurance. Indirect costs related to lost income totaled three times the direct medical costs, averaging $7,711 among wage earners and $3,958 among housewives. Studies also show that economic stresses of chronic rheumatoid arthritis are not restricted to lower socioeconomic groups, but spread evenly over a broad range of social class and income. While attempts have been made at the national level to cope with the rising direct costs of medical care, little effort has so far been made to alleviate the related, but equally costly, problems involving employment of the disabled.

Another factor complicating the delivery of care to arthritis sufferers is that most internists and family practitioners lack formal training in rheumatology, and the approximately 3000 rheumatology specialists now practicing in the United States are mostly clustered in major urban centers out of reach of many who need their services. Expansion of rheumatology training programs and national support for their activities merit a high legislative priority.

Facts About Arthritis

Definition

Arthritis means inflammation of a joint. A joint is the meeting point, usually movable, between two or more bones. The most familiar joints are those of the small bones of the hands and feet and of the larger bones of the wrists, elbows, shoulders, hips, knees, and ankles. Other joints are located in the jaw (*temporomandibular*), along the spine between the vertebrae, and in the front of the chest where the ribs join the breast bone. The ends of the bones are covered by smooth cartilage that provides a low friction surface for motion and weight bearing. The joint is lined by a thin membrane, the *synovium,* that produces a lubricating fluid and nourishes the cartilage. A normal functioning joint requires the structural integrity of all key elements including the synovium, cartilage, bone, and the *capsule* surrounding the joint.

Rheumatism is an indefinite term used to describe various painful conditions in the joints, muscles, and fibrous connective tissues. Even rheumatologists do not agree on a precise definition. In Great Britain, for example, "rheumatism" includes most forms of arthritis. In the United States, however, "arthritis" is the more general term, and includes rheumatism as well as other conditions.

Whenever a joint is injured or inflamed, it may swell and become painful, warm, and stiff. The general term "arthritis" reveals little about the specific cause or form. More than one hundred separate varieties of arthritis are now differentiated according to combinations of patient age, the pattern of affected joints, associated medical features, X-ray appearances, and laboratory tests. Arthritis can be episodic, unpredictable, and chronic. An attack may come with no warning or precipitating event, and years may elapse between recurrences. For many victims, arthritis is little more than an occasional nuisance, while others must endure years of almost continuous suffering and disability. The skilled rheumatologist and internist can distinguish the specific nature of the illness from its onset, progression, related clinical features, and appropriate tests.

Inflammation is an important process that occurs in most forms of arthritis, representing the body's mobilization of its defenses in response to injury. The cardinal signs of inflammation are heat, redness (*erythema*), tenderness, pain, and loss of joint mobility. In arthritis due to bacterial infection, the body's responses help to contain and kill the bacteria, while for many other types of arthritis, the cause and its relation to inflammation are unknown. It is clear, however, that prolonged inflammation liberates substances that harm the joint. The damage may result in more pain, stiffness, and restricted motion.

People often compare their own symptoms with those of a relative or friend with diagnosed arthritis and assume that they have the same disease and that it will take the same course or respond to the same treatment. Such generalizations are misleading. Just as it is foolhardy to look for a number in a telephone directory without knowing the spelling of a name, it is inadvisable to treat arthritis without first making a specific diagnosis. Several rheumatic processes can produce similar symptoms in a joint but are actually different disorders affecting surrounding structures such as tendons, bursae, and ligaments. The familiar bursitis and tendinitis are usually local afflictions, often related to overuse of a joint or minor injury, and will not exhibit the progression, spread, and deformity of some forms of arthritis.

For example, viruses can generate an acute but transient arthritis of several joints at once that subsides spontaneously without harmful aftereffects. There are no specific treatments, since antibiotics are ineffective for viruses. Arthritis may also accompany other viral infections such as *rubella* (German measles), *rubeola* (measles), mumps, and hepatitis B. Vaccines specific for particular viruses may reduce the frequency of associated arthritis. Arthritis associated with bacterial infection is a more serious problem and a medical emergency because delay in accurate diagnosis and treatment may allow the products of inflammation to irreversibly injure the cartilage and bony surfaces of a joint. However, prompt treatment with appropriate antibiotics usually results in permanent cure.

In other instances, arthritis may be a clue to an undiagnosed medical condition that requires separate analysis and treatment. For example, arthritis may accompany inflammatory bowel disease (ulcerative colitis), sickle cell disease, endocrine disorders such as hypothyroidism and hyperparathyroidism, or may be the first indication of an undetected tumor. On the other hand, certain forms of arthritis may produce inflammation in other organs such as the skin, mucous membranes, eyes, lungs, bowel, and kidney. The rheumatologist must elicit a complete history and perform a detailed physical examination to arrive at an accurate diagnosis. X rays and laboratory tests such as analysis of synovial fluid taken from the joint also help to establish a diagnosis. A joint tap for synovial fluid should be routine for most types of arthritis when fluid is available. Someone with an apparently isolated rheumatic problem should not be surprised or perturbed if the physician directs a great deal of attention to the overall medical picture.

Misconceptions

Although arthritis may begin insidiously with minor discomforts, gradual but irreversible deformity is possible, often developing so slowly that the victim is unaware of it. For this reason, a rheumatologist - internist should be consulted to detect the subtle changes and to guide therapy.

Some people fail to seek medical attention because "it is widely known that there is no cure for arthritis." This is untrue. For infectious arthritis, a total cure is possible. For gouty arthritis, symptoms can be relieved and recurrences prevented. Even chronic rheumatoid arthritis is subject to spontaneous remission. Rest, a supporting splint, and the use of anti-inflammatory drugs often ease the discomfort. The beneficial effects of a new class of drug—slow-acting anti-rheumatics—may closely resemble spontaneous remission of rheumatoid arthritis in up to 60 percent of patients.

Early treatment and faithful adherence to home therapy programs give the best chance for success. Even if joints are significantly damaged, a variety of rehabilitative measures including reconstructive surgery can restore function in many cases.

"Diet is the answer for arthritis." Considering the many forms of arthritis, diet is hardly a panacea. Except in gouty arthritis, there is no proof that an excess or deficiency of any substance is a critical factor in making the disease better or worse. Even in gout, diet alone sometimes contributes to rather than causes acute attacks. Nothing that is eaten will cause arthritis or do harm to joints, nor will fad diets, vitamins, honey, or vinegar help arthritis sufferers except as a placebo.

"Arthritics should move to a warm and dry climate." Most rheumatologists discourage such a move, although many people with rheumatic diseases are good barometers and feel more achey and stiff when damp weather approaches. However, there is no proof that weather and climate influence the course of arthritis. If the disease is active and progressive, it is likely to be so anywhere.

"It is proper to treat oneself for arthritis." This is dangerous. Quack remedies are not effective and merely allow serious joint damage to proceed unchecked. Also, the interaction between drugs will not be monitored. Anti-inflammatory drugs can interfere with diuretics, anticoagulants, and oral diabetes medications, and may be harmful to patients with heart disease or peptic ulcers. The best course is to seek proper medical care and to do so early.

Arthritis Warning Signals

Several warning signs may indicate a rheumatic disease. Among them are the following:

- Persistent pain or stiffness in a joint or the spine.

- Pronounced stiffness in the morning or after a period of sitting or lying in one position

- Swelling or redness of a joint

- Recurrent pains in joints or muscles

- Joint discomfort accompanied by other general symptoms such as fever, weakness, lassitude, poor appetite, and weight loss

Types and Treatment of Arthritis

Rheumatoid Arthritis

Rheumatoid arthritis (RA) is the most common of the inflammatory types. It strikes women much more than it does men. The incidence of onset rises to a peak at two age periods, the 30's and the 50's, but the disease can occur at any age from early childhood to extreme old age. It is a relatively recent disease in mankind's experience, and was relatively unknown before the 18th century.

The onset is usually gradual and deceptive. Pain, stiffness, and swelling may occur in a joint, last just a few days, then reappear later in the same or a different place. After a brief period, the disease becomes established, primarily in the small joints of the hands and feet, and in the wrists, shoulders, hips, and knees, usually in the same joints on both sides of the body. Most joints are vulnerable, including those in the neck and jaw, but joints in the lower spine and ends of the fingers are spared. In some victims it is explosively acute, and in others it involves only one joint (monoarthritis) for a long time before the more characteristic features appear. A period of six weeks is usually required before diagnosis can exclude transient forms of arthritis.

Above all, rheumatoid arthritis is a systemic disease, meaning that patients feel generally unwell, and often have a low-grade fever, malaise, diminished appetite, anemia, and weight loss. Pronounced morning stiffness and pain lasting at least one hour are common. Joint tissues also stiffen following a period of inactivity during the day, for example, making it difficult to rise from a chair after long sitting. This eases with resumption of activity.

The course of rheumatoid arthritis is largely unpredictable. Ten percent of all patients experience only one prolonged attack during a lifetime, but most develop a chronic arthritis subject to spontaneous remission and exacerbation. No two cases are ever exactly the same. In juvenile rheumatoid arthritis, the remission rate is much greater, and many young victims enter adulthood with only minor residual effects.

Parts of the body other than the joints may be affected. Approximately 20 percent of rheumatoid arthritics develop firm nodules under the skin, especially over the elbows or other bony prominences, or in tendon sheaths of the hands and feet. These are esthetically unpleasant and sometimes ulcerate or become infected, but usually do not lead to disability. Infrequently, rheumatoid inflammation may affect the eyes, lungs, and peripheral nervous system and enlarge lymph glands, the liver, and the spleen.

Although several factors have been known to precede its onset, the ultimate cause of rheumatoid arthritis remains unknown. Many of its victims have a history of severe emotional disturbance or physical injury, while others have enjoyed good health and a stable emotional background before the onset of the disease. Infections by viruses, bacteria, and other organisms have been suspected, but research has not supported the suspicions. There has been speculation that the cause may be a slow-acting virus not detectable by current test methods because it merges with the genetic elements of the body's cells. In recent studies a genetic tendency has emerged in the development of rheumatoid arthritis. This tendency, coupled with certain as yet unknown environmental factors, may trigger the expression of the disease.

Whatever the cause, physicians and scientists can describe in detail the steps leading to joint damage. it appears that the inflammation in the joint lining (synovium) is self-perpetuating. An immune reaction in the lining produces certain proteins—antibodies—which react with other proteins—antigens—to form complexes that attract white blood cells to the joint. The accumulating mass can be felt as boggy, swollen synovial tissue in the joint. The white blood cells that engulf the antibody-antigen complex release enzymes that can damage cartilage, bone, tendon, and the joint capsule. The result is loss of function, partial dislocation (*subluxation*), and deformity, appearing as loss of grip strength in the hand, improper alignment of joints, a drawing back of the fingers, inability to extend a hip or knee, and painful prominences over the balls of the feet. Inflammation, normally protective, becomes destructive and attacks the body's own tissues.

For this reason, rheumatoid arthritis is classified as an autoimmune disease. The inflammation involves a bewildering series of chain reactions in which several classes of immune competent cells (*lymphocytes*) participate. Two destructive chemicals formed in the process are *collagenases* (enzymes that degrade the structural protein *collagen*) and *prosta-glandins* (fatty acid molecules that increase inflammation and dissolve the mineral of bone). By identifying these substances, scientists hope to learn enough about rheumatoid arthritis to intervene with new drug therapy.

Although rheumatoid arthritis is not directly inherited, the misguided immune system may be genetically determined, predisposing some people to rheumatoid disease when certain environmental factors are present. Genetic susceptibility to rheumatic disease was first detected in studies of *ankylosing spondylitis,* a disease in which over 95 percent of patients were found to have the genetic marker HLA B27 on their white blood cells, as measured by a simple blood test. A different HLA marker has now been detected in 40 percent of rheumatoid arthritics. This test is still experimental and not yet routinely available to physicians. Caution is necessary because not all patients with rheumatoid arthritis have the marker, nor does everyone with the marker develop arthritis. However, a blood test can reveal a possible susceptibility to the disease. The susceptible individual can then be more alert to the onset of symptoms and seek early treatment.

Treatment of Rheumatoid Arthritis and Related Disorders

Therapy for rheumatoid arthritis involves a comprehensive plan to reduce the inflammation, relieve pain, prevent deformity, and restore joint function. Many of the principles applied to rheumatoid arthritis are also applicable to other types of arthritis.

Treatment involves professional teamwork. Basic care begins with the family physician or internist and extends to rheumatologists and orthopedic surgeons for primary treatment or consultation. Physical and occupational therapists and visiting nurses help with exercise, muscle strengthening, mechanical aids, and nursing services. Social workers help with home arrangements, homemaker services, transportation to physicians' offices, clinics, and therapy sessions, and advise patients about medical insurance coverage. A vocational counselor can assist in job retraining programs. Many large medical centers have arthritis or rheumatology clinics to meet all the needs of rheumatoid arthritics, thus saving them many extra trips for comprehensive care. The Arthritis Foundation has organized an Allied Health Professions Section to train members and disseminate information throughout the country.

Rest is important for all types of arthritis, whether bedrest for the systemically ill who have fever, weakness, and stiffness, or rest of a single inflamed joint supported by a temporary splint. The physician may advise hospitalization for a first onset of rheumatoid disease or for subsequent severe episodes. Merely removing someone with rheumatoid arthritis from the stresses of everyday life can help to ease symptoms. Hospitalization also offers an opportunity for patient education. Most rheumatologists agree that patients who understand the nature of their illness and its treatment are better able to deal with the disease activity. Highly motivated patients deal more effectively with their disease and generally gain better results than those who are neglectful and apathetic.

Aspirin (acetylsalicylic acid) is the single most effective drug for rheumatoid arthritis and many related illnesses. However, a misunderstanding of this simple, time-tested drug often causes it to be misused or overlooked. Some skeptics ask, How can it be useful if everyone can obtain it without a prescription? Isn't aspirin dangerous for the stomach? Since the primary goal in treating rheumatoid arthritis is to reduce inflammation and to alleviate pain, aspirin is an excellent drug because it is both anti-inflammatory and pain-relieving. Although low doses are suitable for a headache or common cold, an anti-inflammatory effect requires 12 to 24 tablets per day to build up an effective aspirin level in the blood.

If the drug is discontinued, it is completely eliminated through the kidneys within 48 hours with no long-term residue. Aspirin treats symptoms and helps arthritics to feel better and to perform exercises more easily. The quantity of aspirin needed varies with the individual and should be decided by a physician. Easy access to aspirin should not be considered an invitation to self-medication. Self-medication is to be avoided because unsupervised administration of large doses of aspirin can be dangerous.

Large doses of aspirin may produce ringing in the ears (*tinnitus*) or a mild hearing loss. This is neither serious nor permanent, and merely indicates that a therapeutic level has been reached. Such symptoms can be diminished by reducing the dosage by a few tablets a day. Unfortunately, the level at which side effects occur tends to be lower in older individuals, who may have toxic reactions at less than a therapeutic dosage. Aspirin may also irritate the stomach, aggravate an ulcer, and, in rare cases, cause internal bleeding. These effects on the stomach can be reduced by taking the aspirin with food or milk, or by using buffered or coated aspirin. Aspirin may also interact with anticoagulant and diabetes medications. Those who cannot tolerate aspirin can take salicylate-related compounds, such as choline or choline magnesium trisalicylate, that seem to have fewer gastric side effects and interfere less with blood clotting.

It is well to ignore advertising claims for effective treatment of arthritis by combination drugs containing "the agent doctors most often prescribe." This is merely aspirin sold at much higher cost. Also, acetominophen compounds may relieve headaches, but lack anti-inflammatory properties and are therefore not a suitable substitute for aspirin in arthritis treatment.

Non-Steroidal Anti-inflammatory Drugs So-called non-steroidal anti-inflammatory drugs (NSAID), developed to treat rheumatoid and other types of arthritis, are safe and effective, and comparative studies show them to be equivalent to high-dose aspirin for this purpose. Their advantages are reduced side effects—less nausea, heartburn, and hearing noises—and they are often effective in lower doses given less often than aspirin. They are sold under the generic names of fenoprofen, ibuprofen, naproxen, sulindac, and tolmetin. Although they have occasionally been marketed with extravagant claims, they are not major breakthroughs in the treatment of arthritis. Since the NSAID's are relatively costly, aspirin is often recommended first, and one of the newer drugs is tried only if aspirin is not effective or is poorly tolerated.

Indomethacin and phenylbutazone are other NSAID's available for treatment of arthritis and some inflammatory rheumatic conditions such as bursitis and tendinitis. Indomethacin in a nightly dose occasionally helps to reduce morning stiffness. Both drugs are effective in treating gout and ankylosing spondylitis, but have potential side effects that should be monitored by a physician.

Corticosteroids When corticosteroids were introduced more than 25 years ago, they were widely believed to be the cure for rheumatoid arthritis. Some arthritics confined to wheelchairs walked for the first time in years, while others experienced dramatic relief of pain, swelling, and stiffness. Time has shown, however, that steroids can be a greater enemy than the disease itself.

Since steroids do not alter the underlying disease, joint damage may continue despite the patient's feeling of well-being. Many patients eventually revert to their original condition while on steroids, but then can not be weaned away from their use. The side effects of long-term use of steroids are numerous and disabling. They may include, among others, excessive weight gain, aggravation of diabetes or hypertension, thinning of bone (*osteoporosis*) and skin, peptic ulcers, and cataracts. Small doses of steroids are occasionally required for disease control, but are always given with caution in minimal doses gradually reduced to zero as soon as possible. Sparing use of steroid injections into an inflamed joint may bring temporary relief, but repeated use is avoided.

Slow-acting Anti-rheumatic Drugs   Slow-acting drugs developed specifically for treatment of rheumatoid arthritis take several months to reach full effectiveness, unlike the faster aspirin, NSAID's, and steroids, but have an effect that resembles a spontaneous remission. Improvement is gradual at a barely perceptible pace, but even after discontinuation of the drugs their benefit may last for months. Because all of the drugs in this category have potential side effects, they are not given routinely at the first sign of rheumatoid arthritis. Only those who fail to respond to a conservative program of rest, physical therapy, and standard anti-inflammatory drugs, are considered eligible, especially if progressive disease threatens new joint erosion or early deformity. About 75 percent benefit from the drugs, but success or failure cannot be predicted beforehand.

Gold Salts   For more than 50 years, gold salts have been used to treat rheumatoid arthritis. Gold seems to be effective at several stages of the inflammation but no one knows exactly how. In the past, dosages and monitoring schedules were not standardized. Today, drug administration is more precise and gold is now a popular and safe medication when given by an experienced physician. Prior to each dose, patients are interviewed for symptoms of a toxic reaction, a blood sample is taken for a cell count, and urine is tested for protein. Gold is withheld if there is an indication of danger.

At present, gold can be given only by weekly injection into a muscle, but an oral preparation is being tested and may become available. A series of injections is given for 20 weeks, and the frequency is then reduced to monthly maintenance injections.

Penicillamine Another newly released slow-acting drug for rheumatoid arthritis is penicillamine, which is similar to gold in action and toxicity. It can be taken by mouth, but must be monitored with frequent blood and urine tests. One out of five patients is unable to complete treatment with gold or penicillamine because of side effects. However, early recognition reduces serious reactions so that the risks are warranted by the potential benefits.

Antimalarials Derived from quinine, antimalarials can be effective in rheumatoid arthritis and are also used to treat systemic *lupus erythematosus*. Use of these drugs is usually monitored with an eye examination every six months because of a rare but possible side effect on the eyes.

Cytotoxic Drugs Cytotoxic drugs are potent suppressors of the body's immune system which have been used in organ transplantation to prevent rejection and in cancer chemotherapy. They have been found effective in selected cases of severely progressive rheumatoid arthritis, but are still classed as experimental because they await formal approval by the Food and Drug Administration. Since they are potent and toxic, they must be given with extreme caution and with fully informed patient consent. They should also be given only by a fully qualified rheumatologist, preferably as part of a properly planned research program.

New drugs for treating rheumatoid arthritis can be expected in the near future. Some are likely to be similar to presently available medication, and others may represent new classes with different physiological effects. Many will probably also be useful for treating osteoarthritis, gout, and such non-joint inflammations as bursitis and tendinitis. One, named levamisole, corrects an imbalance in the body's immune system. However, no matter how eagerly arthritis sufferers greet each new medication and its typically exaggerated initial claims, the true wonder drug for arthritis is unlikely to appear until more fundamental knowledge is acquired about the causes of these diseases.

Physical Therapy Physical therapy has become an integral part of the treatment for most forms of arthritis and rheumatism because arthritic joints require a judicious blend of rest and exercise. Paradoxically, much of the pain around an inflamed joint stems from spasms of muscles which tighten defensively to restrict movement and so minimize pain. A painful, swollen joint must be protected from undue stresses and irritation that can make matters worse. This is done by correcting poor sitting, standing, and climbing postures to reduce the forces transmitted to the inflamed joint.

Too much rest and too little motion of the joint can also be harmful. Some joints, such as the hip and the knee, feel better in a bent position because this makes the joint volume larger and reduces internal pressure. If a joint is not worked regularly, it becomes stiff or even frozen as a result of muscle spasm, tendon shortening, and shrinking of the joint capsule. The joint may not become free even after the inflammation subsides. Daily physiotherapy helps to protect the joint and keep it functioning.

Exercise for arthritics need not involve jogging, riding an exercise bicycle, or strenous athletics. It can be done reclining or sitting, and consists essentially of bending the joint through its maximum range of motion twice daily and performing isometric exercises to strengthen weakened muscles. This preserves muscle tone and joint action. A proper balance of rest and gradually varied exercises helps to prevent deformity and allows reuse of joints when acute inflammation subsides. The program should be designed by a physican in consultation with a physical therapist according to individual patient needs and capabilities and the stage of the disease. Excessive, unsupervised exercise can damage the joint and perpetuate inflammation.

The specific modalities of physical therapy include physical measures, therapeutic exercises, and assistive devices. Heat applications soothe inflamed joints by reducing stiffness. Most patients with arthritis prefer moist heat in the form of whirlpool, hot packs, and paraffin dips to the hands and feet. The superficial heat diverts blood flow to the skin, allowing dissipation of heat. In fact, the destructive enzymes in rheumatoid arthritis are less efficient at lower temperatures. Because joint temperatures may rise, the use of deep heat in the form of diathermy or ultrasound is not recommended in inflammatory joint disease. These programs can be carried out in the home setting, but many patients find it convenient to attend outpatient physical therapy sessions several times weekly.

Prescribed exercises are first performed isometrically, then later more actively against a gradually increased resistance. Canes and crutches may be used to lighten the weight on inflamed joints. In many cases, these are only temporary aids, not permanent handicaps. Braces help to support a joint if its ligaments and muscles are weak. Simple, lightweight splints on wrists and knees help to reduce muscle spasm and to minimize, but not entirely prevent, deformity. If severe muscle contraction freezes a knee in a bent position, a series of splints can be used with gradually increasing angles, unbending the joint step by step until the limb is straightened.

Surgery Whether surgery is used to treat joint disease depends on the relative amounts of inflammation and mechanical damage. Swelling, heat, and tenderness are treated largely with drugs and physical therapy. Irreversible damage, pain, and restricted joint action due to mechanical changes that can not be remedied by drugs and exercise alone may require surgery. Surgery used to include removal of inflamed joint tissue (*synovectomy*), but this practice has declined because the diseased tissue grows back. It is still sometimes recommended for control of arthritis that is limited to one large joint, such as a knee, when other measures have failed.

Dramatic progress has been made in reconstructive surgery during the past decade. Of special value are total hip and knee replacements by artificial joints with one surface made of metal and the other of high-density polyethylene plastic held in place by a powerful cement. About 80,000 hip replacements are performed in the United States each year, and most patients can walk a few days after surgery. Artificial finger, elbow, shoulder, and ankle joints are installed less often and the techniques are still being perfected.

Artificial joints do not completely restore normal action. They are not emplaced with the expectation that they will allow their owners to resume tennis, golf, or running. They must be protected from abnormal stress to prevent loosening or fracture. At best (a very good best), they relieve pain and enable a previously chair-ridden arthritic to walk with some freedom.

Osteoarthritis

Osteoarthritis, or degenerative joint disease, is the most prevalent of all types of arthritis and appears in everyone sooner or later. Studies have found it in 97 percent of people over 60. It is usually mild and seldom cripples, but can sometimes cause severe disability. It differs from rheumatoid arthritis in that it affects mainly the large weight-bearing joints— hips and knees—and is not accompanied by systemic symptoms of fatigue, fever, or generalized stiffness. It also does not affect internal organs and inflammation is rare.

Osteoarthritis is often called the wear-and-tear form of arthritis because cartilage and bone surfaces become roughened and frayed. The cartilage may be worn down to the underlying bone, causing bony spurs to form. The bone surfaces no longer glide smoothly over each other, the structure and shape of the joint change, and ligaments may slacken as the joint becomes unstable.

Tissue degeneration is a natural consequence of aging, but this does not explain why some people get degenerative arthritis earlier or more severely than others, while some escape with none at all. Part of the reason is that a perfectly functioning joint is least likely to develop osteoarthritis, while one that is abnormally aligned or unduly stressed is more likely to degenerate faster. Also, forms of osteoarthritis are known to develop after severe joint injuries (especially in sports), in congenitally abnormal joints, and in weight-bearing joints of overweight people. Heredity also plays a part in a form of osteoarthritis that starts in middle age and is not associated with wear and tear. This form primarily affects women and tends to run in families. It appears in the middle and end finger joints and produces bony enlargements (*Heberden's nodes*) near the fingertips. Degenerative changes may also appear in the intervertebral discs of the spine and in the small jointed links (*articulating facet joints*) between vertebrae. These changes are a leading cause of chronic back pain.

Several metabolic conditions or disorders of glandular structures that affect the growth of cartilage may accompany forms of degenerative arthritis. Because of potential complication, even apparently ordinary cases of osteoarthritis require thorough evaluation and diagnosis.

Osteoarthritis sometimes produces minimal symptoms or none at all and may often first be discovered on an X ray taken for another purpose. The severity or lack of symptoms may not correlate at all with the degree of degeneration revealed by the X ray.

People who do have symptoms find that movement causes soreness and inactivity brings stiffness that can be overcome by a gentle limbering-up. If large, weight-bearing joints are affected, prolonged walking, standing, and stair climbing may cause pain. Sitting in a low chair or bending over to slip on shoes may irritate an arthritic hip. Knee deformity, if present, may bow the legs. Finger and knee joints may develop bony enlargements. Grating (*crepitus*) may be felt and heard when the roughened joint surfaces move over each other. Osteoarthritis is diagnosed by the history of such symptoms, physical examination, and X ray.

Treatment for osteoarthritis is very similar to that for rheumatoid arthritis. The main elements include the removal or reduction of stress on affected joints and relief of pain. Although there is no cure, the disease can be controlled.

Stress removal may involve merely the use of a cane or crutches to lighten the load on a joint, especially a hip or knee. Heat and exercise relieve muscle spasms, improve muscle tone, and preserve range of motion. A brace may give needed support to a painful and unstable joint.

Because the joint damage is predominantly mechanical, special anti-inflammatory drugs are not likely to be any more successful than more commonplace treatment. Osteoarthritics too often spend large sums of money trying one antirheumatic after another in the hope of finding a miracle cure, when 8 to 12 aspirin tablets daily will give the maximum possible relief. Drug side effects may also outweigh benefits. Local injections of corticosteroid may help temporarily, but should not be routinely repeated. Oral steroids should never be taken for osteoarthritis.

Advanced degeneration, especially of the hip or knee, may require total joint replacement when the surface of cartilage is completely worn off the bone and the joint hurts with the slightest movement or even when at rest. The artificial joint will relieve the pain and improve joint movement, but requires caution against overstress.

Intensive research is in progress to identify the abnormalities in cartilage that cause it to degenerate. The future may bring the means to alter the biochemistry of this tissue and so slow down the development of the disease.

Ankylosing Spondylitis

Ankylosing spondylitis is primarily an inflammatory disease of the spine, sacroiliac, and peripheral joints, affecting young men in their late teens or early twenties and producing back pain, stiffness after rest, and pain with sudden movements. Various bony and soft tissues become sensitive to touch. The inflammation heals with the growth of new bone, so the spine gradually stiffens and becomes rigid. The disease has a strong familial pattern. Relatives of someone who has it are ten times more likely than others to develop the disease. It is now known that 95 percent of those with ankylosing spondylitis carry a genetic blood marker, HLA B27, detectable by routine laboratory tests. Only 25 percent of those who have the genetic marker develop the disease, and random sampling of healthy Caucasian populations shows that 8 percent have the marker. Under appropriate circumstances, a positive test for the marker can be a useful diagnostic tool, especially in detecting early cases. Although the disease has a greater effect on men, studies show it to be equally common among women.

Inflammation may appear elsewhere than in the joints, for example, in the eye (*uveitis*) and occasionally the aorta. Treatment aims to reduce inflammation, but primarily emphasizes physical therapy. Although there is no sure way to stop the inflammation, its effects are less disabling if correct posture is maintained even with a stiffened spine. The disease often ceases by itself after several years. Although stiffness remains, pain becomes minimal.

Systemic Lupus Erythematosus

Systemic lupus erythematosus (SLE), or lupus, is an inflammatory connective tissue disease that can affect several organ systems. It strikes women between 15 and 45 most often, but all ages are susceptible. The name lupus is derived from the Latin word for wolf, and refers to the characteristic "butterfly" facial rash that resembles a wolf bite. One variety, called *discoid lupus*, affects only the skin and generally heals fairly quickly, but systemic lupus is chronic and subject to flare-ups and remissions. Its exact cause is unknown, but substantial evidence indicates that immune abnormalities play a crucial role.

Lupus is a prime example of an autoimmune disease. There is evidence that a virus may either initiate the abnormal immune reactions or alter the body's natural defenses. Episodes of the disease can be triggered in susceptible people by emotional stress, infection, and excessive exposure to sunlight. Certain drugs, such as hydralazine, an antihypertensive, procainamide, used to treat cardiac arrhythmias, and diphenylhydantoin, an anticonvulsive, can produce lupus symptoms that fortunately vanish when the drugs are discontinued.

Years ago, lupus was considered rare and fatal because only serious cases were recognized. Better tests now detect a broad range of lupus severity. Most victims do well, over 85 percent surviving for at least 15 years after diagnosis. Earlier diagnosis, better treatment—especially antibiotics to control infection that once took a high toll—and a broader understanding of the various manifestations of lupus have contributed to the brighter outlook.

Systemic lupus can produce inflammation in skin, joints, lungs, heart, kidneys, and brain, often accompanied by fever and fatigue. The arthritis of lupus tends not to be deforming. Kidney inflammation is potentially serious but variable, some patients requiring no special treatment while others need strong anti-inflammatory or immunosuppressive medication. Severe kidney damage can be managed with dialysis in most cases, but others may require eventual transplantation.

There is no single cure for lupus, and treatment is directed to the affected areas. Fever, joint pains, and a mild rash can often be managed by rest and aspirin alone. Rash can also be controlled with antimalarial drugs. Steroids effectively suppress inflammation in more severe cases. The many variations in lupus symptoms receive varied treatment that cannot be adequately described in general terms. Avoidance of sun exposure is strongly urged, especially when sensitivity is known to have caused previous rashes. A wide-brimmed hat, long sleeves, and protective skin lotions are advised. Sun bathing is not recommended for anyone, but individuals who are not sensitive can often tolerate normal daily exposure with no apparent harm.

Gout

Gout, or gouty arthritis dates from antiquity. It is a metabolic disorder of body chemistry associated with elevated amounts of uric acid, a normal body substance. The elevation is caused by either excess production in body cells or inadequate elimination by the kidneys. Among the many famous gout sufferers were Benjamin Franklin, Martin Luther, Charles Darwin, Isaac Newton, Samuel Johnson, and Michelangelo. Because of these illustrious examples, gout was thought to be related to high living and intelligence. Today, we know that gout cuts across all social and economic classes and affects over 1.5 million people annually. Nine out of 10 victims are men.

In susceptible individuals, deposits of excess uric acid accumulate in the form of needle-like crystals in joints and kidneys where they produce inflammation. Joints commonly afflicted are the big toe, instep, ankle, and knee. Acute attacks are accompanied by intense pain, swelling, warmth, and redness. Slight pressure—even the weight of a bed sheet— can cause great pain. Symptoms usually disappear between attacks. Large deposits of uric acid *(tophi)* can also occur in tendons and in the cartilages of the ear.

Acute episodes can be triggered by injury, overindulgence in certain foods which the body converts into uric acid, reaction to too much alcohol, the use of diuretics, and low doses of aspirin which reduce the kidney's ability to eliminate uric acid. Overeating by itself is not the primary cause of gout. Gouty kidney disease can result from the formation of uric acid stones or inflammation of certain kidney tissue, and are often accompanied by high blood pressure.

In diagnosis, gout is suspected in an acute onset of arthritis, especially in a big toe or ankle, and is confirmed by finding excessive uric acid in blood or urate crystals in fluid taken from the inflamed joint. People who suffer one attack of confirmed gout remain susceptible to recurring attacks for the rest of their lives, although years may lapse between episodes.

Although there is no permanent cure for gout, it is one arthritic disorder that can be completely controlled with medication. Acute attacks are countered with strong anti-inflammatory drugs. Colchicine is popular, but since it may produce undesirable side effects of nausea and diarrhea before the attack subsides, other drugs such as indomethacin, phenylbutazone, naproxen, or sulindac may be employed. When the attack subsides, the excess uric acid in the body is reduced by either a uricosuric drug that increases kidney excretion of uric acid, or allopurinol which decreases uric acid production. Because of the effectiveness of drug therapy, rigid dietary restrictions are no longer required in most cases.

Fibrositis

Fibrositis is a form of rheumatism that does not attack joints. It also does not appear as a single entity, but rather as a vague pain and stiffness in various parts of the body, most often in the deep soft tissues and muscles around the neck, shoulders, back, and hips. Sharply defined "trigger zones" are sensitive to the touch, but bones and joints remain normal. Routine laboratory tests and X rays are also normal.

The condition seems to affect emotionally tense individuals, and symptoms tend to correlate with periods of fatigue. Recent investigations have shown that many fibrositis patients complain of sleep disturbances followed by increased pain and stiffness when they awake. The disturbances often occur at certain key levels of normal sleep, especially the non-rem (non-rapid eye movement) phase, and may respond favorably to drug therapy. Mild analgesics and moist heat also effectively relieve pain. Patients are assured that fibrositis is never crippling.

It is clear that arthritis and rheumatism are complex problems that cannot be defined simply or treated uniformly. The evaluation, treatment, and rehabilitation of the arthritic is a highly individualized effort that involves a long-range program. There should be no preconceived diagnosis, and there is no instantaneous cure. Since arthritis can be serious, prompt diagnosis and treatment are mandatory.

ORTHOPEDIC DISORDERS

Robert E. Booth, Jr., M.D.

Assistant Professor of Orthopedics
Pennsylvania Hospital

It is estimated that the number of elderly Americans will rise from 23 million today to 55 million in the next fifty years. This fact alone will demand increasing emphasis upon the special orthopedic problems of the elderly—problems which up to now have not been given appropriate separate consideration.

Pediatric orthopedics is virtually a specialty in itself, for it has long been recognized that it is improper to treat children simply as little adults. By the same token, the increasing lifespan of our citizens is creating an expanding pool of individuals whose orthopedic problems are unique in terms of physiologic response, psychological implications, and financial impact.

It has long been recognized that elderly bones and joints heal more slowly than young ones after injury, even though the potential for full recovery is probably not significantly reduced. Indeed, the medical and metabolic complications of a fracture in the older individual routinely cause more difficulty than the physical injury itself. It is thus more important to keep an elderly person mobile and active immediately after an injury or operation, than it is for a child or professional athlete!

Psychological differences between geriatric and other orthopedic disorders are also quite apparent. Many older individuals conceal an injury because they fear hospitalization, surgery, or placement in a nursing home. Even those who successfully recover from some physical breakdown may become emotionally crippled by their fear of a recurrence, a situation analogous to that of the well-known "cardiac cripple." Most people know the typical example of the elderly woman who recovers nicely from her fractured hip, but never again leaves the house or gives up her walker lest she suffer another injury. The critical factor here is fear of the potential loss of independence, physical integrity, and self-determination. Unless this is understood and dealt with properly, the older person with an orthopedic problem has received less than full treatment.

The financial impact of geriatric orthopedic disorders is significant, since these problems may hinder walking and reduce independence in the activities of daily life. Unless more of these individuals can be helped to remain self-sufficient, the cost of their care will soon become more than our society can bear without being forced into unconscionable choices.

As the life expectancy of the average person comes closer to the biblical three score years and ten, the overwhelming majority of orthopedic disorders result from degeneration of otherwise normal parts. This is simply wear and tear, the consequence of countless miles and hours of use. Tendons fray and snap just like a rope run too long over a pulley. *Bursae* (sacs of liquid) and joints dry out, much as appliances lose their lubrication. Cartilage caps over joints erode the way the plastic coating wears off a skillet and allows food to stick. Bones lose their calcium and their resiliency, just as the mortar crumbles in a wall. Spinal discs dry out and develop fissures that mimic the wrinkles we see in our faces each morning.

The sum of these changes does not constitute a disease, merely normal aging. Only when they generate symptoms do we honor them with the unfortunate label of "degenerative disease." A fuller understanding of these processes and their possible consequences should encourage more elderly persons to seek orthopedic help early, reduce their fear about what is happening to their bodies, and encourage them to remain as active and self-sufficient as possible. Understanding that not every "hurt" implies a "harm" is the first step to a small victory over advancing age.

Neck

The neck—or cervical spine—is basically a short flexible stem supporting the head, which permits us to turn our eyes or ears toward a sight or sound. The bones of the neck resemble a stack of seven spools (vertebrae), separated by shock absorbers or discs, held together by ligaments and muscles. Since the neck's range of motion is generous, and since the average adult head weighs 15–17 pounds, stress upon the bones and discs is quite severe. The spinal cord runs along and within the vertebrae, and the individual nerves to the arms and upper body exit at each level to supply sensation and muscle control.

The discs between the vertebrae are the key to disorders of the cervical spine. Each disc resembles a jelly doughnut, with a soft liquid center and a firm outer ring. In younger individuals, the most common problem is an acute disc herniation, in which the liquid center of the disc bulges out through a fissure in the outer ring and compresses a nerve. The pain is sharp and severe. It follows the course of whichever nerve is compressed, out of the neck and down into the arm, and the arm pain often exceeds the neck pain. The motion of the neck is only partially limited, but numbness and weakness may be found in the arms and hands. This problem often does not respond to conservative therapy of rest, support, heat, and drugs. It may require a cervical laminectomy and disc excision (surgical removal of the disc and part of a vertebra) to relieve pressure on the nerve. Known as a "soft disc," acute disc herniation is fortunately somewhat rare, especially as one gets older.

One of the compensations of growing older is that the discs are no longer susceptible to acute disc herniation because they dry out and lose their ability to retain water. This is a gradual process, but by the fifties or sixties most discs resemble wet cardboard. However, the more insidious and relentless process of degenerative arthritis of the neck then becomes apparent. As the discs deteriorate and collapse, the bones of the cervical spine come to rest against one another. Motion in the neck is reduced, and creaking or snapping is often heard. Bone spurs develop, and the space is narrowed further (Figure 1).

Arthritic degeneration is almost universal in the elderly. Careful studies have shown that after age 55, over 51 percent of the population will complain of neck and arm pain. Eighty-two percent will show X-ray evidence of degenerative arthritic changes in the cervical spine. Thus, the many abnormalities seen on an X ray should not cause undue alarm.

Only when these degenerative changes produce symptoms should they be considered a disease. A common pattern is acute disc degenera-

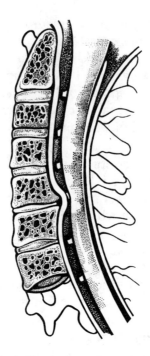

Figure 1. A narrowed cervical disc and resultant bone spurs push backward into the nerves to produce symptoms.

tion, in which a person develops sudden neck pain, usually on one side only, which extends into the shoulder or between the shoulder blades. The pain is often worst in the morning, and there may also be vague aching in the arm. Neck pain exceeds the discomfort in other areas and may be accompanied by blurred vision, nausea, headaches centered at the back of the head, or other symptoms. These symptoms are probably the result of one or more of the cervical nerves being bruised or squeezed where it emerges from the spine.

This is rarely a permanent injury, so treatment should be conservative. Mechanical devices such as a soft cervical collar reduce the likelihood of recurrent nerve irritation if worn as prescribed. The most important time—unhappily the most difficult time—to wear a collar is at night. The brain quickly learns to restrict painful neck motions while we are awake, but this defense mechanism shuts off when we go to sleep. It is thus no mystery that those who fail to wear a collar at night wake up with neck pain.

Inflammation of the squeezed nerve root should be treated with pain-relieving and anti-inflammatory medication. Simple aspirin, taken regularly, is probably the most effective anti-inflammatory drug. Heat and rest are also important, and cervical traction may occasionally be beneficial. Surgery is rarely indicated, and should be considered only after many months of conservative therapy.

After the age of 55, chronic disc degeneration is even more common than the acute form. This usually involves a long history of neck and arm pains that wax and wane with activity. The pain rarely goes below the shoulder, although the chest muscles may occasionally ache as they do in some forms of heart disease. Range of motion of the neck is significantly reduced, particularly in bending. The rear neck muscles are often tender to the touch. ''Trigger zones'' of exceptional tenderness may be found over the back shoulder muscles, although usually no true nerve deficiency can be detected.

Here again, the appropriate therapy is conservative, including anti-inflammatory and analgesic drugs, support, and heat. The symptoms tend to come and go. Remissions can be prolonged by a program of appropriate neck-muscle exercises when pain has eased. Lack of improvement despite adequate therapy should always raise the suspicion of a tumor or infection of the cervical spine, although these are fortunately rare.

The bone spurs typical of degenerative cervical arthritis can also grow forward to compress the esophagus and cause swallowing difficulty. This is called *dysphagia*, and can be diagnosed with a barium-swallow X ray. When the bone spurs extend sideways or toward the rear from the vertebrae, they can compress two of the four arteries that supply blood to the brain. This is known as vertebral insufficiency, and is usually marked by dizziness or blurred vision brought on by turning the head from side to side. It is a potentially serious disorder which should be confirmed with a special X ray called an *arteriogram*.

Fractures and dislocations of the neck seem to be less common over 55, probably because of the greater caution in sports and driving that comes with age. Automobiles remain the greatest cause of neck injury in our society, and head supports, seat belts, and careful attention are even more important when our aging necks are stiffer and less flexible than when we were young.

Most neck fractures are either lethal or obvious, and generally get the attention they require. It is the whiplash injury which is both more common and less successfully treated. Basically, a whiplash is a sprain of the ligaments which support the neck, and may not be apparent for 12–24 hours after the accident. Symptoms such as dizziness, ringing in the ears, or blurred vision are usually only temporary. On the other hand, difficulty in swallowing or veering to one side when walking are ominous symptoms which require prompt medical evaluation.

Just as with a severe ankle sprain, the injured neck must be immobilized and protected for weeks, occasionally months. A cervical collar and extreme patience—also known as ''tincture of time''—are the most effective remedies. Nonetheless, the symptoms are usually long-lasting, and 12 percent of all whiplash victims remain permanently disabled. If a victim sues for damages, litigation should be concluded as promptly as possible, since it is rare for patients to improve while legal actions are still in progress.

Shoulder

The shoulder is the joint with the greatest range of motion in the body, for its function is to keep the arm out and away from the body, allowing placement of the hand in an enormous variety of positions. The price we pay for this mobility is less stability and early deterioration of the soft tissues which hold the shoulder together. Dislocations of the shoulder are common in the young but rarely seen beyond the age of 50. Gradual stiffening of joints with age prevents dislocation, but also reduces motion and makes fracture more common.

Falling on the outstretched arm causes many fractures, primarily of the wrist. The second most frequent injury seen in the emergency room from such falls is impaction of the shaft of the *humerus*, the bone that extends from the shoulder to the elbow (Figure 2). This injury is very painful and may severely restrict arm movement. Also, when the bone is weakened by age, the shaft can fairly easily be driven up into the globe, or head, of the humerus at the shoulder joint.

Despite the pain, this fracture is stable and needs only a sling to support the arm. Early movement after two weeks of rest is the key to successful recovery since the prevention of lasting stiffness of the shoulder joint

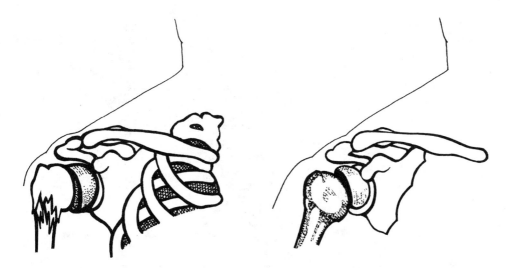

Figure 2. Left: Fracture of humerus near the shoulder. Right: Normal shoulder joint.

is of greater concern than the risk of failure to heal. Substantial internal bleeding and discoloration of arms and chest are to be expected.

Degenerative arthritis of the junction between the *clavicle* (collar bone) and the *acromion* (top of the shoulder blade) is also quite common in the elderly. This is mildly painful in most instances, producing discomfort or creaking when the arm is lifted fully away from the side, as in the follow-through of a golf swing. It may be marked by a painless bony prominence on the topmost part of the shoulder.

In most instances, local heat and anti-inflammatory drugs will relieve the discomfort. Injections of steroid are also helpful. Some stubborn cases may require minor surgery. Pain in this joint causes no harm, however, and the "separated shoulder" of youth is quite unusual.

The most common shoulder problems in older people involve the soft tissues that surround this joint, specifically the tendons (Figure 3). The biceps tendon runs through a bony groove across the front of the shoulder joint. Chronic wear and tear produce inflammation, called *bicipital tendinitis*, with tenderness over the front of the shoulder and pain during flexing of the elbow or turning of a key. The inflammation diminishes with rest and heat, although steroid injection may be neces-

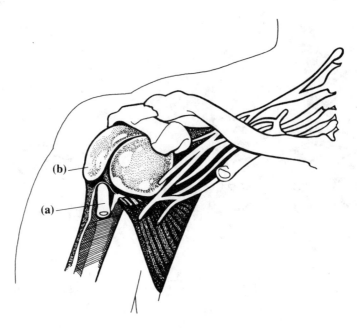

Figure 3. Shoulder joint showing biceps tendon (a) and bursae (b) overlying rotator cuff tendons.

sary. One can occasionally rupture this tendon, leaving a weakened arm and an obvious bulge in the upper arm.

The tendon subjected to perhaps the greatest stress is the broad "rotator cuff," which has the job of lifting the arm away from the side and rotating it outward. Autopsy studies have shown that 50 percent of men over 50 years old have a frayed and worn rotator-cuff tendon. A great deal of friction occurs where this tendon runs between the bones of the outer shoulder joint. Here, as in other high-friction areas, there is a bursa serving as a fluid-filled cushion. When inflammation of the tendon extends to the bursa, a bursitis develops, which is both painful and persistent. Conservative measures such as rest, heat, slings, and anti-inflammatory drugs are frequently effective in reducing the pain, but the condition is usually chronic. The discomfort is often most severe at night, even awakening its victims. Calcium may deposit in the tendon or bursa. Steroid injections or surgical excision of the calcium or bone spurs are frequently necessary.

The shoulder is also a conduit for the nerves and blood vessels that supply the arm. Occasionally, minor injuries will be followed by a progressive increase in pain and decrease in motion in the shoulder, known as the "frozen shoulder syndrome." Its exact nature is unknown, but the end result is a stiff or immobile shoulder and a withered arm. This condition occurs most frequently in the dominant shoulder of slim females, and is often accompanied by psychological disturbances. It must be treated with a very aggressive program of physical therapy and manipulation to prevent a disastrous outcome.

THORACIC OUTLET

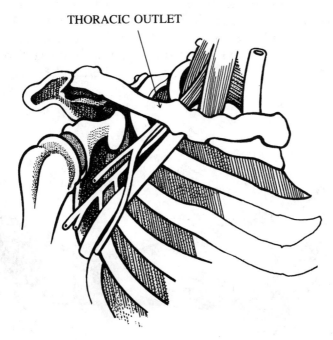

Figure 4. Healed clavicle (collar-bone) fracture at arrow compressing nerves and blood vessels leaving the shoulder.

A final, but related, shoulder problem is that of the "thoracic outlet syndrome," a compression of the nerves and blood vessels where they leave the chest and shoulder and enter the arm. This condition typically evokes such complaints as general numbness and tingling, hot and cold sensations, or just pervasive aching. Although the syndrome occasionally results from congenital abnormalities or the healing of a fractured clavicle (Figure 4), its most common cause in the over-55 group is sagging shoulder girdles due to poor posture and weakening muscles. Correction of posture, often supplemented by a shoulder-strap brace, is normally sufficient to eliminate the symptoms.

Elbow

The elbow is a complex joint, since it is formed by the articulation of three bones. Fortunately, elbow fractures are not common over 55 because the more vulnerable wrist and shoulder joints give way first. However, a direct blow to the point of the elbow (*olecranon*) can produce a painful fracture which generally requires surgery to restore use of the arm. The less common radial-head fracture (the *radius* is the forearm bone in line with the thumb) is produced by a fall on the outstretched arm, and causes tenderness over the thumb side of the upper forearm. Pain is produced when the hand is turned palm up or palm down. Most of these fractures require only a sling to allow them to heal.

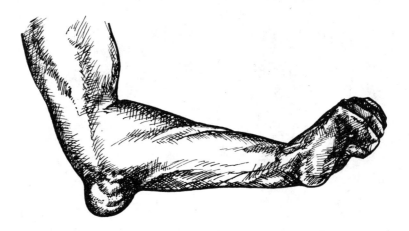

Figure 5. Enlarged olecranon bursa over elbow.

Pain in the elbow or upper forearm often develops as the result of soft-tissue inflammation without a specific injury. For example, olecranon bursitis is an inflammation of the bursa that protects the point of the elbow from pressure. It usually begins as a painless thickening of the elbow tissues which is followed by a large cystic (bag-like) swelling that can become as large as an orange (Figure 5). The cyst may sometimes disappear by itself, but more often the fluid contents must be drained with a needle and syringe. Since the bone rests directly beneath the bursa, one should not puncture the cyst for fear of infection. A swollen bursa can also be a sign of arthritis or gout.

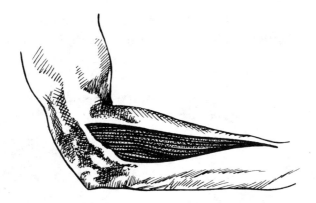

Figure 6. Inflammation *(tendinitis)* of tendons along the side of the elbow is called "tennis elbow."

Pain may also appear over the bony prominence on the outside of the elbow, known as the *humeral epicondyle*, where the strong tendons that extend the wrist and fingers begin. Chronic use and wear cause an inflammation in these tendons known as *lateral humeral epicondylitis*, or tennis elbow (Figure 6). As a sports-related injury, this tendinitis most commonly results from an improper backhand swing, too small a racquet grip, or just too much tennis. The pain will be felt during such movements as shaking hands, extending the wrist backward, and turning a key in a lock. Rest and warm soaks are often enough to quiet the inflammation, but anti-inflammatory drugs, steroid injections, and an arm cast are sometimes required.

Wrist

Fractures of the wrist are probably the most common injury over 55. As we grow older, the strength and calcium content of our bones decrease, especially in the spine and ends of the long bones. A fall on the outstretched hand can crush the weakened bone at the wrist, producing the common "Colles' fracture" (Figure 7). The wrist will be swollen and painful, and a deformity or swelling will be noted over the displaced bone at the back of the wrist. Occasionally, the nerves to the hand will be bruised, causing numbness and tingling in the thumb, index, and middle fingers. A Colles' fracture is a severe injury, and the wrist anatomy must be made normal again to restore full use of the hand. This usually means a cast, often supplemented by metal pins drilled into the wrist bones under anesthesia. The prognosis for this injury is quite good if early motion is begun to combat swelling and stiffness.

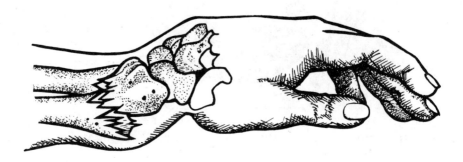

Figure 7. Displaced wrist bones in typical Colles' fracture.

A permanent arthritis may develop after the fracture, but most older adults will already have suffered some loss of mobility and occasional aching in their wrists due to the degenerative arthritis that affects us all in our later years. Little can be done for this beyond the well-known meas-ures of anti-inflammatory drugs and heat. It is quite common for an in-jury or a degenerative arthritis to produce aching pain whenever bad weather is coming. When the barometric pressure drops outside, joints and joint fluids expand and produce the discomfort that so often causes older people to say "It's going to rain, I can feel it in my bones."

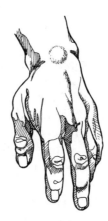

Figure 8. Ganglion cyst on back of wrist.

All joints have lubricating fluid within them, but friction from arthritic or damaged joint surfaces rubbing on one another may cause fluid to bulge or escape. This typically produces on one of the wrist surfaces a small painless cystic mass known as a *ganglion* (Figure 8), or "Bible cyst," from the days when it was the custom to crush it with the thickest book within reach. Nowadays, ganglia are drained with a needle and syringe, injected with steroids, or surgically removed. They are harmless, however, and one should be wary lest the treatment be worse than the disease.

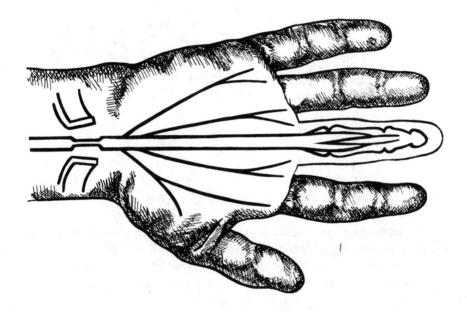

Figure 9. Wrist ligament cut to show compressed median nerve of carpal tunnel syndrome.

Several nerves supply the hand. The most important—the median nerve—crosses the wrist joint through a tight tunnel of bone and ligament. Any extra pressure in this tunnel compresses the nerve, producing the *carpal tunnel syndrome* (Figure 9). This is marked by numbness or "pins and needles" in the thumb, index, and middle fingers and half of the ring finger. It is worse at night and may even awaken people from sleep when it becomes painful. Weakness of pinch strength may cause coffee cups to slip from the fingers or keys to resist turning in their locks. The muscles at the base of the thumb may be visibly atrophied.

Although degenerative arthritis and injury are the most common causes of the carpal tunnel syndrome, sometimes diabetes, hypothyroidism, rheumatoid arthritis, and gout may be at fault. An electrical nerve-conduction test will confirm the diagnosis. Early treatment consists of anti-inflammatory drugs, soaks, and splints. Steroid injections are effective, and surgical release of the ligament compressing the nerves is always successful.

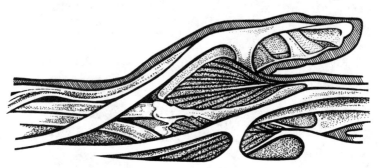

Figure 10. Thumb tendons inflamed in *DeQuervain's tenosynovitis.*

Another area of great stress and friction in the wrist is along the powerful tendons which control the base of the thumb. Tendinitis here, known as *DeQuervain's tenosynovitis* (Figure 10), is usually the result of excessive use. Pain or creaking will be produced by extending the thumb into the hitchhiker's position, or by curling the thumb forcefully into the palm. The tendons may become tender and swollen, and the pain can be severe. Splinting, warm soaks, and anti-inflammatory drugs are the first line of treatment, followed by steroid injection and possibly minor surgery if the pain persists.

Hand

It is often taught that pain and stiffness are the two biggest obstacles to hand rehabilitation after injury. For the aging hands, these twin curses are like Scylla and Charybdis. As joints wear and bones begin to rub one another, joint movements cause pain. However, avoiding pain by not moving joints causes them to become stiff and useless. Thus, a balance must be sought between two perils.

Degenerative arthritis is often noticed first in the hands, usually as hard lumps that form around the last joint in each finger (Figure 11) and at the base of the thumb. While this process occurs to some degree in all

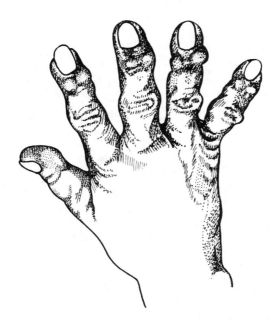

Figure 11. Hard nodules near ends of fingers typical of degenerative arthritis.

of us, it is defined as a disease only when it markedly limits hand or finger movements. Anti-inflammatory drugs are mildly effective, but most victims are best advised to keep their joints supple and mobile at all cost. Since the thumb works in opposition to all the fingers, it often degenerates sooner than the others. However, a rigid thumb in good position is still quite functional as a post against which to pinch and grasp, so surgical fusion of the thumb is an excellent salvage procedure that can provide many years of painless use.

Rheumatoid arthritis ravages the soft tissues as well as the bones and joints of the hands, producing the dramatic deformities that come to most people's minds when they think of arthritis of the hands. Fortunately, it is far less common than simple degenerative arthritis. Rheumatoid arthritis starts as pain and swelling of the knuckles closest to the palm, and rarely affects the last joint in the fingers until late in the disease. The disease literally eats away the joints and their ligaments, and the fingers and the hand itself will "drift" away from the thumb (Figure 12). The knuckles appear to swell as joints slip out of place, and ultimately the tendons are eroded to produce severe finger deformities.

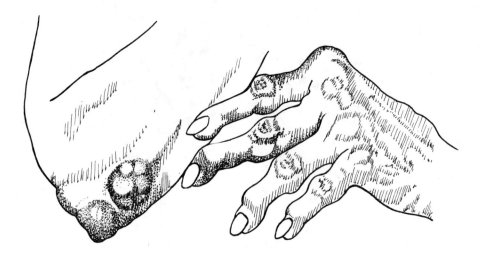

Figure 12. Nodules on elbow and knuckles (nearest palm) and "drift" of fingers away from thumb due to rheumatoid arthritis.

Early treatment—both medical and surgical—is the key to maintaining hand function, and it is truly sad to see how many people wait until only salvage procedures can be performed. Just as keeping blood sugar under control doesn't really halt the course of diabetes, so the use of anti-inflammatory drugs arrests only some of the symptoms of rheumatoid arthritis. Joint injections, removal of inflamed tissues (*synovectomy*), tendon repairs, joint fusions, and actual replacement of hand joints with plastic substitutes are highly successful when done early by competent surgeons.

A peculiar phenomenon of unknown cause, called *Dupuytren's contracture* (Figure 13), affects the hands of some individuals over 55. The tissues and tendons of the palm contract, curling first the ring finger, and later the others rigidly down to the palm. The onset is frequently associated with alcoholism and liver disease. It is typically painless, although later attempts to uncurl the fingers may bring discomfort. The best treatment is surgical release of the scar tissue followed by physical therapy to restore mobility to the fingers.

These same flexor (finger-bending) tendons, worn and frayed by years of hard use, may develop a scar or nodule where they pass through their pulleys over the joints. A finger will produce a snapping sound or sensation, often accompanied by pain, when it is bent into the palm or

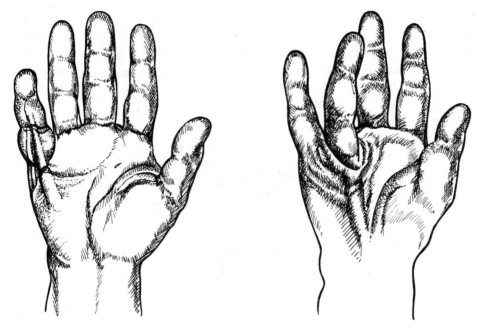

Figure 13. *Dupuytren's contracture* of flexor tendons of the ring finger and palm.

straightened. Some people will awake from sleep with the fingers curled and must use the other hand to straighten them out. This is called a "trigger finger." Help is typically not sought until a true painful tendinitis has developed. Steroid injections are effective when supplemented by splints and rest, and release of tendons by minor surgery is almost always curative.

Back

There is a saying in medicine that "ninety percent of the people get ten percent of the diseases." This is nowhere more true than in problems of the lumbar spine (the lower vertebrae). The overwhelming majority of clinical problems in this area for people over 55 are related to degeneration of the discs between the vertebrae.

With age, these discs dry out and wrinkle so that they no longer evenly distribute the weight they carry. Their fluid center then begins to push through the outer ring. This tends to produce episodes, called *acute disc degeneration*, which recur every year or so accompanied by pain in the lower back but not the legs. They are usually brought on by some strenuous physical exertion that causes one's back to "go out." Although the episodes are normally self-limiting, they also respond to bedrest, salicylates (aspirin), and mechanical support. Heat, massage, and pain medication also help.

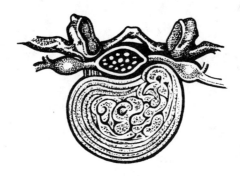

Figure 14. Spine cross section showing disc slipping backward to the right, compressing the sciatic nerve.

When the liquid nucleus finally ruptures all the way through the outer ring, the condition is known as a "slipped disc," or *herniated nucleus pulposus.* This produces severe pain, often worse in the legs than in the back. When the sciatic nerve is irritated, the pain is called sciatica (Figure 14). The symptoms may also be numbness or "pins and needles," weakness or leg collapse, or muscle cramps in the lower legs. People with herniated discs usually feel worse when sitting, as opposed to standing or lying down. They may get "stuck" in a bent position afraid to move for fear of inducing pain, and pain will increase during straining, coughing, or sneezing.

Even in severe cases, a program of ten days of absolute bedrest, aspirin, and pain medications will bring relief to 80 percent of all victims. Although the disc never goes back into place, the nerve recovers from the bruise it has suffered and symptoms disappear. Those who fail to improve or whose symptoms become progressively worse may require surgical removal of the disc and part of a vertebra. Surgery is usually preceded by an X-ray test called a myelogram in which a needle is used to inject dye around the nerves of the spine to outline and locate the herniated disc. Most patients do well following disc surgery when its indications are clear, but also face a higher risk of another disc herniation at a different level of the spine.

All those who suffer from low back pain should be aware of the factors that seem to contribute to disc disease in our society, since in most instances the problem is preventable. Of all predictive factors, prolonged sitting and riding in cars appear to impose the worst stress on our spines. Pressure tests have shown that good posture is every bit as important as our mothers told us. Obesity and poor abdominal muscle tone also predispose a person to disc disease. It should also be clear—especially to those involved in litigation—that injury to the spine is a precipitating but not a causative factor in disc disease. The poorest risks are those who have already had a disc problem and consciously avoid exertion thereafter for fear of stirring up more trouble. Their sedentary lifestyle leads to weight and weakness problems that make recurrent episodes almost inevitable.

Eighty-two percent of all Americans suffer from back pain at some time, mostly in the later years of life. As its discs slowly dry out and settle, the spine shortens and becomes stiff. This is the normal part of aging which is prevalent rather than evidence of disease. Most of the acute episodes of pain represent sprains of the supporting soft tissues of the spine, which resolve with rest, support, and patience. Many individuals develop a "round-back" deformity (*kyphosis*) as they age, which typically represents collapse of the vertebrae as well as of the discs.

Particularly in post-menopausal women, the bones lose calcium and become soft, making them susceptible to compression fracture or wedge-shaped settling of the vertebrae. This softening of the bones is called *osteoporosis* (Figure 15), and is best combatted by adequate calcium in the diet, sunshine, good posture, and exercise. Calcium supplements are rarely required if one has a good diet, and braces or corsets actually tend to weaken the spine when worn for long periods of time. When back pains persist for months, a tumor may sometimes be the cause, especially in cases of prostate cancer in older men.

Unquestionably, the greatest advance in the diagnosis and treatment of back pain in the elderly has been a better understanding of a condition called *spinal stenosis*. This is the end stage of degenerative disc disease in which the bones surrounding the spinal cord settle irregularly, slipping and developing large bone spurs which narrow the space available for the nerves (Figure 16). Its first symptom is apparently ordinary

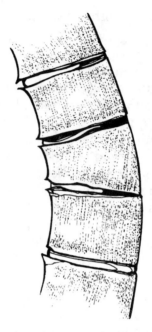

Figure 15. Narrowed discs and wedge-shaped vertebrae of osteoporotic spine.

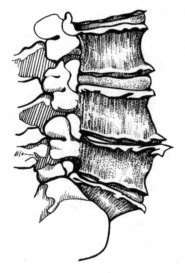

Figure 16. Degenerative *stenosis* (narrowing) of spinal discs and nerve spaces with large bone spurs.

persistent low back pain. However, victims then begin to develop a wide

variety of symptoms—previously considered bizarre or unexplainable—
such as aching in the front of the thighs, numbness and tingling in the
legs or feet, and cramps in the lower legs and feet after a long walk. The
last complaint is called *claudication,* characterized by the ability to walk
only a certain distance before having to stop because of aching calves or
lower leg pains. A few minutes rest then allows the victim to walk the
same distance again. It should be distinguished from identical symptoms
caused by poor blood circulation.

Spinal stenosis occurs almost exclusively in the elderly in whom the
intervertebral discs are too dried out and degenerated to slip any further.
It is rarely improved by bedrest, and most individuals should be kept
moving with the aid of a corset and medication such as aspirin. Where
there is no improvement, the injection of steroids deep into the spine
around the swollen and irritated nerves is about 70 percent effective. Surgery can successfully remove bone and create more space for the nerves,
and should not be withheld merely because of a patient's advanced age.

Hip

In the lower extremities, degenerative arthritis (*osteoarthritis*) is still
the primary offender in the over-55 population. An additional factor is
the effect of body weight on the degenerating joints. Most of our bones
are covered by a cap of smooth, shiny cartilage which slides freely against
a matching structure on the other side of the joint. Years of wear thin the
cartilage cap, causing bones to grind against each other. This is accentuated in lower-extremity joints by the weight of the body they must carry
(Figure 17). Sadly, arthritis in these joints limits the ability to move
about freely and makes the elderly less independent.

Degenerative arthritis in the hip will occur in everyone who lives
long enough, for loss of joint mobility inexorably accompanies aging.
When we are infants, we can put our toes in our mouths; at 75, it is hard
to tie our shoelaces.

The hip is a very mobile ball-and-socket joint, and the first sign of
degeneration is usually gradual loss of mobility. Initial aching is followed
by more severe pain, which increases with activity. As the arthritis
worsens, pain persists even at rest and limbs shorten and become less
stable. As with most degenerative conditions, hurt does not imply harm.
As long as one can continue to be active, the life pattern need not be

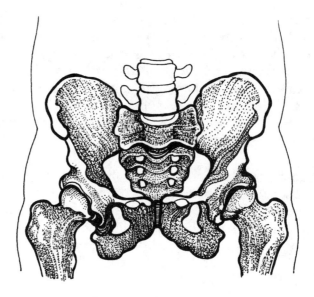

Figure 17. Irregular and eroded hip joints typical of degenerative arthritis.

altered. Nonetheless, most individuals experience gradual weight gain, leg weakness, and a more limited sphere of activities.

Treatment of most hip arthritis should begin with anti-inflammatory medications and a lightening of the forces on the hip. Weight reduction is critical, for each pound lost reduces the force on the hip joint by three pounds. Similarly, the use of a cane in the hand opposite the affected hip will produce an equivalent force reduction, minimizing current symptoms and future deterioration. Crutches or a walker are the final resort in conservative therapy. Steroid injections into the joint are endorsed by some physicians, but condemned by others. Certainly they should be used sparingly and with proper precautions, as should all the more potent anti-inflammatory medications.

Rheumatoid arthritis and hip injuries cause a progressive arthritis whose end stage is indistinguishable from that of degenerative arthritis. Another less common problem with a similar end result is called *avascular necrosis*. In this disorder, the blood supply to the hip joint is reduced, and the bone slowly crumbles and degenerates. The most common causes of this problem in older citizens in our society are excessive alcohol intake, hip fractures, and oral steroid medications.

Until fifteen years ago, the only therapeutic alternatives for the degenerated hip joint were pain medications, supports, hip fusions, or deforming operations in which the joint was surgically removed, leaving an unstable hip. The revolution in reconstructive orthopedic surgery came with the popularization of joint replacement (*total hip arthroplasty*) by Sir John Charnley of England. For the first time, pain elimination was combined with stability and mobility of the hip in one operation. A plastic (high density polyethylene) hip socket and a metal (stainless steel alloy) femoral ball were substituted for the diseased bone and glued into place with a special cement called methyl methacrylate. The success rate of this procedure is now as high as its complications are low, and similar techniques have been devised for other degenerated joints.

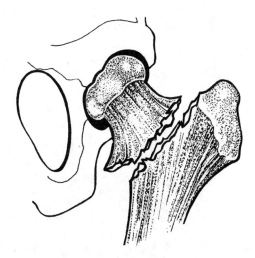

Figure 18. Hip fracture just below ball-and-socket joint.

However, fractures of the aging hip (Figure 18) remain a problem. The loss of calcium and resiliency in our bones makes them susceptible to breaking when we fall, and fractures of the hip are in all too many instances disabling and even lethal events. The problem is not so much the fracture itself, for most of these breaks will heal in time. It is the loss of mobility that leads to a general collapse and accelerated demise in the older patient.

A patient put at prolonged bedrest for a hip fracture tends to develop bedsores that often become infected. Calcium leaches out of immobilized bones, weakening them further and, worse yet, forming painful kidney stones. The characteristic constipation of the elderly is aggravated by pain, bed confinement, and the bowel-slowing effect of narcotic pain medications required for comfort. Lungs are not fully expanded, frequently leading to *atelectasis* (lung collapse) and pneumonia. Blood circulation slows in the legs, promoting the development of phlebitis (vein inflammation) and blood clots in the lungs (*pulmonary embolism*). It is therefore no surprise that only 65 percent of those over the age of 60 used to survive a hip fracture by more than six months.

Today, the keystone of fractured-hip treatment is keeping the patient mobile. Surgery to pin or replace broken hip bones is now standard treatment, regardless of the patient's age. Most patients will be up and standing the day after a hip fracture, even though the bones may take six months to heal. With this treatment, the morbidity and mortality of the adult fractured hip have dropped to very low levels.

A final hip condition seen with great frequency in those over 55 is *trochanteric bursitis*. At the widest point of our hips there is a bone prominence which can be felt just under the skin. When the tendons about the hip move back and forth over this bone (*trochanter*), friction and irritation are produced. This can result either in aching pain while walking, or a persistent tenderness over the area. Inflammation of the bursa located here is best treated with warm soaks and rest, although steroid injections are frequently necessary in severe or chronic cases.

Knee

The knee is a hinge joint in which the bones are held together by ligaments and separated by rubbery shock absorbers called *menisci*. Although older people rarely suffer the acute torn meniscus that locks and clicks in the knee of a young athlete, the inevitable degeneration of this weight-bearing joint causes fraying of the menisci and erosion of the underlying bone and cartilage (Figure 19). Clicking and creaking of the bones are then both audible and palpable, and bending of the joint often causes pain. In typical degenerative arthritis, the inside of the knee wears out first, producing a bow-legged deformity with increasing age. Knock-kneed misalignment of the knees may also be seen (Figure 20), but is more common in rheumatoid arthritis.

Regardless of the cause of arthritis, the knee joint experiences this rubbing and increased friction as insufficient lubrication. It then secretes extra joint, often known as "water on the knee." This is the knee's at-

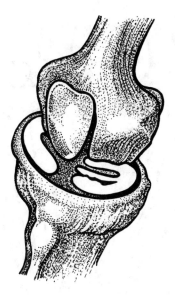

Figure 19. Normal (left) and torn (right) *menisci* within knee joint.

tempt to help itself and is not harmful. However, it may contribute to aching discomfort in the knee, especially when the barometer falls and bad weather arrives. It should not be routinely drained with a needle, as was the practice in years past, for it will merely reaccumulate. Only when the fluid bulges at the back of the knee, producing what is known as a Baker's cyst, should treatment other than anti-inflammatory drugs, heat, and supports be considered. If loose fragments of bone produce clicking or locking of the joint, these should be removed before further damage is done. Steroid injections are usually reserved for severe problems, since there is a chance that they may actually hasten the deterioration of the joint.

The arthroscope is a new device for inspecting the knee joint to aid in diagnosis. A fiberoptic tube the size of a pencil is pushed into a water-inflated knee joint and the contents are inspected under direct vision. This tool even allows the removal of small loose fragments, often forestalling a formal knee operation.

Vanity or pride should not stand in the way when the use of a cane is indicated. Cane support reduces the stress on the knee joint as much as on the hip. The single most important factor in treating almost any knee problem is to maintain the strength of the quadriceps muscles at the front of the thigh which straighten and support the knee. When a knee is favored because of pain, these muscles atrophy, increasing the load on

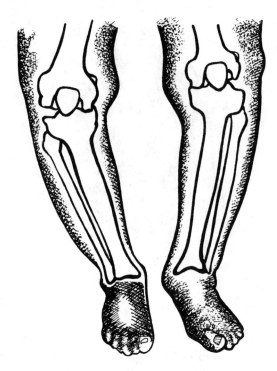

Figure 20. Knock-kneed deformity with degenerative arthritis of inner side of knee.

the kneecap and other bones. This actually aggravates arthritis and leads to further disease and atrophy, establishing a vicious cycle. Only regular straight-leg-raising and weight-lifting exercise can rehabilitate these muscles and improve knee function.

Ankle and Foot

Unlike the ligaments of the knee, which dry out and tighten with age and are thus seldom sprained, the ankle ligaments are subjected to sprains (Figure 21) throughout life. Although far more common in women than in men, sprains almost always result from turning the ankle in or "going over" on the outside of the foot. These injuries range from minor pulls to truly destabilizing ligament disruptions, and can be more acutely painful than the ankle fractures they mimic. Most ankle sprains are undertreated, as people try to ignore them or walk them off. The ankle should be given adequate support ranging from Ace bandages to casts. They permit the initial damage to heal more quickly and reduce the chance of recurrent sprains. Ice helps to reduce bleeding and swelling for the first 24 hours, but thereafter, wet heat is preferable to dilate blood vessels and accelerate healing.

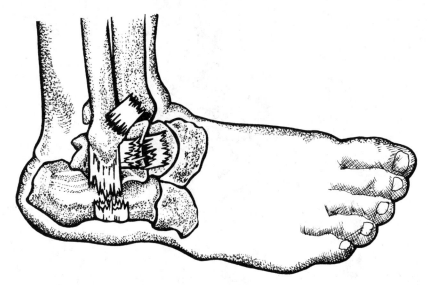

Figure 21. Torn ankle ligaments from severe sprain.

Ankle fractures (Figure 22) in the elderly are rarely minor injuries since the ankle joint must be completely stable to support body weight. True fractures are best diagnosed with X rays taken early and should be fixed definitively, whether a cast or internal fixation with screws and pins is required. Here again, the principle of early treatment followed by early mobility is the key to good results.

Our feet are comprised of many small bones, yet they support great forces over many miles and years of use. Nonetheless, degenerative changes in foot joints are, surprisingly, less troublesome than similar disease in hips and knees because of the foot's small range of movement. The heel takes the first and heaviest blow when we walk, and its tip may develop bony protuberances (heel spurs) which are quite painful (Figure 23). These are treated with cut-out heel supports and an easing of the weight on the foot. If a persistent bursitis develops, steroid injections or surgical excision may be required.

Perhaps the primary change in our feet as we age is a splaying or widening of the forefoot and flattening of the arch. In most individuals

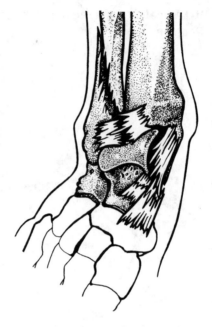

Figure 22. Torn ankle ligaments and bone fractures.

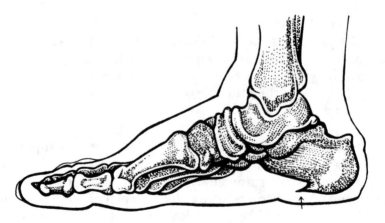

Figure 23. Painful spur under heel bone.

this is a harmless process, causing no pain and little deformity. Wider shoes are often required to accommodate the splayed foot, and as long as vanity doesn't overcome common sense, few problems will result. Tight or weak shoes may produce aching pain (*metatarsalgia*) across the ball of the foot, which usually responds to conservative measures. Occasionally, nerves between the second and third or the third and fourth toes become compressed, irritated, and scarred, creating a sharp pain in the toes. This is called a *Morton's neuroma.* Steroid injection and wider shoes are usually curative, but excision of the neuroma by minor surgery is common in chronic cases.

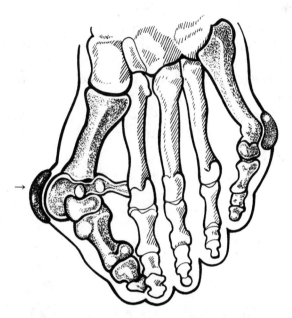

Figure 24. *Hallux valgus* foot deformity with large bunion (arrow).

As the foot widens, the toes are further compressed, particularly in women whose more flexible feet are usually confined by shoes with elevated heels and pointed toes—the opposite of the foot's natural configuration. The result of years of walking and weight bearing under this condition is a sideways shift of the big toe with a tender prominence over its junction with the foot. The deformity is called a *hallux valgus;* the calloused prominence is a bunion (Figure 24). The smaller toes must make room for the big toe, so they ride up on top or become hammered (curled). A bunionette, a small version of the larger bunion, may develop at the junction of the fifth toe and the foot.

Initial treatment of these deformities consists of padding and enlarging the shoes in the areas of friction. A small metatarsal pad, obtainable at most drugstores, placed inside the shoe under the ball of the foot may reduce pressure on the toes. Lengthwise or crosswise bars, or sole supports, reduce motion and pressure along the toes, and may make more aggressive therapy unnecessary. Persistent pain may require steroid injections or corrective surgery. Surgery generally gives excellent results, correcting deformities and alleviating pain.

As with all such orthopedic disorders, however, lasting improvement requires that the patient wear sensible shoes, reduce weight, and exercise to maximize the surgical result. Indeed, most of the musculoskeletal problems of the aging are benign deteriorations of otherwise normal bones, joints, and muscles. Self-help techniques to reduce discomfort and preserve function may be all that is needed to ensure many years of productive activity.

THE HEART AND CIRCULATION

Norman Makous, M.D.

Clinical Assistant Professor of Cardiology,
Pennsylvania Hospital

How the Heart Works

Anatomy

The heart is a four-chambered muscle that pumps blood to all parts of the body. It is located in the center of the chest behind the lower part of the breastbone *(sternum)*. Roughly the size of two clenched fists, it extends from the right edge of the breastbone halfway across the left side of the chest. The heartbeat can normally be felt near the nipple of the left breast. When empty of blood, the heart weighs 200 to 350 grams (one-half to two-thirds of a pound) (Figure 1).

Figure 2 shows the main structures. There are two major and two minor chambers. The two muscular *ventricles* are the major pumping chambers that eject blood from the heart. The two *atria* are minor pumping chambers that receive blood flowing to the heart and relay it to the ventricles. Blood from all parts of the body, darkened because body tissues have depleted it of oxygen, flows through two large veins (*vena cavae*)to the right atrium. It is delivered to the right ventricle which pumps it into the pulmonary artery to the lungs where it is cleansed of carbon dioxide and resupplied with oxygen. The lung's veins collect the now bright red, reoxygenated blood and return it to the left atrium which passes it on to the left ventricle where it is propelled under pressure into the aorta for distribution throughout the body.

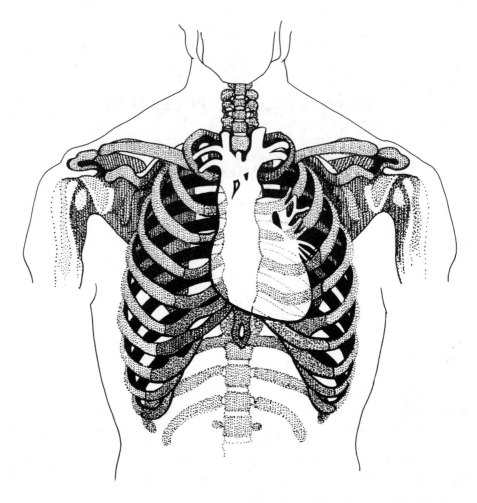

Figure 1. Location of the heart in the chest.

Like any pump, the heart requires valves to insure that blood is pumped in only one direction. The *tricuspid* valve, named for its three leaflets or cusps that come together to seal the passage, lies between the right atrium and right ventricle. It closes when the ventricle contracts to keep blood from being pumped back into the atrium. The *mitral* valve, named for its resemblance to a bishop's mitered hat, is bicuspid (two leaflets) and performs the same function between the left atrium and left ventricle. When the ventricles relax, *semilunar* (half-moon) valves with three leaflets close the openings into the aorta and pulmonary artery and keep blood from flowing back into the heart after being pumped out.

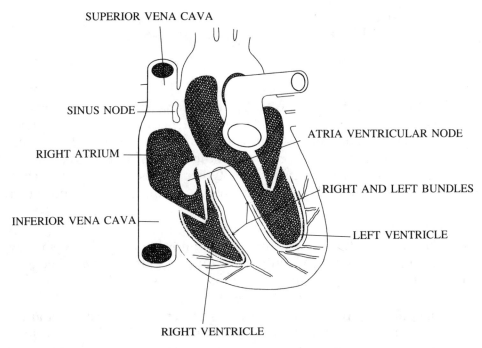

Figure 2. Main structures of the heart.

Blood is also prevented from flowing between the two atria and between the two ventricles by fibrous muscular walls called *septa*.

Like all organs of the body, the heart also requires the fuel carried in the blood. However, although 5 to 25 quarts of blood flow through the heart every minute, none of the blood within the chambers is available for the heart's use as a source of fuel. Instead, some of the blood pumped into the aorta is diverted to the left and right coronary arteries, two small, fragile fuel lines that extend over the heart's surface and penetrate down into the heart muscle where they branch into smaller and smaller vessels.

Three layers of tissue make up the heart. The thickest is a specialized muscle, the *myocardium*. This is covered on the outside by a double layer of very thin tissue, the *pericardium*. One of the thin layers is fixed to the muscle; the other folds back over the first and is separated from it by a small amount of lubricating fluid which permits heart movement with little friction. The third layer is a thin inner lining, the *endo-cardium*, from which the heart valves are constructed.

Physiology

Signals sent from the base of the brain along the autonomic nervous system coordinate the heart's function with demands from other parts of the body. They modify intrinsic mechanisms within the heart that permit the heart to continue beating even when the nervous system has been disconnected, as after a heart transplant. Other factors, such as the oxygen level in the blood and hormones such as adrenalin, also influence heart activity.

When the body is at rest, the heart pumps five to six liters (slightly more than 5–6 quarts) of blood every minute. Vigorous physical activity can increase the flow to more than 40 liters per minute.

The pumping period or *systole*, lasts about 0.2–0.3 seconds, and repeats an average of 72 times (beats) per minute when the body is at rest. However, the heart rate varies widely from person to person and may change from moment to moment, often for no apparent reason. During vigorous exercise, the normal rate may exceed 200 beats per minute, and in a highly conditioned athlete at rest may be slower than 40 beats per minute.

The split second (0.09–0.2 sec) between heart beats is called *diastole*. During this period, the ventricles fill with blood and the resting heart muscles are resupplied with oxygen and nutrients from blood flowing through the coronary arteries.

Following each diastole, the heartbeat is restarted automatically by the *sinus node*. This is a collection of specialized muscle cells located at the junction of the right atrium and the superior vena cava, the large vein that collects blood from the upper part of the body. Arising spontaneously from the sinus node, a wave of electrical excitation pervades the heart muscle, speeding through the thin atrial wall to the *atrioventricular*, or AV, node between the atria and ventricles and the tricuspid and mitral valves of the right and left heart. The electrical impulse hesitates here before it is conducted by modified cells resembling nerve tissue to the *right ventricular* by way of the *right bundle,* and to the *left ventricular* by way of the *left bundle.* Because this specialized tissue transmits the impulse through the heart faster than regular ventricular muscle, the heart is able to contract all over almost simultaneously, permitting efficient ejection of blood.

The nutrients required by the heart muscle are similar to those needed by other body tissues, but the proportions are different. The heart muscle extracts more oxygen from the blood than does any other tissue in the body, and its primary fuel is derived from fatty substances rather than from carbohydrates (sugars).

Circulation

Blood is distributed to the tissues throughout the body by the arteries. Distribution is as important as heart action. Arteries first divide into smaller vessels, called *arterioles,* then into still smaller vessels, the capillaries. The capillaries are so narrow that only one red cell at a time can pass through. On leaving the tissues, capillary blood is collected by small veins which join to form increasingly larger vessels until they reach the superior and inferior vena cava, the body's two largest veins, which return the blood to the right atrium of the heart.

The weight of blood in the body equals about eight percent of the total body weight corresponding to a volume of five to six liters, about 5½ to 6½ quarts. The capacity of all the blood vessels is greater than five times the volume of blood present. Survival thus depends on the efficiency with which the blood is distributed to the body tissues.

Local tissue and organ requirements determine the distribution and utilization of the blood. The fulfillment of these requirements is in turn regulated by local mechanisms and through integrated control exercised by the central nervous system. Blood flow and pressure from the larger arteries are regulated by the ability of smaller arteries to expand and contract. When these controls fail, blood pressure drops, reducing the supply of blood to the tissues. Prolonged reduction of supply produces shock.

Blood pressure is produced by the left ventricle pumping blood into the aorta against arterial resistance to flow. The peak pressure is called the systolic blood pressure and equals the higher number measured with a cuff and a sphygmomanometer. The minimum to which the pressure in the arteries falls between heartbeats is termed the diastolic pressure. Contraction of the elastic arteries after previous expansion keeps the blood pressure from falling to zero. The high systolic pressure is essential to force blood into the tissues. Blood pressure is measured in millimeters of mercury and is written as systolic over diastolic pressure. Pressures between 90–140/60–90 mm are within the normal range.

Each heartbeat generates a pressure wave which travels through the arteries about one hundred times faster than the blood flows. It can be felt as a pulse where arteries pass near the body surface, for example, in front of the ears *(temporal)*, under and in front of the diagonal muscle on the side of the neck *(carotid)*, inside the bend of the arm opposite the elbow *(brachial)*, at the wrist in line with the thumb *(radial)*, in the groin *(femoral)*, behind the knee *(popliteal)*, and on top of the ankle *(dorsalis pedis)*. Since each heartbeat generates only one major pulse, the pulse indicates heart rate no matter which artery is felt.

To measure heart rate in beats per minute, count the number of pulse beats in a convenient time and multiply as follows:

Time in seconds	Multiply by:
10	6
15	4
20	3

Effect of Exercise

The exertion of exercise increases the body's energy needs. Active muscles require more blood, which demands a greater output from the heart. This demand is met mainly by an increase in heart rate, and the rise in blood flow will generally be proportional to the rate increase. However, athletes and other physically trained people have more vigorous heart contractions which expel more blood with each beat. Systolic pressure also rises but not diastolic pressure.

The distribution of blood throughout the body changes with exercise, especially in the physically well-trained individual. Initially, blood flow to the skin, intestinal tract, and kidneys decreases and a larger share flows to the exercising muscles. Later, as the need to regulate body temperature develops, blood flow to the skin increases to release heat to the surroundings. The efficiency of these responses improves with sustained physical training.

Heart Disease

Heart diseases have a variety of forms and affect the heart in different ways and at different times of life. They range from infections, such as viral and bacterial, through metabolic problems stemming from thyroid disorders, to toxic reactions, for example, to drugs such as alcohol. Disease may alter heart structures such as the muscles, valves, and arteries, and may also cause pathologic tissue reactions such as inflammation, infection, and various manifestations of *atherosclerosis* (fatty deposits on arterial walls commonly known as hardening of the arteries).

Diagnosis of heart disease aims to answer three questions: What is causing heart damage? How much is the heart damaged and functionally impaired? To what degree does the disease limit the patient's activities?

Adequate evaluation of the heart usually involves a combination of procedures, beginning with a thorough historical review and including a physical examination, electrocardiogram, and an X ray or echocardiogram (ultrasonic scan) of the heart. It should be noted that many people with heart disease show no symptoms, almost half have normal electrocardiograms, and three-fourths have normal X rays. For these reasons, special procedures may be required to complete a satisfactory diagnosis. Such procedures may be modifications of the above noninvasive examinations or invasive techniques such as heart catheterization requiring hospitalization.

Few symptoms are unique to heart disease. For example, a persistent cough may be caused by heart disease, but is much more commonly due to other conditions not involving the heart. However, some symptoms are more heart-specific and indicate a need for medical attention. Among these are:

- Usual shortness of breath following exertion

- Chest pain, especially if accompanied by discomfort, pressure, choking, or gaseous indigestion

- Consciousness of the heart pounding or skipping, a momentary empty feeling in the chest, choking, or coughing

- Fluid retention with bloating, fullness or soreness of the upper and middle abdomen, or frequent sleep interruption to empty a full bladder

- Sleep interruption by shortness of breath, cough, or heart pounding

Because symptoms alone do not signify the presence of heart disease, the circumstances associated with the symptoms are important. The mode of onset and disappearance of symptoms; their localization in the body or extension to the back, abdomen, shoulders, arms, throat, or jaws; whether the symptoms change with a change of posture or activity; and their relation to gastrointestinal habits—should all be noted and reported to the physician.

Diagnostic Methods

Physical Examination

The physical examination should include the entire body, beginning with overall appearance. Does this suggest illness or distress? Is there evidence of weight loss, pallor, blue lips or fingers, pain, neck vein distension, or troubled breathing? Are blood vessels and pulse normal?

The small blood vessels in the retina at the back of the eye are the only ones in the body that can be observed directly. Visible changes in these arteries observed through an ophthalmoscope often indicate similar changes in other less accessible parts of the circulatory system, including the heart. Pulsations felt in veins and arteries in the neck reflect some features of heart action. Also, measurement of blood pressure in the arms and legs gives useful information about the heart and circulation.

The stethoscope amplifies sound and is used to monitor breathing and other chest sounds. Often, the physician can determine whether heart function is abnormal and affecting the lungs or lung function is abnormal and affecting the heart. Fluid congestion in the lungs due to a weakened heart, for example, produces crackling sounds (rales) in the lower chest.

The visible and palpable pulsation of the heart on the chest wall provides information about possible enlargement of parts of the heart. Turbulence in the blood flow, suggesting valve obstruction, produces a vibration called a thrill that resembles a cat's purring. Also, impulses related to the opening and closing of the heart valves may occasionally be felt.

The heartbeat produces apparently normal sounds when no disease is present. The short sounds normally heard at the beginning and end of each heartbeat (systole) are referred to as the first and second sounds. Often, third and fourth sounds related to the low pressure part of the cycle (diastole) are heard. These may be normal in children, but indicate an abnormality in adults characterized by a change in the elasticity of the ventricular muscle.

Heart murmurs are sounds of longer duration than normal heart sounds, and may occur in either systole or diastole. They are often described as high pitched and blowing, or low pitched and rumbling. Such murmurs may be harmless sounds of a normal heart, or may indicate abnormality such as a leaking or obstructing valve in a diseased heart.

Physical examination may disclose other signs of impaired heart function caused by excess fluids in the body. An enlarged liver or an accumulation of fluid in the abdominal cavity *(ascites)* may be a clue to a heart problem. Fluid may cause a non-tender swelling *(edema)* of the ankles and feet which retains a temporary indentation when prodded with a finger.

However, as with heart sounds or murmurs, any one of these findings, even in connection with other unfavorable signs, does not certify a diagnosis of heart disease. Edematous swelling of the feet, for example, can occur with venous insufficiency, varicose veins, liver or kidney disease, hypothyroidism, or simply as a result of prolonged sitting in hot weather.

Electrocardiography

The electrocardiogram is a graphic recording of the heart-generated electrical activity that spreads throughout the heart and can be detected all through the body and on the skin. This activity triggers the muscle contraction that produces each heartbeat. Two metal plates—-electrodes—are placed on the skin surface and connected to an instrument that measures and records the electric signal between the two points on the skin. Different pairs of points (leads) give different views of the heart's activity. There is no danger of shock since the machine does not send electrical impulses into the body. It merely measures the impulses that the body itself produces. Although the heart's rhythmic electrical activity is the only certain diagnostic evidence provided by an electrocardiogram, other information may be inferred, such as the size of the atria, the condition of the heart's electrical pathways, enlargement of right or left ventricular muscles or chambers, and loss of heart muscle by myocardial infarction with scar formation.

The standard electrocardiogram records only a small sample of heartbeats. In cases of heart attack or other life-threatening illnesses, it may be necessary to monitor every heartbeat (more than 100,000 per day). This is commonly done in coronary or intensive care units, and also in hospital operating rooms. In these situations, the electrocardiogram is continuously displayed on an oscilloscopic screen to permit minute-by-minute observation and to monitor changes in rhythm which may precede serious or even fatal disturbances.

Constant heart monitoring during normal daily activity is possible with a small battery-powered tape recorder, a technique known as Holter monitoring or dynamic electrocardiography. The completed tape is rapidly scanned for abnormalities with special equipment. This method permits a study of past heart action that accompanied episodes of dizziness, fainting, or chest symptoms to determine whether an abnormal heart rhythm is involved. For the special problems presented by cardiac pacemakers (battery devices implanted in the chest to maintain normal heart rhythm), attachments are available to transmit an electrocardiogram by telephone to a physician's office or special facility where diagnosis and treatment can sometimes be established during the call.

Echocardiography

Echocardiography is a non-invasive study of the heart with a beam of sound waves, much as sonar is used to detect underwater objects. It provides with greater safety much of the information previously obtainable only by heart catheterization. There is no need to puncture the skin or blood vessels since no injection is required. A small pencil-like probe merely rests on the skin in a daub of gel or paste added to enhance contact (Figure 3).

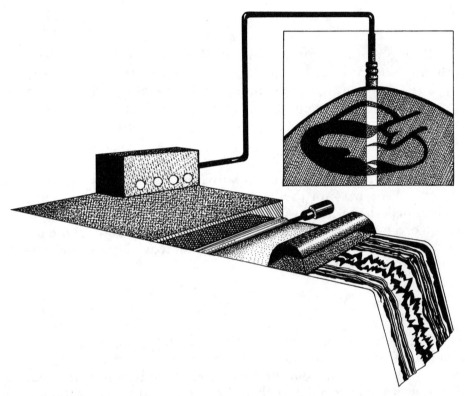

Figure 3. Echocardiograph.

Two echocardiographic modes are currently in use. One, the *m* mode, reveals structures along a one-dimensional (ice-pick-like) line. The other, the *2D* mode, reveals structures in a two-dimensional (cross-section) slice.

The echocardiogram reveals the anatomical and functional relationships of structures within the heart with great accuracy. Echocardiography is the best method for detecting excess fluid in the sac around the heart *(pericardium)* and for measuring thickening of the sac wall. It also permits measurement of the thickness of the heart valves, the sizes of heart muscle walls, and chamber volume. These measurements disclose dynamic features of heart action, including moment-to-moment changes of motion in the heart walls and valves, insufficient or excessive valve movement, and impaired mobility of the left ventricular mass.

X rays

X-ray examination of the heart involves several different techniques, including standard chest X rays and fluoroscopy. The standard chest X ray shows a still outline of the heart, while fluoroscopy shows a moving image on a TV-type screen. An X-ray study is like examining a forest as a whole, compared to echocardiography which is like examining individual trees.

The X ray reveals such information as gross enlargement or bulges—*aneurysms*—of the heart and its separate chambers, and large calcium deposits in heart valves, coronary arteries, and pericardium. Injection of a radio-opaque material helps to outline features of the back of the heart. Variations in the lungs' fluid content also give information about heart function.

Nuclear Cardiology

Radioactive isotopes injected into the bloodstream and scanned with a radiation detector outline the heart chambers and the large vessels carrying blood to and from the heart, and reveal regions where reduced flow causes blood to pool. This technique provides information about chamber enlargement or deformation, blood flow, and heart action. Other isotopes temporarily taken up by heart muscle indicate muscle areas inadequately supplied with blood. Reduction in blood flow to muscle may be an impairment due to myocardial infarction or a temporary response to physical exertion or drugs.

Exercise Stress Testing

In the broadest sense, exercise stress testing consists of a cardio-respiratory examination conducted during and after exertion. Exercise tolerance is measured, symptoms are clarified, and the heart and lungs are examined. Blood pressure, heart rate, and respiratory rate are recorded, and electrocardiograms are taken at regular intervals. The test should not be limited to electrocardiography.

Stress testing is useful for patitients who have known heart disease or symptoms of unknown origin, or who are well but worried. Its most common application is interpretation of chest symptoms.

Stress testing should not be performed if the subject has uncontrolled severe or active heart disease, such as impending myocardial infarction, active inflammation of the heart, or congestive heart failure. The information obtained in these circumstances is generally useless. Other contraindications depend on the information needed, how useful it may be, and how carefully the test can be performed.

The risk of an acute heart event in the 24-hour period following the test is one and one-half to two and one-half times that of a non-test period. This is less a reflection of the test's danger than of the fact that those tested are more likely to have had unstable hearts before the test, and therefore were at risk for an acute attack that could not be readily predicted. In a carefully conducted test, the exertion adds no danger.

The procedure varies, but stress test equipment usually consists of steps, a stationary bicycle, or a treadmill. Exercise may be continuous or interrupted by stopping and restarting. It may be ungraded at one level of exertion, or graded, starting at a low level and building gradually to higher levels. The test may be stopped at a predetermined heart rate, representing a certain percentage of the estimated maximum exercise tolerance, or at the appearance of a warning symptom or event. An electrocardiogram is taken and blood pressure measured every minute or at each level of exercise.

Testing should be under the supervision of a physician who has evaluated the subject's medical history and made a physical examination. The actual test may be conducted by a technician, but a physician should be within easy call. Emergency equipment to administer oxygen and support respiration, drugs, and a heart defibrillator should be at hand.

The information disclosed by stress testing ranges from an assessment of exercise motivation to an evaluation of the electrocardiogram. Normal walking rate is estimated, and symptom type, time of onset, and other relevant factors are clarified. Among the latter are the onset or increase in dryness of mouth that commonly develops at about 80 percent of maximal exercise tolerance, with or without heart disease. Changes in skin color, sweating, and temperature are noted. Air movement in the lungs and blood pressure are checked. Normally, systolic pressure will not exceed 210 mm, an increase of roughly 50 percent above the level at rest. If appropriate, the adequacy of treatment for high blood pressure can be assessed. A falling systolic pressure or heart rate signals the need to end the test. A rising diastolic pressure indicates that the limit of cardio-circulatory tolerance to exertion has been reached, possibly because of the presence of heart disease. Changes in heart sound and the appearance of murmur are also noted.

While various electrocardiographic changes, such as heart rate and regularity are important, most attention is given to a portion of the displayed heart beat called the ST-T segment which is sensitive to changes in muscle cell metabolism. A change here induced by exercise usually indicates inadequate blood flow and oxygen supply to a part of the heart muscle, a condition that commonly develops with coronary artery arterio-sclerosis.

Cardiac Catheterization

Cardiac catheterization is an invasive method of heart study used when other methods fail to provide specific information. Its most common application is in evaluating coronary arteries.

The procedure is done under local anesthesia and sedation. A thin, wire-like tube—the catheter—is inserted into a blood vessel through a needle puncture or surgical incision and threaded into and beyond the heart, guided by fluoroscopy. The choice of an artery or vein depends on the information required, and the insertion point may be the inside of the upper arm, opposite the elbow, the groin, or occasionally a superficial jugular vein in the neck.

Pressures are recorded, blood samples may be taken, and X-ray contrast material may be injected. X-ray motion pictures outline the inner walls of the blood vessels and heart chambers and show the movement of the injected material through the circulation. A dye or cold salt solution may be injected into parts of the heart or its blood vessels, and measurements made of the subsequent change in dye concentration or temperature in blood samples drawn from other parts of the heart or blood vessels. These give an estimate of blood flow rates, leakage through or around the heart valves, and the volume of blood in various parts of the circulation.

Heart catheterization is justified when the threat of undiagnosed and untreated heart disease appears to be greater than the risk of the procedure itself. Safety requires hospitalization. The threat to life is very slight, but possible complications include bleeding, infection, perforation, allergic reactions to the dye, and heart irregularity. Heart catheterization is also indicated when precise diagnosis is needed prior to surgery. Conditions most often requiring such study include congenital heart disease, valvular disease, and pain—*angina pectoris*—suggesting coronary insufficiency resulting from atherosclerosis.

Treatment of Heart Disease

Reasonable certainty that treatment will be effective depends heavily on accurate diagnosis. While some diseases can be cured if heart damage is reversible or minimal, cure may be impossible if the cause of disease cannot be determined, or if damage is irreversible.

Management of a heart condition involves direct and indirect medical and surgical treatment. Treatment may directly affect the heart itself, as when digitalis is administered to strengthen heart muscle contraction, or another part of the body, as when a diuretic acts on the kidneys to relieve fluid overload.

Personal Habits and Diet

Prudent changes in the personal habits are often necessary to promote heart health. Since excess weight may lead to high blood pressure, diabetes, and elevated cholesterol, and tends to hasten the development of atherosclerosis, the diet may have to be reduced in calories. To the extent possible, saturated animal fats should be replaced by unsaturated vegetable fats, and intake of salt should be restricted.

Dieting is a lifelong pursuit, with the goal of maintaining proper weight. The prudent diet advocated by the American Heart Association lowers total blood cholesterol. Evidence suggests that strict dieting helps to reabsorb cholesterol deposits in arterial walls, decreasing the risk of complications such as myocardial infarction.

Salt (sodium chloride), which tends to be excessive in most diets, acts to raise blood pressure. A family history of high blood pressure should be a warning of strong susceptibility to the pressure-elevating effects of sodium. Sodium also causes the system to retain water, which aggravates inadequate heart function and increases the risk of congestive heart failure. Reduction of daily sodium intake by limiting salt in cooking and at the table, and by eliminating foods with large amounts of sodium—lunch meat, canned soups, baked goods, condiments—often permits as much as a 50 percent reduction of medication for high blood pressure and congestive heart failure.

The use of tobacco, especially cigarettes, increases the risk of developing atherosclerosis. Smoking also aggravates and even causes chronic bronchitis, which contributes to the impairment of heart function. While it is not known how tobacco harms the coronary arteries, the effect completely disappears when tobacco use is stopped, and the risk of atherosclerosis is lessened.

Occasional use of alcohol in moderate amounts is not harmful, but it should be kept in mind that alcohol is a poison. The ingestion of several ounces will depress muscle action in both normal and abnormal hearts. In medicinal use, alcohol acts as a tranquilizer and depressant; overuse by those with diseases such as angina pectoris can be harmful. Impaired judgment may encourage imprudent activity, and a drinker may then fail to heed the warning symptoms of heart stress. However, alcohol in moderation does reduce anxiety and enhances the apparently beneficial high density lipoprotein component in cholesterol blood levels.

Caffeine-containing liquids such as coffee, tea, and colas are not inherently harmful. Caffeine is a mild heart stimulant, and its use should be reduced or eliminated when cardiac irritability and irregularity are experienced. Because the heart is highly irritable following acute myocardial infarction, some physicians prohibit coffee in such circumstances. Consumed in large amounts, caffeine may overstimulate the nervous system, resulting in overeating, excessive smoking, or overwork. Thus, heavy coffee consumption can be a sign of other bad habits more injurious to the heart than caffeine itself.

Because vitamin deficiencies can adversely affect the heart, vitamins are as essential to a healthy heart as to other organs and body tissues. Vitamin B-1 (thiamine) deficiency causes heart enlargement, which may lead to congestive heart failure. There is no good evidence that large amounts of vitamins E or C have any therapeutic value for the heart in healthy adults.

Stress and anxiety unquestionably affect health, though it is impossible to predict with any consistency what different individuals will find stressful. Anxiety plays a significant role in responses to health problems.

Those who ignore or deny threats to their health are often suppressing anxiety about their heart; impending illness intensifies such anxiety. The pain of angina pectoris, for example, often causes a response that is out of proportion to its intensity, leading the sufferer to seek surgical relief. Therapy failures and problems of heart health often result from refusal to modify activities or life styles as recommended by a physician. Those with sufficient emotional strength to respond calmly to heart disease will often find that only minimal changes in their lives are required, and that they can live longer and more satisfying lives.

A diagnosis of heart disease does not automatically demand curtailment of exercise or work. In fact, the reverse is true for many heart conditions. An increase in activity is especially desirable for coronary heart disease. For many heart valve conditions in many individuals, however, the heart is already working at capacity, so the condition does not benefit from increased activity, although some improvement in muscle strength and training of the circulatory system may bring improved efficiency and a feeling of well being. Stress testing helps to determine a safe level of activity.

Exercise has important benefits apart from improvement of cardio-circulatory efficiency. It helps to heal the damaged self-image, relieves depression, and raises self-esteem. Occasionally it improves collateral artery circulation.

Although some modification of workload is indicated in 10 to 20 percent of all cases of heart disease, such a diagnosis is not an automatic call for retirement. Most jobs in American industry are more or less sedentary, and 90 percent of all individuals who have suffered heart attacks return to work. Most should be able to return to work in six to ten weeks following an acute myocardial infarction, with full recovery in three to four months. Failure to return to normal activity is often a sign of poor management of the rehabilitation program, perhaps because of a lack of needed information.

Individuals who are able to resume other normal activities need not curtail sexual activity. If a heart rate of up to 130 per minute during physical exercise is tolerated, sexual intercourse can also be tolerated, since the heart rate does not exceed this level in the middle-aged. The impotence commonly experienced following a heart attack may reflect both partners' fear, but is more often due to the depression that accompanies acute heart episodes. Sexual activity can usually be adjusted to the satisfaction of both partners without imposing cardiocirculatory risk.

Drugs

Like most medications, drugs for the heart and circulation have both direct and indirect effects, wanted and unwanted. These classifications may change as the goal of treatment changes.

There is no ideal drug that is absolutely safe in all circumstances. The justification for administering a drug depends on the expected benefit, the risk of reaction, and the prognosis if the drug is withheld. Whether prescribed by a physician or purchased over the counter, a drug is a kind of experiment, a therapeutic trial. It may be likened to buying a new suit, which is not taken home before it has been tried for fit and possible alterations. In a similar way, a drug is first taken in a standard dosage before alterations are made if needed.

Surgery

Except when a permanent pacemaker is to be placed, heart surgery is a major operation. Pacemaker placement normally requires only local anesthesia; the chest is not opened. A tube is threaded through a vein in the neck or under the collarbone, and a battery pack is placed under the skin and tissues of the upper chest outside of the ribs. Almost all other cardiac surgery requires opening the chest.

A diseased pericardium can be surgically removed without opening the heart itself if pericardial fluid persists in forming or if the pericardium has become scarred and is constricting the heart. However, when the heart or coronary circulation is surgically invaded, special support of the heart, lungs, and circulation by a heart-lung machine is required. In coronary artery bypass surgery, a vein is removed from the thigh and connected between the aorta and a coronary artery beyond any severe atherosclerotic obstruction. The heart must be stopped for this procedure, and the circulation artificially maintained, but the heart chambers are not entered. Occasionally, a bulging scar from a previous infarction must be cut away, but this is usually deferred until the heart shows signs of failing or exhibits a severe arrhythmia (abnormal electrocardiogram). The removal of such a bulge, known as an aneurysm, improves the efficiency of heart function.

Valve surgery requires invasion of the heart chambers. Occasionally, diseased heart valves can be corrected by removal of calcium deposits and cutting of scar tissue to free the valve. This is most effective for *mitral stenosis* (narrowing of the mitral valve). Usually, however, heart valves must be replaced because of irreparable damage. The replacement valve may be an artificial one made of a plastic-covered metal frame, a natural valve from an animal heart, or a combination of both.

Valve surgery entails a considerable risk of complications, especially from clot formation. Unless anticoagulants ("blood thinners") are used, a clot may form on a new valve and break away, causing stroke or other problems in the systemic circulation. Anticoagulants help to prevent clot formation, but also involve an unavoidable risk of bleeding. Additional risks in valve surgery include infection, mechanical failure, and detachment from supporting tissues.

Abnormal Conditions

Arrhythmias

A heart arrhythmia is a disorder in the origin or propagation of the heartbeat. It may or may not appear as a complication of known heart disease. Its significance depends on the cardiocirculatory insufficiency inherent in the arrhythmia itself and in impairment caused by the underlying disease. The capacity of the heart and circulation to compensate for impairment depends on the nature and extent of damage from the disease.

Arrhythmias have three general origins: the atrial portion of the heart above the ventricles, the ventricles themselves, and a reduction in electrical contact between the atria and ventricles. The most common arrhythmias, premature or extra heartbeats, stem from irritability of the heart muscle. There may be one or a succession of ectopic out-of-place beats. A succession is called *tachycardia* (rapid heart rate).

Another type of tachycardia is the result of *fibrillation*, a very rapid, grossly irregular beating confined to either the atrial or the ventricular muscles. Atrial fibrillation only slightly diminishes the heart's efficiency, but ventricular fibrillation is lethal. The fibrillating ventricle is able to pump very little blood into the circulation. Drugs or a modified electric shock are used to correct atrial fibrillation, but controlled electric shock (electrocardioversion) is the only treatment that will terminate ventricular fibrillation. Light anesthesia is given for non-emergency cardioversion. Electrical contact is made with paddles pressed to the middle and the left side of the chest, and a jolt of high DC voltage is administered.

Reduced electrical conduction between the atria and the ventricles indicates the presence of a heart block. When this is complete, the ventricles beat independently at a rate of less than 40 per minute. If no heart or circulatory disease is present, a complete heart block may be tolerated, but sudden onset may cause fainting (Stokes-Adams attacks).

The heart may also beat irregularly without other symptoms. When symptoms are present, they range from the pounding in the chest caused by a rapid heartbeat to sensations of the heart stopping, a sudden fullness in the chest or throat, and occasionally a slight cough.

An arrhythmia may be eliminated by correction of underlying disease, suppression with drugs, or, for an abnormally fast beat, electric shock. When the heart rate is too slow, a pacemaker is used to speed it up. Pacemakers supply an electrical impulse which initiates the heartbeat at preset intervals, and can be made to work constantly or only when the normal heart rate falls below a particular level.

Abnormal Blood Pressure

In general, high or low blood pressure produces no symptoms unless severely abnormal. When symptoms do appear, they are often erroneously attributed to the abnormal pressure but are more likely to be due to the underlying cause of the abnormality.

The "normal" blood pressure range can be quite wide. Some people function normally with systolic pressures as low as 70 mm, while vigorous exertion in others may raise their pressures above 200 mm. However, a systolic pressure of 120 mm, ordinarily considered normal for the body at rest, may be too low in cases of long-standing high pressure and advanced arteriosclerosis. A higher pressure may be necessary to force blood through the narrowed arteries. If the pressure is so low that an inadequate blood supply reaches body tissues (a condition called hypotension), shock may result.

Congestive Heart Failure

Congestive heart failure is the inability of the heart to pump suffi-cient blood for the body's needs. It may be due to a weakening of the heart muscle or obstruction of a valve. If the left side of the heart cannot eject all the blood returning from the lungs, blood backs up into the lungs, fluid leaks into the lungs' air sacs, and breath becomes short and makes crackling sounds (rales). If the right side of the heart cannot ade-quately accommodate the blood returning from all parts of the body through the veins, blood backs up into the veins. Neck veins distend, the liver enlarges, fluid may accumulate in the abdomen, the feet swell, and body weight increases. Also, the body often retains salt and water because of effects on the nervous sytem, endocrine glands, and kidneys. Excess fluids overload the heart and the circulatory system and make them even more inadequate.

Treatment consists of drugs such as digitalis to strengthen and slow heart action and diuretics that cause the kidney to excrete more salt and water. It may also include supplementary oxygen to ease breathing, dietary limitations on salt and fluids, and restrictions on physical activity. Several other older drugs, as well as new ones, are used for treatment.

Common Heart Diseases

Coronary Heart Disease

Heart disease resulting from atheroscelerosis of the coronary arteries is variously called coronary, arteriosclerotic, or ischemic heart disease. It displays five major patterns (syndromes) which include sudden death, acute myocardial infarction, angina pectoris, an intermediate syndrome of acute coronary insufficiency, and *cardiomegaly* (enlargement of the heart).

Coronary *heart* disease and coronary *artery* disease are not identical and should not be used interchangeably in diagnosis. Almost everybody develops coronary artery disease (atherosclerosis) at some time. This is a narrowing of the arterial opening by fatty deposits of cholesterol which also cause scarring and calcium deposition. Certain diagnosis is possible only by autopsy, but clinically acceptable diagnosis can be made by ex-amination of the arteries during heart surgery or cardiac catheterization.

Coronary artery disease progresses to coronary heart disease only when the arterial opening is at least 50 percent obstructed and the reduced blood supply to the heart muscles significantly affects heart action and produces symptoms that require a reduction in physical activity. The body then compensates to some extent through *collateral circulation,* the opening of very small blood vessels, nonfunctioning at birth, that parallel the arteries and supply blood to the deprived muscle.

The extent and rate at which coronary artery blood flow falls and collateral circulation grows are major determinants of the symptoms of coronary heart disease. Heart pain *(angina pectoris)* usually appears when the blood supply to a particular heart muscle area falls by 50 to 70 percent. Typically, pain in the early stages is felt only after a strong exertion that makes heavy demands on the blood supply flowing through the coronary arteries. As the obstruction grows, heart pain appears after less and less exertion, eventually even when the body is almost at rest.

If the progressive reduction of blood flow to the heart muscle is gradual and partly compensated by collateral circulation, and the heart pain varies in frequency and duration with minimal death of muscle cells, the condition is called the *intermediate syndrome of coronary insufficiency.* When blood circulation to some of the muscle is cut off, whether due to sudden blockage by a clot *(coronary artery thrombosis)* or progressive reduction of blood flow to the area *(coronary artery insufficiency),* part of the muscle dies *(myocardial infarction)* and the dead muscle is replaced by scar tissue.

Half the deaths of the sudden death syndrome from coronary artery disease occur within 15 minutes of the onset of an attack. Death is not necessarily due to clot obstruction, but is more likely to be caused by a temporary instability in the heart's blood supply that precipitates the erratic beat of ventricular fibrillation. Unless electric shock is administered within four minutes, irreversible brain damage and then death will follow.

Occasionally the heart will gradually enlarge (cardiomegaly) without apparent myocardial infarctions or heart pain. This is presumably the result of a slow reduction of blood flow to the heart muscle caused by chronic coronary insufficiency.

Symptoms: How the pain of angina pectoris develops is not understood, in part because the heart lacks nerve fibers specific for pain. Even a myocardial infarction due to the sudden obstruction of an artery does not necessarily cause pain. Victims describe their discomfort as pressure, tightness, choking, or merely shortness of breath. Discomfort lasts just a few moments if caused by angina, but twenty minutes or more if caused by myocardial infarction.

The discomfort or pain is typically located in the middle of the chest, but on rare occasions is limited to the left side. Pain may radiate to the neck, lower jaws, shoulders, and down the upper arms, especially on the left side, or may appear as indigestion in the stomach. Occasionally, it shoots directly through the chest to the left side of the back. Chest pain that is sharp, brief, confined to a very small area, or affected by deep breathing, twisting, or moving the shoulders, head, or neck, is not ischemic heart pain.

Angina pectoris is triggered by exertion or emotion and grows worse if the stimulus continues. Infrequently, it is mild and steady for a while and then vanishes spontaneously, a condition known as "walk through" angina pectoris. A sense of alarm, apart from anxiety over chest pain, is common, together with sweating, pallor, and lightheadedness.

Most chest discomfort or pain—including that which mimics heart pain—originates in the muscles, bones, and cartilages of the chest wall and back. A disorder of the esophagus, stomach, gall bladder, and even the bowel may also cause discomfort that mimics heart pain. Paradoxically, some heart attacks cause no pain at all. Victims may feel generally ill, fatigued, weak, and sweaty, as if infected by a virus.

However, chest discomfort that lasts 20 minutes or more with increasing severity is a signal to go directly to an emergency facility without delay for a diagnosis. Because delay may prove fatal, a personal physician need not be called until the patient is under proper medical supervision in an emergency station.

Risk factors of Latent Disease: A disease is latent if causative factors are present but have not yet produced overt symptoms or examination findings. Atherosclerotic coronary artery disease is latent coronary heart disease. Although the latent disease can be detected with reasonable certainty by heart catheterization, the risk and expense of catheterization make it inappropriate for the person who is still apparently well. It is preferable, if possible, to eliminate the factors that cause or aggravate the latent disease even without a firm diagnosis.

Unfortunately, many of the sources that contribute to atherosclerosis are not well defined. Those that have been identified are termed risk factors. Some are correctable but others are not.

Uncorrectable risk factors are sex, an inherited predisposition, and aging. Women are relatively protected against atherosclerosis until menopause, after which their incidence of coronary heart disease rivals that of men.

Correctable risk factors include high blood pressure, smoking, and blood cholesterol levels. Cholesterol level assumes its greatest importance for men in their forties, followed by high blood pressure and smoking. By the time men reach their seventies, the importance of cholesterol level recedes and the risks from hypertension and smoking are greater.

High blood pressure and cholesterol level are of equal importance for women in their forties and fifties, when smoking is less significant. By the seventies, high blood pressure still presents the same risk, but cholesterol and smoking have minimal significance. Although absolute levels are less important at this advanced age, an increase of 10 mm in pressure or 10 mg of cholesterol per 100 cc of blood is more significant for women than for men.

Minor risk factors include, but are not limited to, obesity, elevated blood sugar and uric acid levels, lack of exercise, and stress. Weight control is essential to effective treatment of coronary disease because obesity, although a minor risk factor by itself, is often associated with high blood pressure, elevated blood cholesterol, and diabetes mellitus. In combination, these are a major risk factor.

Restless, aggressive competitors and compulsive achievers (Type A personality traits) are also especially prone to coronary attack.

Accumulating evidence indicates that reduction or elimination of risk factors reduces the likelihood of coronary heart disease. The evidence suggests that atherosclerosis can be slowed and possibly stopped or reversed, even at an advanced state. Although scar tissue and calcium deposits cannot be reduced, clots and cholesterol can.

Treatment: The treatment of coronary heart disease is essentially medical management in which habits, diet, working conditions, attitudes, and even life goals may have to be changed if they are detrimental. Reduced consumption of alcohol and caffeine is normally obligatory. Smoking should be stopped and physical exercise increased to or continued at a desirable level. Heart pain can usually be controlled with appropriate drugs and the required dosage tends to decrease as treatment proceeds.

In the past, nitroglycerine preparations were the primary elements in drug therapy, in part because of their rapid effect. Nitroglycerine in a tablet placed under the tongue passes into the bloodstream in less than a minute and acts on the heart and circulation in at least three ways: widening the coronary arteries and relaxing other arteries to reduce the left ventricle's workload, but mostly by relaxing the veins to reduce the return blood flow to the heart. The effect lasts 10–20 minutes. Nitroglycerine also passes rapidly through the skin and can be used in the form of an ointment with longer lasting results. Longer acting preparations can also be taken by mouth, but most of the drug is prevented from entering the circulation by the liver.

More recently, beta-blocking agents have become the mainstay in the treatment of angina pectoris. These drugs block the stimulatory effects of the sympathetic nervous system and adrenalin-like substances on the heart and blood vessels, thus reducing the blood pressure, the heart rate, and the vigor of heart contraction. Lightening the heart's workload and oxygen requirements often makes the limited blood flow permitted by diseased coronary arteries adequate for increased physical activity with fewer pain episodes.

If angina pectoris becomes intolerable, surgery is required. In certain situations, coronary bypass surgery not only relieves the angina, but also improves heart function and reduces the threat of heart attack or death. However, the kinds of pain-free coronary heart disease that might benefit from surgery remain to be identified.

While there is no firm evidence that coronary bypass surgery is superior to medical treatment in increasing life expectancy, it does improve the quality of life. One reason for the failure of surgery to prolong life is that many who undergo it do not afterward modify their lifestyle to reduce risk.

Hypertensive Cardiovascular Disease

High blood pressure overworks the left ventricle, causing the heart muscle first to thicken, then to enlarge and weaken, with the result that activity brings shortness of breath. Early enlargement is best measured by ultrasonic echocardiography; X-ray evidence appears later.

A secondary effect of high blood pressure is its contribution to the development of coronary artery atherosclerosis. If left untreated, high blood pressure can lead to congestive heart failure. The electrocardiogram is studied for evidence of heart involvement.

Effective treatment of high blood pressure prevents or reduces heart enlargement, and also delays recurrent acute coronary heart disease. If congestive heart failure is present, a reduction of pressure lightens the heart load. Digitalis acts to improve muscle strength, and diuretics reduce the pressure and the heart's fluid load.

Valvular Heart Disease

Heart murmurs are a sign of valvular heart disease. However, a vigorously beating normal heart may sometimes produce an innocent murmur, and such murmurs are common during childhood. Organic or abnormal heart murmurs are most often produced by valve abnormalities such as a leaky valve that permits blood to flow back into a chamber from which it has just been pumped, a narrowed or obstructed valve, and a deformed valve that otherwise functions adequately.

The significance of a murmur depends on the severity of the valve deformity, the degree of malfunction, and the overload it places on the heart. Obstructed valves cause more problems than leaky ones. Heart enlargement is directly proportional to the severity of valve deformity.

Damaged heart valves may be present at birth or the result of later illness or injury. Rheumatic fever during childhood is the most common later cause, about equal in incidence to congenital deformities. Although its cause is unknown, rheumatic fever is normally preceded by a specific streptococcal infection (group A). Since the streptococcus bacteria and the heart valves contain similar proteins (antigens), antibodies formed to fight the infection also attack the valves, causing them to swell, scar, and malfunction. A myocardial infarction in later life can disturb the attachment of the mitral valve to the left ventricle and cause abnormal valve function and a systolic murmur. Viral infections and a sharp blow or other chest injury may also harm the heart valves.

About one out of ten adults has a systolic murmur that persists from childhood. It is a clicking sound due to a leaking mitral valve which allows some blood to regurgitate back into the left atrium near the end of the systolic contraction of the left ventricular muscle. The condition is known as a click murmur, mitral valve prolapse, or Barlow's syndrome, and is often associated with unusual bone structure such as spinal curvature or depression of the breastbone. It is usually harmless, but occasionally accompanies a serious but poorly understood heart muscle disorder.

Bacterial endocarditis is an infection that produces wart-like lesions on the heart valves. The bacteria enter the blood stream from respiratory or genitourinary infections or during dental work and are detected by cultures of blood samples. Two to six weeks of antibiotic treatment usually cures the infection, but may not prevent additional valve damage. Endocarditis can be prevented by prompt antibiotic treatment of the original infection.

Specific treatment of valvular heart disease is usually unnecessary, but surgical repair or replacement with an artifical valve may be required when the disease is advanced. Such surgery helps to improve and prolong life, but involves unavoidable new risks and does not eliminate all old ones. In general, valve surgery is justified only when the disease has made life intolerable or further delay creates a greater risk than immediate surgery. Selecting the proper time can be a difficult decision.

Heart Muscle Disease

A number of conditions—many poorly understood or unknown—-can weaken the heart muscle. Chronic conditions without inflammations are called *myocardiopathy*. Acute inflammations, as with diphtheria or viral infections, are called *myocarditis*. When the muscle has been poisoned, as by arsenic, it may thicken, enlarge, or both. In some susceptible individuals, this condition may be caused by alcohol.

Some of these disorders have genetic bases. The muscle of the left ventricle may grow so thick that it obstructs the ejection of blood from the ventricle into the aorta. Such conditions are known as *idiopathic* (unknown) *subaortic hypertrophic stenosis* and *asymmetric septal hypertrophy*.

Pericardial Disease

Because of associated pain, inflammation of the pericardium (sac around the heart) can be alarming. It often occurs as an isolated condition in younger persons and is thought to be due to a virus. The site of the pain is apt to be higher in the chest and shoulders than for angina pectoris, and sitting and leaning forward provide some relief. The two pericardial surfaces rubbing over each other as the heart muscles move usually produce a grating sound. Also, an echocardiogram will reveal excess fluid in the pericardium, and an electrocardiogram will often show an abnormality. The condition is usually self-limiting, but its tendency to recur throughout the year following the first episode can be unsettling.

Occasionally, a tumor or a disease such as tuberculosis may cause unusually large amounts of fluid to collect in the pericardial sac. Also, a sudden accumulation of fluid, for example, when an injury penetrates the heart and releases blood into the pericardium, may inhibit muscle action, causing a "choking" of the heart known as *tamponade*. Removal of fluid with a syringe and needle gives immediate relief, and surgery is usually not required.

CHEST AND LUNG DISEASES

Robert L. Honish, M.D.

Clinical Assistant Professor, Pulmonary Section
Pennsylvania Hospital

The lung is a large, spongy, pyramid-shaped mass suspended in the chest cavity that communicates with outside air through the mouth and nose by way of the interconnecting windpipe (*trachea*) and smaller channels (*bronchi*). The airway can be visualized as an inverted tree, with the mouth as the base and the windpipe as the trunk branching repeatedly into smaller and smaller twigs down to fine *bronchioles*. The bronchioles lead to small air ducts that end in tiny sacs, called *aveoli*, where the exchange takes place between new air and exhaust gases from the body. (See Figure 1.)

Alveoli are uniquely linked with three different types of cells, each with a different function. One type is a kind of housekeeper which literally "eats" microorganisms and other foreign matter to keep the lungs clean. Another produces a detergent-like substance that keeps the alveolar walls from sticking together when the air sacs collapse like deflated balloons during exhalation. This makes them easier to inflate with newly inhaled air. The third type of cell provides the supporting wall structure of the air sac.

Within the tracheobronchial tree are complex cell families which serve important functions. One group of cells in the upper airway is covered with fine hairlike strands, called *cilia*, which wave rhythmically and sweep mucus and entrapped foreign matter upward to be coughed away or swallowed into the stomach (Figure 2). Another group of cells secretes the mucus. A third group makes up the spiral muscle tissue that gives the airway the ability to contract suddenly and produce a cough which ejects accumulated mucus and debris. Thus, the airway is normally kept clear to allow fresh air to reach the remotest alveoli and to allow waste gases to be vented to the atmosphere.

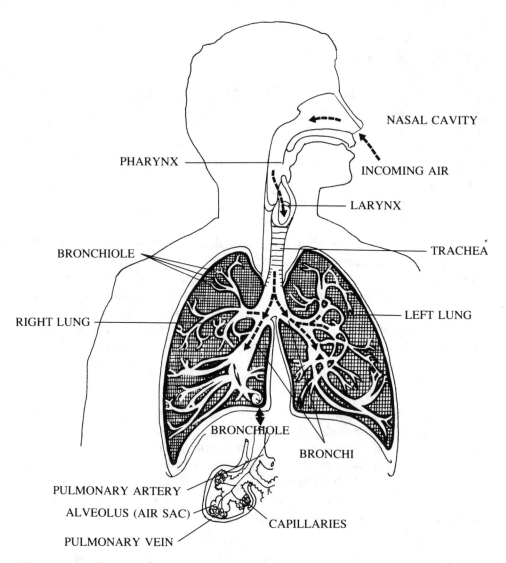

Figure 1. As the lungs expand during inspiration the outside air passes from the nose, pharynx, trachea, bronchi, and bronchioles to the smallest units — the aveoli. Here the oxygen of the air passes through a thin membrane into the blood stream. During expiration (breathing out) the carbon dioxide diffused from the blood into the aveoli is expelled from the body.

accumulated mucus and debris. Thus, the airway is normally kept clear to allow fresh air to reach the remotest alveoli and to allow waste gases to be vented to the atmosphere.

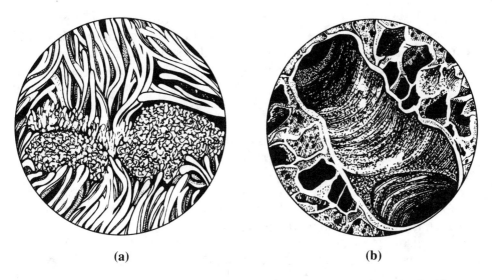

(a)   (b)

Figure 2. (a) The cilia, many short hair-like processes, located on the inside surface of the airway, move in a coordinated wave-like motion to cleanse secretions
and foreign material from the breathing tubes. (b) Cross-section of a small bronchus or airway and surrounding alveoli.

The other major component of the lung system is the blood supply
to the alveoli. Dark blood, rich in carbon dioxide (byproduct of the
body's metabolism of food) and depleted in oxygen, returns through
veins to the right side of the heart. The right side of the heart pumps the
dark venous blood to the lungs to be cleansed of carbon dioxide and replenished with oxygen. The gas exchange takes place between the alveoli
and the network of fine capillaries surrounding them. The lungs also alter
the chemical composition of the blood by reactions with enzymes se-
creted by lung tissues. Now bright red, the blood returns to the left side
of the heart which pumps it out to all parts of the body.

The right side of the heart pumps venous blood to the lungs at a relatively low pressure, 20/10 millimeters of mercury, compared with the
pressure of 120/80 millimeters of mercury at which the heart normally
pumps clean blood into the arteries. (The upper number is the pressure
at the peak of the pumping action; the lower number is the pressure
when the heart has relaxed. In people with high blood pressure, these
pressures can be much greater.)

Unlike any other organ in the body, the lungs receive two blood supplies. They not only receive venous blood from the right side of the heart for cleaning and oxygenation, but also share in the high-pressure arterial blood pumped from the left side of the heart. Part of this oxygen-rich supply, called the bronchial circulation, is distributed to the bronchi and the lungs to nourish these tissues so that they can perform their tasks.

If the millions of tiny air sacs in the lung were thinly spread over a single plane, they would cover an area the size of a tennis court. Thus, they provide an enormous surface—100 times as great as the surface of the body itself—through which gases can be exchanged between the blood and inhaled air. Except for the heart, the lungs are the only organ to which the entire blood volume is exposed.

Pneumonia

Pneumonia is an inflammation of the lungs accompanied by accumulation of fluid which can seriously diminish respiratory capacity (Figure 3). It can be caused by infectious agents such as bacteria, viruses, fungi, and some other less common microorganisms. Despite potent antibiotic drugs effective against bacterial infection, and efficient, lifesaving, mechanical breathing devices, pneumonia remains the major cause of all deaths in the elderly today.

This apparent contradiction stems from the tendency of pneumonia to complicate other underlying diseases. Whether the underlying disease is a malignancy or extensive heart disease with a primary problem of heart failure, pneumonia is the terminal event. In addition, pneumonias are much more prevalent in vulnerable individuals such as the diabetic and the patient who has been weakened by radiation or chemotherapy or severely debilitated by bowel disease or kidney failure.

The symptoms of bacterial pneumonia can be quite varied. If defense mechanisms are depressed, the onset may go completely unnoticed. However, if the patient is otherwise in good health, the symptoms may include high fever, a productive and persistent cough, night sweats, loss of appetite, and, late in the course of the disease, chest pain. A less frequent but equally important complaint is a sensation of breathlessness.

Although antibiotics are the mainstay in treating patients with bacterial pneumonias, the medication itself does not cure. The patient's own

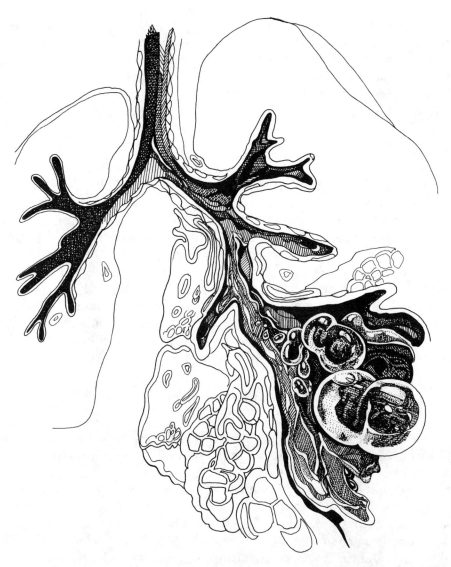

Figure 3. The airways affected by pneumonia are congested, inflamed, and partially filled with purulent thick fluid. The surrounding lung tissue is infected. The diseased area cannot perform the normal function of transporting oxygen into the blood stream.

defense mechanisms really terminate the disease process; antibiotics only help to overcome the infection. Rest, adequate nutrition, and the control of coexisting disease such as diabetes and heart or kidney failure are essential therapeutic supplements.

Characteristic indications of viral pneumonia are a dry, non-productive cough, a low-grade fever usually no higher than 102°F (38.9°C), moderate muscle ache, and a general feeling of lassitude. The extreme exhaustion that often comes with bacterial pneumonia is absent. Occasionally, a person with viral pneumonia will continue with normal daily activities, suspecting at most a severe cold or a mild bronchitis. When medical help is sought, a lung X ray may present an alarming picture that belies a relatively healthy outward appearance.

In most instances, antibiotic therapy is not appropriate for viral pneumonia because it will have little effect on the virus and may enhance the growth of bacteria resistant to the antibiotic used. If the patient is in relatively good general health, supportive measures are best, including rest, adequate nutrition, expectorants where applicable, aspirin or other mild analgesics for pain, and careful monitoring to detect complications. The most serious complication of viral pneumonia is involvement of the sac around the heart (*viral pericarditis*). Rarely, the pneumonia patient may also develop viral meningitis or severe pleurisy. Ironically, bacterial pneumonia is often superimposed on the viral infection in patients with respiratory difficulty or chronic lung disease.

Tuberculosis

Modern medical treatment has reduced the incidence of tuberculosis (TB) to a level that no longer warrants the expense of maintaining isolation facilities for TB patients. However, TB is again appearing in the general community hospital rather than in a sanitarium or other TB center, and doctors must once more be alert to the possible presence of TB in patients with lung problems. It is most likely to arise in patients treated with steroids or chemotherapy, both of which increase susceptibility to TB bacteria and the risk of reactivating a healed tubercular site.

An example is the 65-year-old patient hospitalized with weight loss, weakness, and an X-ray shadow in the upper lobe of the right lung. He has received steroid therapy intermittently for Crohn's disease (inflammation of part of the small intestine), and inspection of the chest X ray reveals calcified lesions that suggest, but do not prove, previous exposure to TB. In this instance, the patient was probably exposed to TB in childhood and recovered, but the microorganism remained dormant in his lung. The steroids given for bowel disease then reactivated the infection.

Reactivated TB is one of the commonest forms of the disease seen in the hospital today.

New TB cases are most frequently discovered during health screening when a skin test is found to be positive (an allergic reaction indicates previous exposure). These people have contracted TB, but their defense mechanisms have successfully contained the disease. In such cases, they are given anti-tuberculosis therapy to reduce the chance of reactivation of the infection later in life when they may become debilitated for any reason and less able to combat the disease. Such therapy is frequently, but incorrectly, called prophylactic, that is, intended only to ward off the disease. These people actually have the disease, contracted through contact (it is highly contagious), but it simply is not active in the sense that they are not discharging the microorganism in their sputum.

TB also appears in some people who were adequately treated in the past when the disease was active, but who now have persisting lung problems. It is then difficult to determine whether the old TB has been reactivated, or if the old infection had weakened natural defenses so that recent exposure has caused a new infection.

Today, unlike years ago, TB is often insidious and without severe symptoms. The ill person does not lose weight, but complains only of night sweats, feeling unwell, and a slight cough. Occasionally, even the cough may be absent. A diagnosis is made by examining the sputum for TB microorganisms and then growing them in a culture to confirm that they are infectious.

Present TB treatment has significantly reduced the financial drain so common in the past. Once infection is recognized and appropriate therapy begun, the patient may return to normal life in ten days to three weeks, depending on the severity of the illness and the speed with which the sputum is cleared of potentially infectious microorganisms. Prolonged hospitalization is no longer necessary.

Atypical TB, caused by less common microorganisms, occurs in people with already diseased lungs and resembles the more severe classic type. For example, it may appear as a complication of severe emphysema or in someone previously treated for classic TB whose lung has developed fibrous tissue (*pulmonary fibrosis*) or chronically enlarged bronchial passages (*bronchiectasis*). The infectious microorganisms of atypical TB are found in soil, dust, and bird droppings. They often feed parasitically on the dead or decomposing tissue in the diseased lung. Unlike classic TB, the atypical varieties are not known to be transmitted from one human to another.

Treatment of atypical TB is difficult because it often does not respond to the usual antibiotic treatment so effective against ordinary TB. In some cases, the only choice is to remove the infected portion of lung.

Fungal and Protozoan Lung Infections

Lung infections by fungi have become more common in the United States as world travel has increased exposure to microorganisms not usually encountered locally. Some of the more frequently seen fungal infections include *histoplasmosis, cryptococcosis,* and *coccidioidomycosis,* some of which may sometimes have symptoms resembling those of other lung diseases such as influenza, pneumonia, tuberculosis, and even cancer. Since treatment of fungal lung infection requires the use of possibly toxic medications, proof that the infection exists and identification of the fungus must precede therapy.

Other lung infections now seen more frequently as complications in lung disease include those due to single-celled animal microorganisms (*protozoa*): *Toxoplasma* and *Pneumocystis carinii.* In adults, they occur most often after the patients have received radiation and chemotherapy for an underlying malignancy. However, infants usually contract the disease while still in the mother's uterus. Early recognition and prompt treatment are essential for the successful control of these unusual lung infections.

Benign Tumors

Nonmalignant lung tumors are relatively infrequent. When present, they appear as solitary nodules on a lung X ray and must be considered malignant until proved otherwise. Tumor types vary widely. They include cell growth from the lining of the airway (*adenomas*), overgrowth of fibrous or scar-like tissue (*fibromas*) at sites of healed inflammation, an abnormal nest of blood vessels anywhere in the lung (vascular tumors), and fatty growths (*lipomas*) most often at the periphery or near the center of lung tissue.

Benign lung tumors seldom create serious problems, but if they bleed, they may obstruct an airway and cause pneumonia. The main problem is to determine if the growth seen on a chest X ray, or the abnormality found while seeking the cause of a persistent wheeze, is truly benign. To minimize the risk of overlooking a malignancy, a suspicious growth is subjected to both direct and indirect examination.

Direct examination is by a bronchoscope inserted down the windpipe, which permits the doctor to scan the airway for abnormalities and facilitates a biopsy (removing tissue samples for microscopic examination). Indirect examination is the collection of sputum for microscopic determination (cytology) of the presence or absence of malignant cells. Occasionally these procedures are insufficient and the chest must be opened for surgical removal of the affected portion of the lung before the diagnosis of a benign tumor can be conclusively demonstrated.

Lung Cancer

Lung cancer is an increasing cause of death worldwide and especially in North America. Twenty-five years ago, cancer of the lung was primarily a disease of males. Now, with more women performing roles previously reserved for men, cancer of the lung in females in increasing at an alarming rate. The widespread use of tobacco is clearly responsible for increasing rates of lung cancer in both sexes. Statistically, the risk of cancer due to cigarette smoking becomes significant when a person has smoked the equivalent of one pack per day for 20 years. That is, the same risk is incurred by smoking two packs per day for 10 years or four per day for only five years.

The cancer most commonly attributable to cigarette smoking is composed of *squamous* (scaly) or *epidermoid* (skin-like) cells found in approximately 55 to 60 percent of all lung cancers. Small cells of *oat-cell carcinoma,* another type of lung cancer, grow from the cells lining the bronchial tree. Other, less frequent, cancer types, which cannot be attributed to particular carcinogenic agents, often arise in patients who have never smoked. Those that sometimes appear in scarred parts of the lung are called scar cancer. A rarer type of cancer involves the cells lining the aveoli.

The only effective known cure for lung cancer is early detection and surgical removal. Chemotherapy and radiation can slow the rate of cancer growth and delay the appearance of complications, but do not cure.

Other factors that contribute to lung cancer, which may work in conjunction with each other and which have only recently been identified as hazardous, include the inhalation of asbestos fibers and exposure to arsenic dust, uranium ore, and chemicals such as polyvinyl chloride and sulfur dioxide. Often, a single causative agent cannot be identified because the patient has been exposed to several over a lifetime. Thus, for example, an asbestos worker who smokes increases his risk of developing lung cancer after twenty to thirty years of exposure by a factor of 29.

The search for potential carcinogens continue and, though the effect of a particular agent may be difficult to prove in humans, a malignant potential in animal tests is a sign that risk is present. While the success rate for cure depends on early detection of the malignant process, prevention can be promoted by avoiding potential carcinogens.

Chronic Lung Diseases

The American Thoracic Society defines chronic bronchitis as a cough which persists for three consecutive months in the year for two consecutive years. The fact that the cough is chronic is of far less concern than its tendency to alter normal lung function and to damage airways by continued inflammation.

There are two forms of chronic bronchitis. In the first, the sufferer produces phlegm (mucus) all day and ejects it by hacking and spitting. In the second, the cough does not bring up phlegm and the sufferer may even be unaware that mucus is accumulating and rattling in the chest.

Victims of chronic bronchitis often underestimate the significance of their cough, blaming it on their inability to stop smoking. The real hazards of this condition include the increased risk of developing more serious lung infections, greater difficulty in clearing upper airway infections such as colds and sinus irritation, and, in time, progression to emphysema. Attacks of wheezing may accompany the coughing up of mucus or occur sporadically in conjunction with an upper respiratory infection or other airway irritation. Ordinary exertions may bring on shortness of breath. Wheezing and breathlessness may respond to treatment for a cold only to recur with the next infection or exposure to an irritant such as smoke, cooking odors, strong perfume, auto or bus exhaust, or changes in temperature or weather.

Emphysema

Examination of the lung of someone with emphysema reveals distinct abnormalities. The tiny air sacs are gone. The delicate alveolar air-exchange mechanism has been replaced by large, limp bags of tissue (*blebs*) or, in severe cases, fluid-filled cyst-like structures. Also, the blood supply to these tissues is reduced or entirely absent so that the surface area formerly available for exchange of carbon dioxide and oxygen is greatly diminished. With fewer channels through which blood can reach the lungs, the flow resistance rises, raising the pulmonary artery pressure and increasing the load on the heart.

The majority of emphysema cases result from bronchial irritation. Mucus builds up in small air passages which are narrowed further by spasms of the wall muscles, thus creating a valve effect. Air can enter the lungs with deep inhalations, but then coughing and forced exhalation collapse the airway so that the air cannot be expelled. Alveolar sacs become overstretched and their membrane walls rupture. If this process continues over a period of years, it gradually destroys the lung surface through which gases are exchanged. Because new tissue cannot grow in the area of destruction, the process is irreversible.

The most successful treatment has been clearing of the airway secretions to prevent progressive deterioration and air entrapment. This is accomplished by thinning the secretions for easier removal, avoiding irritants, promptly treating infections, strengthening the breathing muscles and improving general body tone through exercise and adequate nutrition, and using medications judiciously to eliminate bronchial muscle spasms and keep the airway open.

A rare variety found in less than one percent of all patients is known as congenital or hereditary emphysema. The condition stems from a genetic defect in the elastic tissue that forms the walls of the alveoli. Victims are found to have an enzyme (*alpha one antitrypsin*) deficiency in their peripheral blood. Congenital emphysema may appear in the very young with no history of bronchial irritation, infection, asthma, or other airway irritation. The usual treatment has no effect. Although an in-

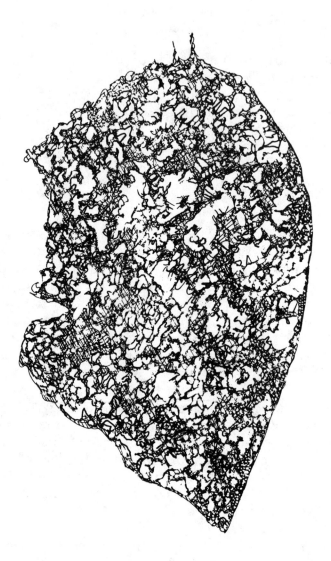

Figure 4. Emphysema — the small delicate aveolar air-exchange units are absent. They have been replaced by overdistended cysts and blebs of accumulated air. The blood supply is decreased. This diseased tissue is ineffective in exchanging oxygen and carbon dioxide for the body's use.

creased risk of infection is common, the airway collapse and air trapping normally associated with emphysema does not occur.

Can emphysema be prevented? The answer for the non-congenital type lies in the extent to which we develop an awareness of its hazards and risks, while recognizing that individuals vary in their response to exposure to irritants. One patient may be incapacitated by a simple cold, while another has no problems except for the discomfort of nasal congestion and a scratchy throat. But if we study large groups, it is clear that emphysematous changes begin to appear in the form of airway closure when smoking has been habitual for 20 years or more. The risk increases when there has been simultaneous exposure to other types of irritants found in the air in most major industrial cities. Thus, prevention involves knowing and avoiding hazards that irritate the airway and recognizing the early signs of emphysema when they first appear so that deterioration can be arrested.

Restrictive Lung Disease

Whereas emphysema represents air entrapment and ballooning of lung tissue, restrictive lung disease is characterized by a reduction in lung volume, or a decrease in the ability of the lung to inflate fully. Restrictive changes refer only to the ability of the lung to inflate normally, not to changes in air flow. For example, the presence of fluid in the lung reduces the lung's ability to expand to its full volume, hence the term, restrictive. More permanent restriction involves fibrosis, that is, scarring of lung tissue. Three predisposing conditions are *bronchiectasis, pneumoconiosis,* and *sarcoidosis.*

Bronchiectasis Bronchiectasis is a scarring process which primarily involves the lung's air passages and usually follows a significant infection. As with any infection, the degree of scarring may vary from patient to patient. More importantly, depending on the virulence of the infecting organism, the healing process itself can produce further destruction and scarring.

Typically, bronchiectasis may develop in a young person who suffers a bacterial pneumonia which damages air passages in a lung segment. Years may pass before progressive scarring reaches the point of actually changing the airway characteristics, commonly widening the ducts. The normal snapping collapse of the lung brought about by a strong cough does not take place in these air ducts because scars prop them open. The physiologic effect is a diminished ability to clear secretions which then begin to stagnate within the scarred lung segments, forming a pool that is highly vulnerable to infection. As the person with this condition ages and suffers recurrent infections in the damaged area, the scarring and stagnation spread, spilling over into neighboring regions. Each infection (pneumonitis) destroys more airway tissue and leaves more scars.

As the condition worsens and becomes chronic, certain characteristics develop. The smoldering infection in the lung produces a foul mucus which gives the breath an offensive odor. If allowed to stand, the mucus separates into layers, a dense pus-laden portion settling to the bottom under a watery overlay.

In its early form, bronchiectasis may be simply a recurrent bronchial infection, producing only small amounts of mucus and no foul-smelling breath. In older people, the disease has had time to spread, perhaps even from one lung to the other. Coughing then brings up large amounts of mucus, breathing becomes more difficult, and the breath becomes malodorous.

Pneumoconiosis   Fibrotic or restrictive lung disease associated with the inhalation of dust and other irritants is characterized by distinctive chest X-ray findings. However, sufferers from asbestosis (due to asbestos fibers), black lung (due to coal dust), and kaolin lung (due to clay dust) often merely feel short of breath and may not even have a cough. What the X rays and direct examination of the lungs show, however, is that exposure to the dust or fibers causes general scarring of the tiny air sacs. This destroys the lung's ability to stretch and fill with air during a normal inhaling effort. As the scarring becomes more widespread, the breathlessness becomes more pronounced.

Unfortunately, the incubation time between exposure to harmful dust and the appearance of symptoms varies widely. Pipefitters and others who work with asbestos, and coal miners and sandhogs who have been inadequately protected by air filters, may inhale irritant particles for 30 years before shortness of breath becomes severe.

Modernization of air filtration systems and the mandatory wearing of protective clothing and respirators have greatly reduced the risk of pneumoconiosis for workers in these industries.

Sarcoidosis Sarcoidosis is a chronic restrictive lung disease of un-known cause, characterized by scarring of the alveolar walls (*interstitial fibrosis*) and the development of scar nodules (*multiple granulomas*). Eighty percent of the people who have sarcoidosis feel no symptoms. The disease usually afflicts young people who may not know they have it until it is detected when a chest X ray is taken for some other reason. In most cases, the only sign of the disease is an enlarged lymph node near the center of the lung. Proper diagnosis is essential because the enlarged node might represent a more serious disorder such as Hodgkin's disease or other cancer of lymph tissue.

It is believed that, as the disease progresses, the enlargement of the lymph node gradually subsides but lung tissue then becomes scarred, making breathing more difficult. Unfortunately, the scarring is not limited to the lung. Sarcoidosis may spread to the skin, joints, parts of the eyes, and other organs such as the liver and one of the body's important defenses called the *reticuloendothelial system*.

The main treatment for sarcoidosis is corticosteroid drugs which slow down the scarring of lung and other tissues.

Asthma

Asthma is a term frequently misused to describe persistent wheezing. True asthma is a specific disease category broadly divided into two groups according to cause, rather than the mere presence of musical sounds in the chest. In the first group, the cause of the chest sounds lies outside the body, and in the second group, it lies within the body.

In adults, the onset of asthma is usually related to an extrinsic cause such as airway sensitivity as an aftermath of a serious infection. For example, someone with chronic bronchitis may have asthma-like symptoms on exposure to irritation by cigarette smoke or other air pollutants. These symptoms consist of fits of wheezing that accompany forceful attempts to draw breath into airways filled with mucus and narrowed by muscle spasms in the walls of small bronchial tubes. Turbulent air rushing through the constricted passages produces a whistling or hissing audible to an ear placed against the chest.

Intrinsic asthma, common in pre-adolescents and children, afflicts someone who is highly allergic, and is sometimes accompanied by other signs of allergy such as eczema, chronic sinus problems, or sensitivity to many foods. The offending substances are identified by trial-and-error and then avoided. Intrinsic asthma rarely develops in the older adult.

Failure of the heart to empty properly with each pump stroke may bring on the symptoms of cardiac asthma. Fluid builds up in the lung, especially in and around the smaller passages, narrows the airway, and causes exhaling difficulty, wheezing, and breathlessness.

Pleural Cavity Problems

The pleural cavity is the space (potential rather than actual since it may be filled by the lung) between the chest wall and the lung. The chest (*thorax*) is lined with a glistening membrane called the *parietal pleura*. A similar covering over the surface of the lung is called the *visceral pleura*. The slippery pleural surfaces allow the lungs to slide over the chest wall as they expand and contract.

Pneumothorax

If a leak develops through which air can escape from the lung, the air will collect in the pleural cavity. This occasionally happens when an air sac, ballooned by emphysema, ruptures on the surface of the lung. With each breath, more air leaks from the lung and increases the pressure in the pleural cavity. This rising pressure squeezes and eventually collapses the lung, a condition called a *pneumothorax.*

With the lung collapsed, blood vessels in the chest are compressed. This can be life-threatening because blood may be trapped and prevented from returning to the heart. Other forms of pneumothorax may occur if the lung ruptures spontaneously or is ruptured by injury, for example, when the chest strikes the steering wheel in a car accident or bone splinters from a broken rib puncture the lung surface.

Bleeding from the lung itself, or from one of the arteries beneath the ribs damaged by a chest injury, can fill the pleural cavity with blood and collapse the lung by liquid pressure. Hemorrhage within the pleural cavity must be drained with a tube or needle to prevent the formation of fibrous tissue and incapacitation of the lung.

Infection

If pneumonia in the lung extends to the surface, the infection can cross from the lung to the pleural cavity. This condition, called *empyema,* is dangerous because it can scar and roughen the pleural linings, creating damaging friction as the lung rubs against the chest wall during breathing. Fluid must be suctioned out through a chest tube or needle to overcome the infection.

Severe pneumonia may also cause the formation of abscesses which are difficult to heal unless drained. A lung abscess sometimes forms a channel, called a *bronchopleural fistula,* through which it drains into the pleural cavity. If the fistula resists antibiotic treatment and proper medical management, surgical intervention may become necessary.

Other infections also occasionally affect the pleural cavity. For example, tuberculosis can surround the lung with thick fibrous tissue, restricting its expansion to the point where surgery is required to free the lung from the trap.

Asbestosis

Several diseases characteristically affect the pleural cavity lining first. In asbestosis, deeply inhaled asbestos fibers frequently penetrate to the lung surface, causing scars to form at the pleural boundary. The scarring appears in X rays as a thickening of the pleural cavity. Calcium deposits in the pleural cavity are a typical indication of the presence of irritating asbestos fibers. These particles may also cause the formation of a tumor (*mesothelioma*) in the cavity. Although a mesothelioma may occur spontaneously, it is usually associated with exposure to asbestos.

Pulmonary Embolism

Because the heart pumps the entire volume of blood in the body through the lung's blood vessels, the lung is particularly vulnerable to foreign bodies, such as blood clots, carried by the blood stream from elsewhere in the body. *Pulmonary embolism,* a clot trapped in the lung, can be a problem at any age but is especially troublesome in the elderly. This is because clots tend to form where blood does not flow freely, and pooling of blood (*venous stasis*) in the arms and legs is more common in older people. For example, the bedridden elderly patient risks formation of clots in the legs and other areas where blood may stagnate.

Symptoms

The risk is sometimes overlooked because clots can be micro-scopically small and pass through the lung's blood vessels without doing significant harm. However, if the clots grow so that relatively large fragments break off and become trapped in the lung, the result can be short-ness of breath, pain, spitting of blood, and wheezing.

In the male, the veins around the prostate are frequent sources of clot fragments; in the female, it is the veins near the womb. Regardless of the site of origin, the critical factor is movement of the clot through the heart to the lung where it may obstruct vital blood flow.

Since the lungs receive not only venous blood but also arterial blood from the bronchial circulation, the arterial blood tends to compensate for deficiencies in the venous flow. However, in older patients with conges-tive heart failure or other heart abnormalities, the compensation may be inadequate and a clot in a vein can then be life-threatening. Insufficient blood flow to a lung segment may cause the death of lung tissue (*pul-monary infarction*).

In the hospital, anticoagulants are given preventively to elderly patients to reduce the risk of clot formation, regardless of the condition being treated. Anticoagulants do not dissolve clots, but they do help to prevent them. The lung's own cleaning mechanism breaks down the clots and reopens blocked vessels.

When several clots occur at once, or when clots are trapped in lungs that already receive a reduced blood circulation, the pressure in the artery supplying the lung may rise (*pulmonary hypertension*). The right side of the heart, which pumps blood to the lungs to be cleansed and returned, normally operates at a relatively low pressure. However, when an obstruc-tion increases the resistance to blood flow through the lungs, the pressure in the blood vessel and in the right side of the heart increases. This condi-tion can cause blood to back up through the entire venous system and enlarge the heart.

Mechanical Pulmonary Care

Mechanical aids to ventilation (delivery of oxygen and removal of carbon dioxide) range from a simple device that facilitates spontaneous respiration to complex electromechanical apparatus. One of the simple devices is used in a technique called *incentive spirometry*. The patient is asked to take a deep breath and blow hard into the device which then displays the degree of effort by the rise of a pingpong ball. The visual display encourages the patient to breathe more deeply and to exercise respiratory muscles. This incentive is valuable when normal breathing has become difficult because of pain, abdominal distention, or other reasons. Deep breathing ventilates lung segments which might otherwise remain collapsed.

Another technique requires the patient to breathe through a tube which traps exhaled carbon dioxide. Accumulation of the gas in the tube causes a feeling of breathlessness and stimulates physiological sensors which urge the patient to breathe more deeply and to blow harder against the minimal resistance presented by the device. The patient is thus helped to achieve a full inspiratory and expiratory effort and to avoid the spontaneous collapse (*atelectasis*) of unventilated parts of the lung. Application of this technique is limited because some patients may already be retaining carbon dioxide in their lungs due to inadequate breathing. However, the technique can be very effective for the vast majority of patients recovering from otherwise uncomplicated pneumonia or surgery.

The *Intermittent Positive Pressure Breathing* (IPPB) machine both disperses medication into the airway and forces a deep inspiration by applying pressure at the right time. With this device, the patient's weak inhaling triggers the mechanism that drives air at a preset pressure into the lungs. The technique is too hazardous for patients with severe emphysema or whenever there is a risk that the pressure will rupture a segment of the lung already expanded and weakened by disease. However, it is effective in cases of severe bronchial spasms for which medication is difficult to administer as a simple mist or by hand-held nebulizer.

When a patient is unable to breathe well enough to achieve adequate air exchange, continuous ventilation with a volume-cycled respirator may be necessary. In this case, a tube is placed in the airway to permit a mechanical apparatus to inflate the lungs for each required breath. In most instances, the patient, although uncomfortable, is greatly relieved by receiving adequate ventilation.

Several other techniques permit investigation of the airway or lungs for more accurate diagnosis and sometimes the improvement of ventilation. Bronchoscopy, for example, does both. A flexible tube inserted through the mouth into the airway allows the suctioning of mucus or other material lodged in the airducts, as well as observation of severe inflammation and obstructions such as tumors and foreign bodies.

Mediastinoscopy enables the diagnosis of tumors growing in the central portion of the lung (mediastinum). A small incision is made at the base of the neck, just above the breastbone, and a lighted instrument is carefully inserted to observe possible abnormal tissue and to take a biopsy sample. Another procedure, known as thoracocentesis and pleural biopsy, withdraws a sample of tissue from the pleural cavity through a needle inserted between the ribs.

Appropriately applied, these procedures are relatively safe and help the physician to make a specific diagnosis with only minor discomfort to the patient. Proper diagnosis can then be followed by the most effective therapy.

PERIPHERAL VASCULAR DISEASE

Dominic A. DeLaurentis, M.D.

Professor of Surgery, University of Pennsylvania
School of Medicine
Director of Surgery, Pennsylvania Hospital

Blood Vessel Disorders

Peripheral vascular disease is a general term that refers to any disorder of the blood vessels of the body. The word "peripheral" indicates that this category does not include the "center," that is, the heart and its associated blood vessels. Although vessels to the brain, kidneys, liver, and other organs are considered peripheral and can be abnormal, most peripheral vascular disease involves the vessels of the extremities, especially the legs and feet. The lower extremities have three kinds of blood vessels: arteries, veins, and lymphatics.

Arteries

Arteries bring fresh oxygenated blood from the heart and lungs to the peripheral tissues (Figure 1) and are responsible for their nourishment. If the arterial supply is interrupted permanently for any reason, the tissue dies. In the extremities, this is called *gangrene*.

Different body tissues differ in their response to a cutoff of blood supply. The most vulnerable is nerve tissue—including the brain—and muscle. The most hardy are skin and bone. Nerve tissue can tolerate the complete loss of its blood supply for only minutes, muscle for three to four hours, and bone and skin much longer.

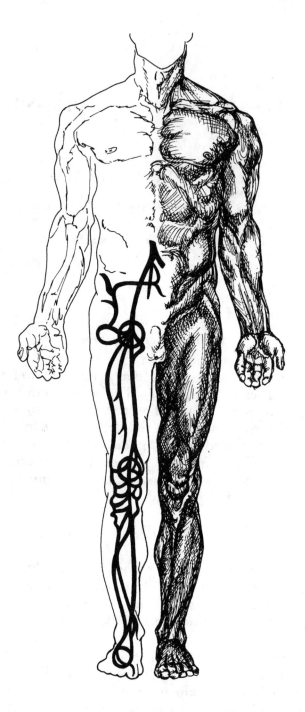

Figure 1. Freshly oxygenated blood flows from the heart through the arteries toward the foot.

Arteriosclerosis

The most common cause of narrowed or obstructed arteries in the lower extremities is *arteriosclerosis* (Figure 2), a disease of the walls and lining of arteries that is more prevalent with advancing age, high blood pressure, metabolic defects such as diabetes mellitus, obesity, smoking, and perhaps diet and stress. Although often called "hardening" of the arteries because calcium deposits appear in the walls, this is not always an accurate description of arteriosclerosis. Some diseased arteries become soft and weak. Degeneration is a more appropriate term than hardening.

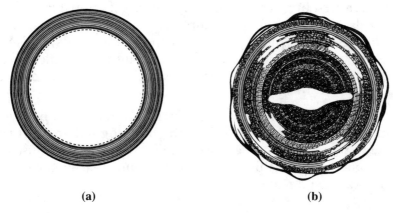

(a) **(b)**

Figure 2. (a) Cross section of normal artery. (b) Arteriosclerosis narrows the passageway open to blood flow.

Aneurysms

When arterial walls become very weak, "blowouts" or "blisters" called *aneurysms* are formed. Aneurysms in the groin and behind the knee are fairly common. They can induce clotting and restrict the flow of blood to an extremity. An abdominal *aortic aneurysm* (an aneurysm in the aorta, the major artery of the abdomen) can be lethal because rupture can cause massive bleeding.

Arterial Insufficiency

Arteries can be occluded (closed or obstructed) in several ways. Most often, a blood clot blocks a passage already narrowed by arteriosclerosis. This process is called *thrombosis*. Arteries can also be occluded by a traveling clot called an *embolus*. Emboli usually originate in the heart chambers when blood stagnates because of an abnormal heart rhythm or comes free, it is immediately propelled by the rapid arterial blood flow to distant arteries. Ninety percent of the emboli come to rest in and occlude arteries feeding the lower extremities. The other 10 percent occlude arteries to the brain, kidney, upper extremities, and other organs.

Another common source of arterial occlusion is injury, particularly fractures. The artery is often cut, pinched, or otherwise damaged so that clots form.

If the arterial supply is only partially restricted, for example, if the artery is narrowed by arteriosclerosis, symptoms of arterial insufficiency or *ischemia* (lack of blood) may develop. These include *intermittent claudication* in the calf or thigh, paleness when the foot is elevated, coolness and absence of perspiration in the foot, a "pins-and-needles" sensation in the foot, and, finally, the most severe symptom, foot pain even at rest.

Intermittent claudication is a pattern of cramps, "charleyhorse," weakness, or discomfort in the calf or thigh during walking that vanishes after a rest. Standing still always brings relief. If the person must sit down to relieve the pain, it is probably due to a muscular or bone-joint disorder, not vascular disease.

Claudication almost always occurs outside the home. Walking fast or uphill brings it on sooner. The discomfort is thought to be due to an inadequate oxygen supply to the muscles being exercised. It is rarely severe and does not require pain medication. It appears most often in the calf muscles because the *femoral* (thigh) artery which supplies the calf is the most likely of all extremity arteries to be narrowed by arteriosclerosis. The condition may improve with time because other vessels sometimes bypass the occluded parts of the femoral artery and partially restore the blood supply.

Intermittent claudication reflects a mild arterial narrowing or obstruction. More severe obstruction causes ischemia, including a lack of blood supply to the nerves in the foot, which produces persistent, intense pain in the resting foot (*rest pain*) requiring narcotics for relief. Raising the foot intensifies the pain; hanging the foot over the side of the bed decreases it. The condition will progress to gangrene unless reversed. Applications of heat, especially hot soaks and skin irritants, should be avoided because these increase the metabolic rate. Faster metabolism

damaged heart tissue (*myocardial infarction*). When an embolus be-
consumes the already inadequate nutrients more quickly and accelerates
the development of gangrene.

In diagnosing arterial insufficiency, the physician looks for the following signs:

- Loss of pulse (heartbeat) in the groin, behind the knee, and in the
  foot
- Paleness when the leg and foot are elevated
- Shrinking of muscles (*atrophy*) in the affected limb
- Loss of toe hair, malnourished toenails, thin shiny skin on the
  bottom of the foot and toes, and small cracks in the skin of
  the foot
- Bright red-to-violet color of the skin of the foot when the foot is
  allowed to hang down (*dependent rubor*)
- Absence of foot perspiration
- Slow filling of veins when foot is lowered from a raised to a
  dangling position

Coldness by itself is not a sign of arterial insufficiency or poor circulation.

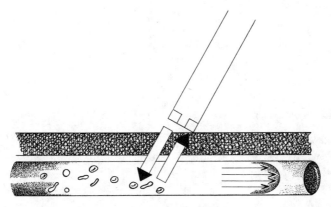

Figure 3. Doppler Flow Detection Probe projects sound waves into an artery.
Reflections from red blood cells are electronically converted into an indication of
blood flow.

In recent years, noninvasive techniques which do not require entering veins and arteries with needles, catheters, and similar devices, have
been developed to augment the physician's examination. One important

noninvasive technique uses the Doppler effect (change in pitch of a sound from a moving source) and ultrasonic waves (sounds too high in pitch to be heard by the ear) to detect arterial disease and blocks (Doppler Flow Detection Probe). In this technique (Figure 3), a pencil-like probe with a sound transmitting-receiving crystal in its tip is held over the artery being studied. Sound waves enter the artery and reflected sound waves are recorded on paper or made audible. The character of the reflected waves indicates the flow rate of blood cells. This apparatus can also detect low blood pressure in a leg or foot that is not receiving enough blood because of a blocked artery (Figure 4).

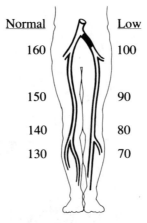

BLOOD PRESSURES

Normal	Low
160	100
150	90
140	80
130	70

Figure 4. Low downstream blood pressures due to a blocked artery can be detected with a Doppler probe.

Veins

The veins and lymphatics return blood from the extremities to the heart and lungs (Figure 5). Vein disorders almost never lead to gangrene.

The most common vein disorders are varicose veins and *thrombophlebitis* (clots).

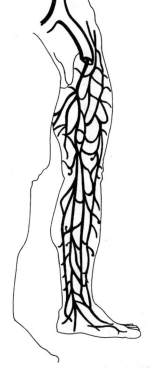

Figure 5. A network of many veins returns blood to the heart from the various parts of the leg.

Varicosities

Mild varicosities rarely cause problems and are best treated with support hose. Severe varicosities (Figure 6) can cause pain, itching, ulceration about the ankles, dark brown discoloration of the skin, edema (swelling), and dryness of skin. They cause foot pain or loss of an extremity due to gangrene. Severe varicosities are best treated by surgical removal of the diseased veins. Because there are many non-diseased veins in the leg which can take over the function of returning blood to the heart, this surgery is relatively simple and safe.

Thrombophlebitis

The cause of thrombophlebitis is not known, but predisposing conditions include the postpartum state (after giving birth), postoperative periods, fractures, cancer, and infection. The disorder is especially preva-

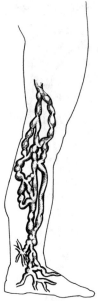

Figure 6. Severely varicose veins.

lent in patients with congestive heart failure. It can be serious and even lethal if a clot breaks off and moves to the lungs.

Although thrombophlebitis can occur without signs or symptoms, common indications are swelling of the leg and discomfort in the calf and inner thigh at rest. It is best diagnosed by noninvasive techniques such as ultrasound and by injecting dye into the veins to outline the clot on X rays (*venogram*). The best treatment is "blood thinners" such as heparin and Coumadin.

Heparin is a naturally occurring anticoagulant produced in many human tissues, including the liver from which it gets its name (*hepar* is Greek for liver). When supplements to the natural supply are needed, heparin extracted from beef lungs and hog intestines is administered by injection. Heparin is short acting (four to eight hours) and its action can be reversed quickly with protamine.

Coumadin, the other popular anticoagulant, is effective when taken orally. It acts by interfering with the liver's ability to produce *pro-thrombin*, a substance essential for clotting. Coumadin was originally used as a rat poison.

Although a pulmonary embolus (clot that has reached the lungs) is the most serious early complication of thrombophlebitis, an important late complication is a varicose or *stasis* (due to reduced blood flow) ulcer. These ulcers usually occur about the ankle (Figure 7) and are invariably associated with swelling, tenderness, skin discoloration, and itching. The cause is inadequate venous blood flow.

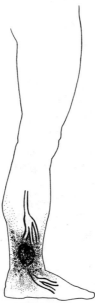

Figure 7. Ankle ulceration due to severe varicosities of blood clot in vein.

When the clots in the veins are finally dissolved and absorbed by the body, the venous valves (which insure that venous blood flows only toward the heart) are destroyed. The venous blood then stagnates in the foot and leg, and the skin is poorly nourished because nutrients in the static blood are depleted and not replenished by new flow.

Approximately 10 million people in the United States have this condition, which is often known as the ''post-phlebitic syndrome.'' It is controlled by preventing swelling with custom-fitted strong support hose worn at all times the patient is up and about. Elevating the foot of the bed four to six inches and avoiding long periods of sitting and standing are also important.

It is essential to keep in mind that local ointments are never curative. Millions of dollars spent on topical ointments and creams are wasted because the ulcer is not primarily a skin problem but one of circulation.

Patients should be made to understand this and to recognize that their condition is lifelong—not life-threatening, but disabling if not managed correctly.

Venous disease is no more prevalent among diabetics than among the general population.

Lymphatics

Lymphatics are microscopic vessels which return to the heart, via major veins, tissue fluid which is delivered by the arteries but not returned by the venous network. Diseases of the lymphatics are not common. The usual symptom is painless swelling of the leg and foot. The common causes of lymphatic obstruction are lymphatic deficiency (a congenital defect), cancer, and injury from surgery, radiation, and infection. Lymphatic obstruction does not cause gangrene, is not more prevalent in diabetics, and is usually treated with surgical support hose, low-salt diet, limb elevation, and weight reduction. Because skin over areas deficient in lymphatics is susceptible to streptococcal infections, all injury should be avoided. If the skin is damaged, penicillin should be taken prophylactically.

Management of Vascular Disease

Although arteriosclerosis remains a major problem, the past twenty years have brought improved treatment and new knowledge to help decrease the incidence of major amputations. Proper diet, cessation of cigarette smoking, sugar control in diabetics, foot hygiene, and regular exercise are all very important prophylactic measures.

No known medicine will increase the blood supply to an arteriosclerotic ischemic (blood-starved) extremity. When symptoms of the disease occur, the patient should be seen by a competent vascular specialist. If the ischemia is significant, the patient should also be evaluated by a vascular surgeon and undergo *angiography* (Figure 8) (X rays of the arteries after injection of opaque dye) to determine the extent of the disease and the feasibility of vascular reconstruction.

The basic vascular surgical technique for a blocked artery is a bypass procedure (Figure 9). One of the patient's own veins, an umbilical vein, or a plastic tube (teflon or dacron) is used to bridge over the obstructed

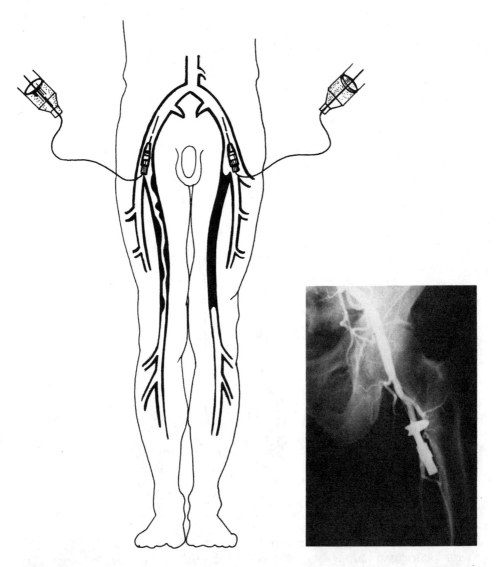

Figure 8. Injection of radiopaque dye into the blood stream reveals narrowing or blockage of arteries in X ray .

portion of the artery. Blood can then flow from the open high-pressure area above the occlusion to the open low-pressure part of the artery below the occlusion (Figure 10). Vascular surgery produces significant improvement in approximately 70 percent of all patients, but the chance of success of bypass grafts to small arteries below the knee is less the smaller the size of the reconstructed artery.

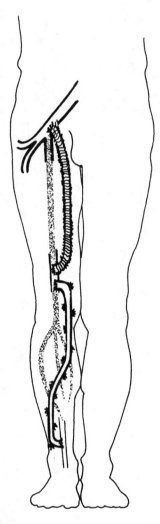

Figure 9. Arterial bypasses. Blocked arteries (shaded in gray) are bypassed by a dacron plastic graft (upper segment) and by a vein graft (lower segment) taken from elsewhere in the patient's body.

The best graft material for use in the lower extremity is the patient's own vein (*saphenous vein*) because it resists infection, is not rejected, and retains a special lining (*endothelium*) necessary to prevent clotting. The umbilical vein is prepared by tanning to prevent rejection, and thus becomes more like an artificial tube such as dacron or expanded teflon (Gortex). The risk is generally low if surgery is limited to the extremities, but the two percent mortality rises to seven percent for diabetics.

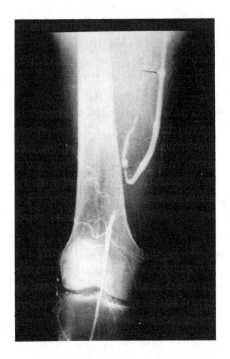 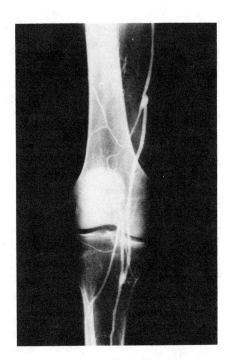

Figure 10. X rays of arterial bypass:(a) Before — blockage appears as a gap in the dye-filled artery.(b) After — a vein taken from the patient's body now carries blood between points above and below the blocked segment.

Although low, the risk is significant, especially for diabetics, so surgery should be avoided in minor cases and applied only when careful evaluation indicates its necessity. For example, mild claudication need not be corrected if it does not interfere with the patient's ability to work. It is more important to realize that stable claudication in a non-diabetic, non-smoking individual rarely implies eventual amputation, but is significantly related to coronary artery heart disease. Although vascular surgery can achieve dramatic results in most cases, the patient and his family must understand that the underlying disease is still present, and that intensive general body care—diet, insulin for diabetics, weight control, proper treatment of infection, and cessation of smoking—is of critical importance.

Often patients with peripheral vascular disease will ask if any medicines or drugs can reverse claudication or dissolve the obstruction in the occluded arteriosclerotic artery. They usually have in mind drugs called vasodilators. There is no evidence that these drugs are effective against peripheral vascular disease due to arteriosclerosis. Physicians often prescribe them and drug companies publish suggestive advertisements, but in fact no drug has ever been demonstrated to "clean out" an obstructed artery or to "increase the collateral circulation" to an ischemic extremity.

The question is then asked, Why do physicians prescribe them? The reasons are several. The absence of improvement demonstrates to the patient that no magic medicine is available. The physician may be applying a placebo effect. The drugs may do good in some cases, for example, Raynaud's disease, when a spastic contraction is involved in the peripheral vascular disease. Finally, the physician may not be aware that the drugs have little value.

Some drugs can modify the metabolism, especially of cholesterol and fats, but still do not reverse the disease in an obstructed, arteriosclerotic artery. Exercise is of value in peripheral vascular disease because of its beneficial effect on the heart, lungs, and general circulation. Walking is excellent and so are bicycling and swimming. However, it is essential that exercise be under the direction of a physician. Although exercise and weight loss help in peripheral vascular disease, they, too, cannot reverse the damage already done to an artery. Of all the non-surgical modes of management, by far *the most important is the cessation of cigarette smoking*! Nicotine and carbon monoxide have been shown repeatedly to damage the walls of arteries.

Another great recent achievement in the surgical management of vascular disease and its complications has to do with amputations which sometimes become necessary when a limb loses its blood supply and tissue dies. For example, leg amputations were commonly above the knee in the past. Now it is known that below-the-knee amputations are sufficient for many patients. Preserving the knee joint makes the fitting and use of a prosthesis much easier, and subsequent rehabilitation is more complete and satisfactory. Also, instead of amputating a foot, the surgeon may remove only one or two dead toes, reducing the disease while salvaging foot function. The decision is often made at the time of vascular surgery. If a diseased vessel cannot be reconstructed and the patient has gangrene or rest pain, a careful evaluation can limit amputation to the minimum required for optimum results. The patient and his family should be assured that a competently performed amputation is often life-saving and should not be regarded as a failure of treatment of the vascular disease.

HIGH BLOOD PRESSURE
AND THE OLDER PERSON

J. Edwin Wood III, M.D.

Professor of Vascular Disease and Hypertension, Pennsylvania Hospital

Professor of Medicine, University of Pennsylvania

High blood pressure by itself is not a serious problem. However, its secondary effects—prolonged exposure of the heart, brain, kidneys, and blood vessels to high pressure—are serious threats to well-being. Fortunately, harm can be minimized by lowering the blood pressure with drugs prescribed by a physician. But effective control requires full awareness of the condition and the aims of therapy. Because treatment may involve some side effects, the hypertensive must learn to deal with them. If necessary, the physician can usually modify the drug program to reduce troublesome reactions, so that therapy need not interfere with the normal enjoyment of life.

What Blood Pressure Is

The term "blood pressure" refers to the pressure in the large arteries of the arms and legs. The measured pressure in millimeters of mercury is expressed in two numbers, the first always higher than the second. The first number is the peak (*systolic*) pressure reached when the heart muscles fully contract. When the heart relaxes, the pressure falls to a low point, the diastolic pressure, preceding the next heartbeat. This is indicated by the second number. Thus, a reading of 130/80 means a systolic pressure of 130 and a diastolic pressure of 80 millimeters of mercury.

Systolic Pressure

Systolic blood pressure is related to the strength of the heart muscle as it pushes blood into the arterial system, and more importantly, to the elasticity of the arteries—their ability to expand and contract with changes in pressure. Thus, if the arteries are flexible and give easily as the heart beats, systolic pressure will not be excessively high. This is characteristic of young persons who often have a systolic pressure of 110, or even less. Such low pressure is not clinically significant. A medical school teacher may remark that the only thing to do for such individuals is to offer congratulations.

As we grow older, the blood vessel walls tend to stiffen, and arteriosclerosis (hardening of the arteries) may aggravate the normal loss of elasticity. Loss of elasticity causes a higher systolic pressure as the heart tries to force a normal amount of blood into the unyielding arteries. After the age of 55, systolic pressure tends to be higher, and a pressure of 150 to 160 is not unusual due solely to the normal loss of elasticity in aging tissues.

Diastolic Pressure

Diastolic blood pressure is controlled primarily by the tiny arteries at the end of the innumerable branches of the arterial tree in the muscles, skin, brain, and other parts of the body. These tiny arteries, or *arterioles,* contract and expand in response to muscle activity in the arterial wall. The muscles are controlled in turn by the autonomic nervous system, influenced by the amount of salt in the muscle. When the arterial muscles are relaxed and the arterioles are open, blood rushes into the arterial system as the heart pumps and out through the arterioles into the veins. Between heart beats, the pressure falls to the lower diastolic pressure. If systolic pressure is low, diastolic pressure will be correspondingly lower.

The inelastic large arteries of the older person with high systolic pressure tend to contribute to high diastolic pressure even if the small arterioles are clear because the pressure doesn't have enough time to fall to a normal low level before the next heart beat raises it again. Thus, an older individual may have a systolic pressure of 160 and a diastolic pressure of 90, yet have completely normal arterioles.

High Blood Pressure

In certain individuals, the muscles in the arterioles contract abnormally, reducing the blood flow from the arterial system into the capillaries and veins, and raising diastolic pressure to high levels. This, in turn, results in higher systolic blood pressure. A diastolic pressure higher than 95 in an older individual is considered abnormal, and usually indicates resistance to the flow of blood out of the arterial system because of constriction of the arterioles.

Causes

Whether young or old, each of us experiences changes in blood pressure throughout the day. It is usually lower at night when we sleep and higher during waking hours. Psychological stress can temporarily increase the pressure, although even a relaxed person in a quiet room may experience increased or decreased pressure for no obvious reason. Blood pressure also varies considerably among different individuals, tending to vary more widely in younger than in older people. This may reflect older persons' greater experience in coping with the contingencies of day-to-day living.

In addition to momentary fluctuations, the average blood pressure over a period of time also varies from one individual to another. It is this average pressure that physicians seek to determine and understand by measuring blood pressure several times during a single visit and again on successive visits, comparing readings to obtain an average. After the age of 40, systolic pressures of 140 or less are normal, pressures of 140 to 159 are considered borderline, and pressures exceeding 160 may signal an abnormality, especially if sustained over a period of time. At these ages, diastolic pressures under 90 are normal, pressures of 90 to 95 are borderline, and pressures greater than 95 are considered abnormal, indicating a need for further evaluation.

For the most part, psychological influences on blood pressure are transitory. Only rarely does psychological stress sustain an elevated pressure, the pressure usually dropping when the source of stress is removed. Excess salt, or sodium, is a more common cause of elevated pressure. Sodium apparently gets into arterioles, increases their contraction, and causes constriction.

Although the association is poorly understood, overweight also significantly contributes to high blood pressure. However, it is clear that when weight raises the blood pressure, reducing the weight also lowers the pressure.

Heredity is the principal contributor to the most common type of high blood pressure, known as essential or familial hypertension, which affects almost 90 percent of all people with excessive diastolic pressure. For this reason, a family history of high blood pressure is significant. This problem often first appears in middle life, but minor elevations in pressure during youth may give early clues. However, the mechanisms by which genes affect blood pressure are unknown.

Evaluation of high blood pressure usually includes a study of the kidneys because kidney disease is frequently associated with pressure problems. While this form of high pressure differs from essential hypertension, the essential type can damage the kidneys. In some cases it is difficult to determine whether high pressure preceded kidney disease, or vice versa.

In rare instances, mostly in young people, tumors of the adrenal gland cause high blood pressure. The possibility must be considered, but is usually quickly ruled out.

Complications

High blood pressure sometimes produces headaches, spots before the eyes, dizzy spells, or nose bleeds, but these symptoms are not major concerns. However, high blood pressure that persists over a period of years accelerates arteriosclerosis, which can be serious because it is a major predisposition to stroke, heart attack, kidney disease, poor circulation in the legs, and heart failure. In response to a long period of high pressure, the heart gradually increases in size as it attempts to do heavier-than-normal work. Eventually the workload becomes too great, pressure cannot be maintained, the heart fails, the lungs become congested, and breathing becomes difficult. Thus, the complications of high blood pressure are much more serious problems than the pressure itself.

Diagnosis and Treatment

Treatment must always be preceded by a clear understanding of the causes of high blood pressure. This is achieved by careful evaluation of the patient's history, a thorough physical examination and appraisal of the status of the heart and circulatory system, laboratory tests, an electrocardiogram, and X rays of the heart and possibly the kidneys. The results are a guide to therapy.

Although help with psychological problems is often beneficial, it usually has little or no effect on the blood pressure. Occasionally, relief from an exceptionally stressful situation brings a temporary reduction in pressure, but only rarely is the improvement permanent. On the other hand, substantial weight reduction and maintenance of the lower weight over a period of time will often reduce borderline pressures to normal levels. This does not hold true for pressures above 160/95 which weight reduction is unlikely to lower to normal.

A substantial reduction in dietary salt, together with weight reduction, can sometimes significantly affect the blood pressure, especially if it is borderline. This can often be achieved merely by omitting the use of salt during meals and avoiding salty foods such as ham, bacon, and soups. Physicians will usually recommend weight loss and reduction of salt intake as initial steps to lower borderline pressure, but are likely to begin drug treatment immediately for very high pressures.

Drug Therapy

Treatment of high blood pressure normally starts with the simplest and least disruptive measures as described above. Similarly, when drug therapy is appropriate, most physicians begin with a mild diuretic such as one of the thiazides. Taken in tablet form, these reduce blood pressure by increasing excretion of salt in the urine. They have minimal side effects and can be taken only once a day. Inconvenience is usually limited to the need to urinate more frequently for two or three hours after swallowing a tablet. The diuretic has the side effect of reducing potassium—a loss which must be compensated by eating fruit or drinking fruit juices. This undesirable effect makes it necessary to check blood potassium at three - to six-month intervals and to add potassium to the diet if needed.

If, after a month or two of thiazide therapy, blood pressure fails to return to normal, Aldomet or an equivalent antihypertensive drug may be added to the thiazide. Especially in the early weeks, Aldomet may cause tiredness, but the reaction is usually short-lived. As with any drug therapy, side effects should be promptly reported to the physician. If the combination of drugs proves ineffective in controlling blood pressure, guanethidine may be substituted for the antihypertensive while the diuretic is continued. The strength of guanethidine is a virtual guarantee of reducing pressure. The physician's main concern is that the pressure should not drop too fast. A slow but steady decrease over a period of months is preferable. The body that has adjusted to high pressure requires time to readjust to lower pressure. Excessively low pressure will be most apparent during any sudden movement such as rising from a prone or sitting position, and causes slight dizziness, lightheadedness, or a feeling of faintness especially when getting out of bed in the morning. Such episodes should be reported to the physician, as they may indicate a need for a reduction of drug dosage.

Reserpine was among the first drugs used to treat high blood pressure. It is a very effective yet mild drug, but unfortunately tends to cause mental depression—an effect that can be more acute in older people because age increases the susceptibility to depression. This may lead to problems such as the inability to sleep well or sudden crying for no apparent reason. The reserpine user should also be alert for abdominal discomfort or indigestion, which may indicate a stomach ulcer.

Apresoline may sometimes be used in combination with other drugs, but only with due precaution as to its potential side effects. It tends to stimulate the heart and is therefore seldom considered appropriate to treat high blood pressure in older individuals.

Inderol is especially useful in the treatment of older patients whose high blood pressure is associated with chest pain caused by coronary artery disease. The drug reduces both blood pressure and chest pain.

Clearly, the risks associated with high blood pressure make the trouble and expense of lifelong treatment acceptable to most hypertensive people. Actually, after the appropriate drug and dosage have been established, only minor adjustments over long periods are usually needed to maintain normal blood pressure. Success depends heavily on a willingness to learn the facts about the condition and the best ways to manage it effectively.

LIPIDS (FATS) AND THE RISK OF HEART ATTACK

Harold L. Rutenberg, M. D.

Head, Section of Cardiology, Pennsylvania Hospital

*Associate Professor of Medicine, University of Pennsylvania
School of Medicine*

The various fats in the body come under the general chemical name of lipids. These are formed from complex chemical reactions and serve essential roles in metabolism. Most people think of fats as "bad." Fats are considered the cause of obesity, the perpetrator of all of the lumps and bumps that we gain with age, and many believe fats to be the cause of premature death from heart disease. These statements are much too simplistic, however, and do not accurately or adequately describe the true role of fats and what they mean to the human organism. For example, cholesterol is an important chemical needed for the normal function of many body cells.

The most frequent causes of death in the United States are diseases of the circulation, primarily circulation to the heart (coronary artery disease), but also include circulation to the brain (cerebrovascular disease, stroke). These disorders are commonly linked with aging and classified under various diagnoses, the most popular having been "hardening of the arteries." In recent decades, it has become clear that stroke and cerebrovascular disease are linked to hypertension (high blood pressure). Better methods of detection and therapy have brought a marked decrease in the incidence of stroke. High blood pressure has been an important risk factor for the development of coronary artery disease as well, but for the last thirty years most people have associated fat intake, especially cholesterol, with the development of this disorder.

In their microscopic examination of diseased coronary blood vessels from patients who had suffered heart attacks, pathologists found that the lining of the vessels was distorted and caked with various chemicals which narrowed the channel. The normal flow of blood supplying essential nourishment to the heart muscle was thus blocked. One of these chemicals was cholesterol, and since this discovery, the role of cholesterol in the development of coronary artery disease (*atherosclerosis*) has been the subject of numerous investigations. However, despite extensive research, the basic cause and operative mechanism involved in the development of atherosclerosis remain unidentified. Levels of cholesterol in the blood may give a clue to the risk that atherosclerosis may develop, but the amount of fat and cholesterol consumed does not necessarily correlate with the level of cholesterol in the body. Regardless of the risk, most of us prefer fat in our foods because it supplies important nourishment and improves taste. Like many other substances, use in moderation probably is not harmful.

Cholesterol

While cholesterol has been a significant factor in premature death from coronary disease, it would be incorrect to assume that dietary cholesterol determines the level of cholesterol in the blood. Epidemiologic studies have shown that cholesterol in the diet has a limited effect on the level of cholesterol in the blood. Subjects put on low cholesterol diets show a decrease in blood cholesterol averaging 10 to 12 percent, a relatively small change which indicates that other factors also contribute to the cholesterol level. It seems likely that our cholesterol levels are determined largely by our genes. This would explain why normal cholesterol levels in a population such as the United States can vary from 150 mg percent to 300 mg percent. Dietary habits alone cannot account for such a wide variation.

The genetic influence on cholesterol levels in the blood is seen most dramatically in the disease, familial homozygous hypercholesterolemia (*hyperbetalipoproteinemia*). These patients have a severe genetic disorder—fortunately rather rare—in which blood cholesterol levels are extremely high, sometimes reaching levels two or three times normal. Victims develop coronary artery disease very early in life, some suffering heart attacks before their twentieth year. This abnormality is not affected by diet, and attempts to lower cholesterol in such subjects have encountered great difficulty.

It is probable that a reciprocal relationship exists between the amount of cholesterol taken in the diet and the amount the body produces on its own. Thus, when a normal individual eats more cholesterol, the rate of body cholesterol production probably falls to keep the total amount unchanged. However, this reciprocal relationship does not prevail in patients with genetic metabolic abnormality, causing their total cholesterol to remain at very high levels.

Lipoproteins

Classes of Lipoproteins

Recent developments in our understanding of the chemistry of body fats emphasize the complexity of their metabolism. Fats in the blood are usually linked to protein, and these molecules are called *lipoproteins*. Lipoproteins are classified according to the relative amounts of fat and protein they contain, which determine the weight and density of the molecule. The four classes of lipoproteins are: (a) chylomicrons, formed primarily from dietary fat; (b) low density lipoproteins, which contain most of the cholesterol in the blood and which may be a risk factor for the development of coronary atherosclerosis; (c) very low density lipoproteins, formed primarily in the liver and an important source of metabolic fuel for the body; and (d) high density lipoproteins, which contain small amounts of fat, including cholesterol, and which may protect against coronary heart disease.

Chylomicrons

Chylomicron molecules consist primarily of fats taken in the diet, digested, and then absorbed into the body. They first pass through intestinal cells, are absorbed into the lymphatic system of the intestines, and are then transferred to the veins which carry them to peripheral cells throughout the body where some fats are burned for energy and the excess is stored in adipose (fatty) tissue. Because chylomicrons are not cleared from the blood for several hours following a meal, any blood test will show abnormally high fats if samples are taken too soon after a meal. For this reason, the physician will instruct a patient under study for blood fat level to fast for 12 to 14 hours before a blood sample is drawn for testing.

Very Low Density Lipoproteins

Biochemists probably know more about the production and metabolism of very low density lipoproteins than of any of the others. This chemical functions as a circulating container carrying fatty substances through the blood to various body tissues. Because fats such as cholesterol and triglycerides cannot exist in the blood in their pure form, they are made more soluble by inclusion in lipoproteins.

The liver serves as a lipoprotein factory which combines the proteins and fats in correct proportions. The very low density lipoprotein package consists of cholesterol, triglycerides, and other fats such as phospholipids. Triglycerides are made up of *glycerol*, a product of glucose (sugar) or carbohydrate metabolism, and a second component derived from the free fatty acids essential to the production of energy in humans. After leaving the liver, very low density lipoproteins move through the blood to body cells that need energy. Here they are broken down (metabolized), allowing free fatty acids to be used immediately for fuel or stored for later use.

Research indicates that triglyceride fats are possible risk factors in the development of heart disease. While there is some disagreement about this, it is important to recognize that triglycerides derive from the metabolism of carbohydrate and glucose not of dietary fats. Thus, one of the most important fats in the blood comes from starch and sugar in the diet. Excessive calorie intake (more than needed for fuel), especially in the form of starches or other carbohydrates, will cause overweight and a high blood triglycerides level. This is often accompanied by abnormalities of glucose tolerance or carbohydrate metabolism, an indication of adult-onset diabetes.

When it was learned some years ago that certain drugs reduce high triglyceride levels, many patients were placed on drug regimens to normalize the triglycerides in their blood. Although this was done with the hope of preventing heart disease, it was overlooked or ignored that metabolic abnormalities in triglycerides levels could be normalized by low-calorie, low-carbohydrate diets without drugs. The new medications were effective, but their safety was not established and even now remains in question.

Elevated blood triglycerides are considered a risk factor in coronary artery disease, although not as statistically significant as an elevated cholesterol level. Since the bulk of the evidence suggests that high triglycerides are really an abnormality in the metabolism of carbohydrates and sugar due to an excessive calorie intake over a long period of time, the most judicious therapy is a low-calorie diet to achieve normal body weight rather than the use of questionable medications.

Low Density Lipoproteins

To date, low density lipoproteins have eluded attempts to understand many aspects of their formation and metabolism. Like cholesterol, the low density lipoproteins level in the blood is known to be an important risk factor in the development of coronary artery disease. Since low density lipoproteins contain the largest proportion of circulating cholesterol in the blood, they may very well be an important chemical agent in the development of the disease.

Low density lipoproteins are, for the most part, products of the metabolism of the *very* low density lipoproteins. As the very low density but large sized molecules break down, lose triglycerides, and become progressively smaller, they end up as molecules of the low density lipoprotein. Small amounts of low density lipoproteins are probably also produced in the liver or the intestine.

Despite incomplete knowledge of the metabolism of low density lipoproteins, many investigators believe they are the most important single factor in the development of atherosclerosis. The exact mechanism and relation to food consumption are unknown and certainly not obvious. Indeed, it seems that the popular view—"diet indiscretion equals heart disease"—is simplistic and becoming more doubtful with each passing year.

High Density Lipoproteins

High density lipoproteins, originally considered less important than some other blood chemicals, have lately come under intense study. More than 25 years ago, some investigators felt that this chemical might offer some protection against coronary artery disease because women tended to have unusually high levels of it and the rates of coronary artery disease were higher for men than for women, especially under the age of 50. Although this theory was then rejected by many medical professionals, the accumulating data do indicate a correlation between the highest levels of high density lipoproteins and a low incidence of coronary artery disease.

The actual mechanism of protection remains unclear. The most interesting but still unproven theory proposes that high density lipoproteins act as collectors or scavengers of cholesterol, removing it from areas of the body where it may do harm and transporting it to other areas where it can be more easily eliminated.

If high density lipoproteins are beneficial, how can their level be kept high or increased? They give most protection to younger women, particularly during child-bearing years. In this group, oral contraceptives and cigarette smoking have been shown to reduce this protection and to increase the risk of coronary artery disease. For older age groups, the protective effect of higher levels of high density lipoproteins can be nurtured by maintaining normal body weight or reducing obesity, keeping physically active and engaging in appropriate exercise programs. A modest daily intake of alcohol (one or two cocktails) also seems to help, but over-indulgence is to be avoided.

Summing Up

Although dietary fats have some effect, abnormally high blood cholesterol levels are probably more related to genetic inheritance. People with family histories of coronary heart disease and high levels of blood cholesterol are well advised to adhere to relatively low-cholesterol diets. However, since such diets lower cholesterol by relatively small amounts, supplementary medication is often advisable. Although the benefits of lowered cholesterol have not been absolutely proven, the combination of diet and medication is the most sensible recommendation for people at risk.

It should be noted that as we age, the blood level of cholesterol becomes a less important risk factor. This may begin after 50, and is especially true after 65.

The controversy continues as to whether triglycerides increase the risk of coronary artery disease. There is no controversy about the fact that overeating, especially of carbohydrates, will elevate triglyceride levels in almost anyone. It is not uncommon for a healthy person to gain significant weight and raise the blood triglyceride level by heavy eating during vacation, and then to quickly reduce both the weight and the triglycerides by a light diet. Although some physicians recommend medication for reducing triglyceride levels, its safety has not been clearly established.

Normally, then, lower triglyceride levels are associated with higher levels of protective high density lipoproteins, and vice versa. Therefore, a diet that reduces triglycerides (and very low density lipoproteins) brings a corresponding increase in high density lipoproteins. Since physical activity accelerates the loss of excess weight, it also tends to increase the level of high density lipoproteins in the blood.

Risk Factors

A discussion of lipids as risk factors in the development of coronary artery disease is incomplete without consideration of others that are equally important. It should be emphasized that the mechanism underlying the disease remains unknown. The correlation between risk factors and disease is statistical rather than cause and effect. The other most important risk factors are blood pressure (hypertension), diabetes, cigarette smoking, and a family history of the disease.

Hypertension

High blood pressure has been known for many years to be a strong risk factor for coronary artery disease and stroke. Although it seemed reasonable that high pressures within the arteries could damage the walls and help to develop obstructions, it is still not known how this happens. High blood pressure also requires the heart to work harder and demand more energy. Obstructions in the arteries to the heart muscle thus both increase the heart's demand for energy and reduce the supply, resulting in a lack of oxygen that can seriously injure the heart muscle.

It has been proven that adequate control of hypertension has contributed greatly to a decline in the incidence of stroke in the United States. Although final returns are not yet in with respect to a similar decline in coronary artery disease and heart attack, physicians treating heart patients have found that control of high blood pressure helps to alleviate or even completely eliminate symptoms.

Because high blood pressure often presents no symptoms that the patient can recognize, it is important that all adults have their blood pressure checked at least once a year. Contrary to a propular belief, headache is not a prominent symptom.

The large amount of salt in the average American diet probably has much to do with the prevalence of high blood pressure. Hypertension is almost nonexistent in cultures where little or no salt is consumed. Although high blood pressure may be genetically influenced, it has been proposed that low salt intake from early childhood may prevent it even in those born with a predisposition to it. Thus, if reducing high blood pressure does significantly reduce the incidence of coronary disease, a low-salt diet may be as important as a low-cholesterol diet.

Diabetes

Diabetics are especially susceptible to blood vessel disease, although the connection is not completely understood. Since diabetes tends to occur in overweight adults, maintaining normal weight should help to ward off the disease. Diabetes and high blood triglyceride levels frequently go together, as might be expected since both are linked to abnormal carbohydrate and glucose metabolism and overweight. This reinforces the desirability of weight control, a prudent diet, and physical exercise to improve triglyceride and glucose metabolism and raise the level of protective high density lipoproteins.

Cigarette Smoking

Cigarette smoking is thought to damage blood vessel walls by producing high levels of carbon monoxide in the blood. Some researchers believe smoking also affects blood platelets and so contributes to clotting abnormalities in the vessels. Although cigarette smoking is certainly harmful, its exact role in the development of arterial disease is still being investigated.

Whether smoking influences the development of the disease or not, it does influence the symptoms after the disease has established itself. Nicotine can provoke abnormal heart rhythms. Long-time smokers have lower blood oxygen levels which are sometimes not adequate for the body's demand. Since oxygen is distributed to body tissue largely by red blood cells, deprivation causes the body to compensate by producing more red cells. In severe cases, the number of red blood cells becomes so high, the blood thickens to sludge in vessels supplying vital organs.

Whatever the underlying biochemistry may be, giving up smoking can be expected to decrease the risk of heart attack. The nonsmoker also receives a bonus in the form of a heightened sense of well-being and greater physical capability.

Family History

The importance of family history as a risk factor in coronary artery disease is increased by its close association with other risk factors—high cholesterol, hypertension, and diabetes. However, a family may have a strong history of arterial disease even without the other risk factors. People with such a heritage should make special efforts to maintain a normal body weight, use salt sparingly if at all, exercise regularly, and stop or never start smoking cigarettes.

After the 55th Year

Reaching the age of 55 with no record of symptoms associated with heart disease implies a strong possibility that good health can be maintained if risks are understood and preventive habits are adopted or continued. If risk factors such as high blood pressure are present, it is never too late to start counteracting them. A physician will supervise a program of diet, giving up smoking, increasing physical activity, and appropriate medication to control blood pressure.

Blood pressure control is also important for relief of symptoms in those over 55 who have suffered heart attacks, myocardial infarction, and other consequences of coronary artery disease, including the chest tightness of angina pectoris. Although such people may be understandably discouraged, all is not lost! Not only can medication bring symptomatic improvement, but heart attack victims who give up smoking have less cause to fear a sudden, fatal onset. Complete cessation of smoking also helps to reverse lung disease. For many, a heart attack is the occasion for renewed interest in achieving good health to a degree they had not known for many years before the attack.

The way we feel is a combination of how we see ourselves in our minds, the image we wish to project to others, and the physical sense of well-being within ourselves. The following guidelines will help the well individual to look forward to many years of healthful activity, and the individual with heart disease to attain an improved sense of well-being.

- Maintain normal body weight appropriate for height and build.

- Eat a normal diet containing a suitable balance of protein, fat, and carbohydrate. Dieters should reduce calories to lose weight by omitting some carbohydrate and fat rather than protein.

- A relatively low-salt diet is probably beneficial to everyone. Avoid table salt and eat fresh rather than packaged, bottled, canned, or other preserved foods.

- Physical activity that creates a good feeling is probably beneficial. It is important to check with a physician before embarking on a new program of physical conditioning. The physician may recommend gradually increasing activity or a preliminary stress test to determine the body's response to exercise, and may also list warning symptoms to report immediately if they occur.

- No smoking!

- A few ounces of alcoholic beverage daily may be helpful, but are not necessary.

- If high blood pressure medications have been prescribed, take them regularly, regardless of the mildness or absence of symptoms. Proper body weight and avoidance of salt will help to minimize the necessary dosage.

KIDNEY DISEASE

Charles J. Wolfe, M.D.

Assistant Professor of Medicine, Head Renal Section
Pennsylvania Hospital

Kidney Anatomy and Function

Anatomy

The kidneys are a pair of organs weighing approximately 150 grams (5 ounces) situated on each side of the body at the back of the upper abdomen. Their characteristic shape can be seen in the aptly named kidney bean. The kidneys receive their blood supply through a large artery branching from the aorta, the main blood vessel of the body. Urine made by a kidney flows to the bladder through the ureter, a long funnel-shaped tube. The bladder stores the urine until it can be conveniently excreted (Figure 1).

Each kidney is loosely held in position by supporting ligaments and surrounded by fat, even in very thin people. It moves quite a bit during breathing or a change in body position, a fact which once led to some confusion. A kidney that moved an unusual distance when its owner stood upright was called a "dropped kidney" and was thought to cause back pain and recurrent urinary infections. This belief has been discarded, and such surgical procedures as "tacking up the kidney" or removing an overly "droopy" kidney are generally no longer practiced.

Kidneys display other less common variations in number, size, shape, and position. Some people are born with only one kidney, which generally enlarges almost to the size of two kidneys. Some pairs of kid-

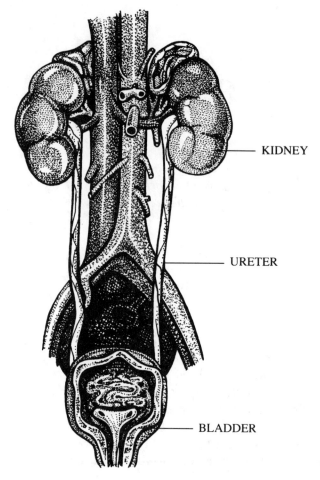

KIDNEY

URETER

BLADDER

Figure 1. Normal kidneys, water and bladder.

neys are joined at their lower ends and resemble a horseshoe (Figure 2). Frequently one or both kidneys have two ureters instead of one, which either empty separately into the bladder or unite before they reach the bladder (Figure 3). None of these variations necessarily causes kidney disease, although some may predispose the kidneys to infection, for example, when more than two ureters empty into the bladder.

Function

Elimination of Waste Products   The kidney's best known function is the elimination of waste, usually the products of body metabolism and

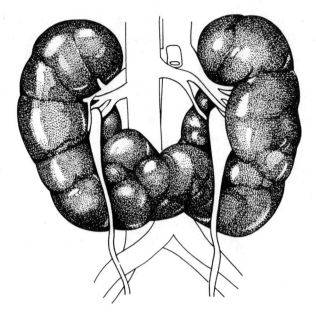

Figure 2. Horseshoe kidney.

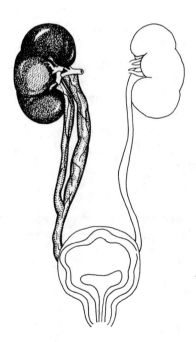

Figure 3. Double Ureter (incomplete).

ingested impurities. It is like a large filter made of millions of tiny sieves, and receives about 20 percent of the body's blood supply to enable it to filter efficiently and keep waste products at a very low level.

Filtering is indirect. Instead of screening out waste products and passing essential elements and nutrients through with the bloodstream, the kidney filters out all the important circulating substances such as salt, sugar, and amino acids along with the waste products. It then reabsorbs the desired ones and returns them to the bloodstream, and discards toxic waste into the urine.

Regulation of Salt and Water   A less appreciated, but perhaps even more important function, is the regulation of salt (minerals) and water. Ordinarily, we pay little attention to how much salt and water we take in each day. We can ignore this because the kidney automatically "senses" the correct quantities and proportions needed for a healthy balance. It maintains this balance by selectively conserving to make up a deficit and excreting to reduce a surplus. A correctly functioning kidney can regulate the amount of water and salt so precisely that body weight fluctuates no more than a pound or two even when the quantities consumed are extremely large or small

Hormones   The kidney is also an endocrine organ and produces important hormones. One is *renin,* which the kidney releases to regulate the blood pressure. Renin also stimulates the production of another hormone, *aldosterone,* by the adrenal gland (located just above the kidneys) which helps to regulate the salt balance. A second kidney hormone, *erythropoetin,* is responsible for regulating the amount of hemoglobin contained in red blood cells in the circulation. Absence of this hormone usually causes severe anemia. The kidney also converts a weak precursor of vitamin D into the active form. Vitamin D acts on calcium to maintain normal bone structure.

Parts of the kidney also produce lesser known hormones, such as the *prostaglandins,* which are known to be important but are not yet thoroughly understood.

Normal Effects of Aging

The healthy kidney has a great deal of reserve capacity. In fact, if one kidney is removed from a young individual because of injury, malformation, or donation to a relative, the remaining kidney will grow and soon assume almost the same load as the original two kidneys did together. After 35, removal of one kidney will not stimulate much growth in the other, but the remaining kidney will still assume approximately 75 percent of the former full load. After 50, the ability of the kidneys to compensate for loss of kidney mass gradually decreases. In fact, a slow reduction in capability starts in the young adult. By the time the kidneys have performed for 70 years, they have lost approximately half their ability to excrete waste products.

This is not very consequential. Since the amount of waste in the bloodstream is normally so low, up to ten times the normal amount might not be noticed. A loss of 50 percent of kidney capacity is equivalent to only doubling the waste level. A more important problem of the aging kidney is its decreasing ability to compensate for further losses.

A 60-or 70-year-old kidney tends to lose its ability to fine-tune the salt and water balance and may not adequately conserve water in times of need (anything from a desert safari to an attack of "tourista" in Mexico City). Consequently, the body is much more dependent on daily water intake. Interestingly, the infantile kidney also does not conserve water very well, so that severe dehydration usually occurs only in the very young and the very old. Much less is known about the effect of aging on the kidney's hormone production.

In contrast to the gradual effects of aging, specific conditions can adversely affect the kidneys in ways that severely impair their ability to regulate waste excretion or salt and water balance. These are hypertension, vascular disease, diabetes (which all damage the blood vessels supplying the kidney), obstruction, and glomerulonephritis.

Hypertension

Severe uncontrolled hypertension can damage the kidney and cause a rapid decrease in function, but more commonly, the decrease is slow and gradual as a result of progressive damage to blood vessels due to long-term, undetected, and moderate increases in blood pressure. The kidney no longer filters out poisons efficiently. More importantly, an impaired ability to regulate salt and water may cause *edema* (swelling) due to a salt-and-water overload or, paradoxically, dehydration due to salt-and-water deprivation. If the kidney damage by severe high blood pressure occurs quickly, it may be partially reversible if the blood pressure is promptly brought under control and the kidney is allowed to heal. However, gradual damage over many years usually produces irreversible scarring. Control of blood pressure at this stage prevents further damage and may preserve enough kidney function for normal requirements.

Blood Vessel Disorders

Any type of atherosclerosis (hardening of the arteries) can affect both the small vessels of the kidney and the large vessels coming directly from the aorta. Such disease of the small vessels is essentially indistinguishable from that caused by high blood pressure, but atherosclerosis of the large vessels may narrow the main kidney artery, reduce the blood flow, and thus cause a unique form of high blood pressure as well as decrease kidney function. This is because the kidney responds to the reduced blood flow by producing renin, the blood-pressure-raising hormone. In some cases, blood pressure can then be significantly lowered by surgical removal of the vessel constriction or special X-ray techniques.

Thus, hypertension and disease of the kidney blood vessels are closely related. High blood pressure can cause hardening of the kidney vessels, and hardening of the kidney vessels can contribute to or greatly aggravate high blood pressure. Treatment aims to break the vicious cycle.

Diabetes

Diabetes mellitus, either juvenile or adult onset can significantly accelerate vascular disease throughout the body, including the kidney. When kidney vessels are affected, the results are essentially those described above. Vascular disease in the kidney takes both forms discussed above, involving small vessels and the large renal arteries, and is essentially identical in its effects. Treatment to relieve obstruction of a large vessel may be undertaken in selected cases of diabetes mellitus. However, the successful control of progressive vascular disease in diabetics by close regulation of blood sugar, as strongly advocated by some diabetologists, is not nearly so well established as is the control of hypertension-induced vascular disease by reduction of high blood pressure.

Obstruction

Obstruction of the ureters or bladder (see *Urologic Problems* for details), if unrelieved, can cause progressive damage to the kidney. The result is backing up of waste products and impaired regulation of salt and water.

Glomerulonephritis

Glomerulonephritis is an inflammation of the kidney by an allergic reaction rather than by bacterial infection. Although it occurs more often in the young, age is no barrier.

In this condition, the inflamed sieve tissue of the kidney leaks, not only small molecules such as salt, water, and the normally eliminated poisons, but also larger molecules such as proteins and even red and white blood cells. Proteins and blood cells pass into the urine. The loss of protein and the decrease in filtering action usually lead to retention of fluid and general swelling. Some cases are treatable with anti-inflammatory agents such as cortisone, but there is no known treatment for the others except for symptomatic relief such as the use of diuretics ("water pills") for swelling. Still other cases of glomerulonephritis may be caused by a non-kidney tumor. (Our bodies can react against a tumor much as they react allergically against foreign substances.) Thus, anyone over the age of 55 with symptoms of glomerulonephritis should be checked thoroughly for a tumor.

Kidney Tests

A suspicion of kidney dysfunction, either in waste excretion or salt regulation, may require diagnostic tests. These range from simple to complex and from inexpensive to costly.

The simplest test is analysis of the blood for substances normally excreted by the kidney. If concentrations exceed the normal low range, they indicate the presence and extent of the kidney's reduced ability to excrete these substances. The two substances most commonly used as indicators are *creatinine* and *blood urea nitrogen* (BUN). Neither is poisonous itself, but both are end products of metabolism normally eliminated by the kidney in the same way as toxic substances. Therefore, an increase in levels of creatinine or BUN signals a diminished ability to excrete toxins.

Other blood studies evaluate concentrations of minerals such as sodium, potassium, phosphate, and magnesium as indirect measures of the kidney's ability to regulate the salt-and-water balance.

Urine Tests

Since the kidney excretes not only toxic products but also excess salt and water, the urine contains important clues to kidney function. For urinalysis the physician may use either a single randomly collected specimen or a 24-hour accumulation. By comparing urine concentrations of waste products normally excreted by the kidney with blood levels of the same substances, the physician can determine how well the kidneys are functioning.

The ability of the kidney to conserve water (concentrate the urine) decreases with age. To measure this ability, the physican may request abstention from drinking any liquids for 12 to 18 hours before taking a urine specimen for test.

X rays

Kidneys are x-rayed in several ways. A routine X ray of the abdomen can reveal most types of kidney and bladder stones, and often shows the kidney's size. Frequently, the kidneys are difficult to see on a routine X ray, and special X rays, known as *tomograms* or *laminograms,* are taken. These more effectively show the size of the kidney, but do not give fine detail.

An intravenous *urogram* (*Intravenous Pyelogram,* or IVP) (Figure 4) is generally more revealing. This involves injection of an iodine compound into the bloodstream which is picked up by the kidneys, concentrated, and excreted in the urine. A series of timed X rays shows the size of the kidneys and details of the ureters and the bladder. Some people have allergic reactions to the injected iodine compound. Although these are usually minor they can also be extremely serious and require emergency treatment. For this reason, as well as the expense and inconvenience of the procedure, the IVP is reserved for specific indications, and the radiologist must be told beforehand of allergies to iodine-containing substances, including shellfish.

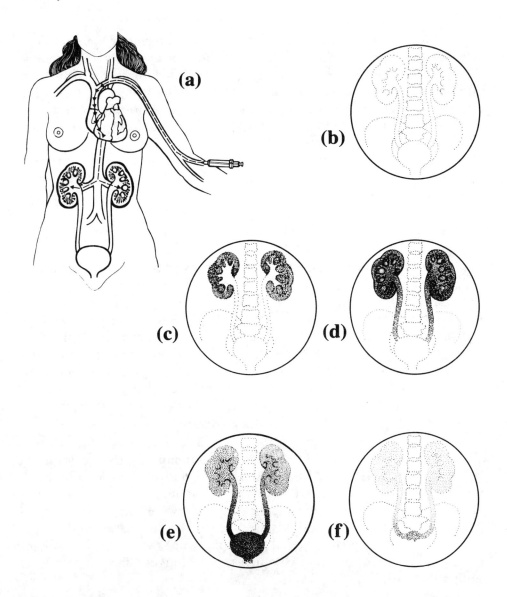

Figure 4. Intravenous Pyelogram (IVP). **(a)** injection of radio-opaque material; **(b)** preliminary film to show relationship of kidneys, bones, etc. (before injection); **(c)** five minutes after injection (kidneys outlined); **(d)** 10 minutes after injection (kidneys and ureters outlined); **(e)** late film, 20 minutes (ureters and bladder outlined); **(f)** after voiding, bladder empty.

For other suspected kidney tumors or certain forms of hypertension, a kidney arteriogram is taken. Enough of the contrast material, similar to that used for an IVP, is injected into the blood flowing to the kidneys to outline the blood vessels in an X ray. The material is injected through a plastic tube (catheter) passed through a blood vessel in the groin up the major artery of the abdomen (the aorta), and in most cases into the main kidney arteries. The risks are similar to those of an IVP with the addition of possible bleeding from the injection site because a high-pressure artery is punctured. For this reason, the procedure usually requires at least overnight hospitalization for observation.

Ultrasound

A different kind of picture of the kidneys is obtained by the use of ultrasonography. Sound waves (similar to sonar) bounce back as they pass through different tissues in the abdomen, and interpretation of the echos yields a display of the kidney's size and shape, obstruction to urine flow and the resultant widening of the ureters, and often cysts in the kidney. This test is convenient and does not require an injection of contrast material. Its shortcoming is the difficulty of correct interpretation; an experienced operator is required to perform the test effectively.

Special Kidney Therapy

The function of the natural kidneys is far superior to that achieved by an artificial kidney machine or a donated transplant, the only therapies now available for failed kidneys. Consequently, every attempt is made to preserve remaining function, and to restore function after temporary impairment. The methods used depend on the disease and are too numerous to be covered in detail. The following is a description only of the two alternatives to kidneys which can no longer function at a level compatible with life.

Dialysis (Artificial Kidney)

Dialysis is currently available in two forms: *peritoneal dialysis* and *hemodialysis*. Peritoneal dialysis involves placing a salt solution inside the abdominal cavity so that the exchange of waste products may occur across the cavity lining. Since the salt solution does not contain waste products, and because of kidney failure—the blood contains a high concentration of them, the wastes diffuse into the salt solution which is then removed. The procedure requires the placement of a plastic catheter in the abdomen for a relative long time. It has the advantage that it is safe, can be performed at home, is effective in patients with serious vascular disease, or even severe diabetes, and requires little supervision. A new technique is now being tested in which the fluid is placed in and drained out of the abdomen at convenient intervals, leaving the patient free to walk in the interim. The present method requires continuous flow of the fluid into and out of the abdomen overnight several nights a week, or for a 35–48-hour period every 7 to 10 days.

Hemodialysis uses the well-known artificial kidney machine in which blood is continuously drawn from the patient, purified, and returned. The time per treatment varies from 3 to 6 hours, depending on the equipment and severity of the problem, and treatments are required 3 times per week in a dialysis center or at home. Home dialysis has the advantage of not requiring long periods away from a familiar environment and permitting greater flexibility in the scheduling. It has the disadvantage that the machinery must be in the home, with additional time needed to set up and clean the machine after dialysis, and requires a partner to help with dialysis since the patient cannot be on dialysis and run the machine at the same time.

The federal government under Medicare covers dialysis for individuals who have the required Social Security or railroad retirement work credits, and their dependent children. Coverage begins 90 days after chronic dialysis has been initiated. The 90-day period not covered by the federal government is usually covered by private health insurance plans or state departments of health and rehabilitation.

Kidney Transplantation

Suitable kidneys for transplantation are obtained from a living relative or from an unrelated donor who has died, who shows no contraindications to organ donation, and expressed such a desire before death. In general, greater success is obtained with a living related donor, the degree of success corresponding to the closeness of the kinship. Because of the unavoidable medical and other complications and the high doses of medication required to maintain a transplanted kidney, people over 55 years are generally not considered good risks to receive kidney transplants. However, the decision is variable, depending on the transplantation center involved and the health of the possible recipient. In general, there is no age requirement for the kidney donor, but obviously donors must be free of kidney disease, tumor, or an infectious disease which may be transmitted to the recipient. There continues to be a short-age of kidneys for transplantation, and all eligible donors should be encouraged to arrange for possible donation prior to death. Many states now include a legally accepted form with driver's licenses with which a person can indicate a desire to donate a kidney in the event of sudden death. Because the number of potential recipients now far exceeds the number of donors, more help of this kind is needed.

UROLOGIC PROBLEMS

Terrence R. Malloy, M.D., F.A.C.S.

Chief, Section of Urology, Pennsylvania Hospital

*Clinical Associate Professor of Urology, University of Pennsylvania
School of Medicine*

Victor Carpiniello, M.D.

Assistant Clinical Professor of Urology,

Pennsylvania Hospital

Alan J. Wein, M.D.

Associate Professor of Urology,

Pennsylvania Hospital

Introduction

Urologic (genitourinary) problems often don't appear before the age of fifty. The genitourinary tract includes the adrenal glands, kidneys, ureters, bladder, urethra, and—in men only—the prostate, seminal vesicles, penis, scrotum, testicles, epididymides, and vas deferens (Figure 1). The following deals with the most common conditions and diseases associated with aging that are seen by a urologist (a surgeon who specializes in treatment of genitourinary problems).

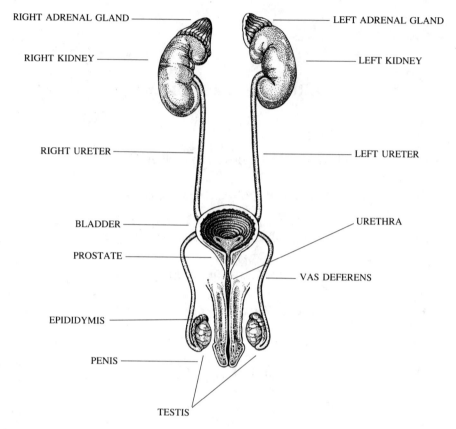

Figure 1. The male genitourinary tract.

Anatomy, Disorders, and Treatments

Adrenal Glands

The adrenal glands, positioned above the kidneys, produce a number of hormones essential to the maintenance of normal body functions. They help to regulate blood pressure, sexual function, and salt levels in the blood. Adrenal malfunction leads to various diseases, such as Cushing's syndrome if the gland produces an excess of hormones, and Addison's disease if it fails or is underactive. Tumors—both benign and malignant—are found at all ages. In general, there is no greater incidence of adrenal problems among the elderly than among the young. Increasing age does not necessarily render the adrenal gland more susceptible to malfunction or disease.

Kidneys

Situated below the chest and behind the intestines, the kidneys filter the blood and excrete waste products, while also conserving essential elements in the blood, such as proteins, minerals, and salts. They filter approximately 180 liters (about 48 gallons) of blood per day, but produce only 1 liter (just over a quart) of urine. The proper functioning of other organ systems depends heavily on the kidneys to keep body fluids in balance.

Infections, kidney stones, cancer, and insufficient blood supply can all cause kidney (*renal*) disease. Symptoms may range from chills, fever, and pain in the back or side to no symptoms at all. The most common signs of kidney cancer are *hematuria* (blood in the urine), pain, and an abdominal mass. Various foods and medications may harmlessly discolor the urine, but the appearance of blood is a warning to see a physician immediately. When in doubt as to the cause of the color, medical advice and examination are in order.

Microscopic examination of a urine specimen (urinalysis) reveals the signs of kidney disease. Further tests may be made to disclose the presence of abnormal amounts of protein, sugar, acetone, and sometimes bilirubin. Many urologic disorders are diagnosed by X ray of the genitourinary tract.

In an X-ray test known as an *intravenous pyelogram* (IVP), a dye opaque to X rays is first injected into a vein and then serves to outline the kidneys, bladder, ureters, and urethra, before being excreted in the urine. This study is essential when blood appears in the urine.

A renal mass found by IVP examination may be either a tumor or a cyst. Further examination by ultrasonic scanning is used to distinguish between them, and a selective arteriogram may be required to verify a diagnosis of cancer. In this test, dye injected into an artery through a small tube outlines the blood supply to the mass on X-ray photographs. The X-ray image is different for cancer than it is for a benign cyst or a stone. The arteriogram is also employed to study narrowing of the blood vessels to the kidneys, a condition which can produce high blood pressure (hypertension). The combined radiologic tests yield reliable diagnoses in up to 98 percent of all cases.

Normal treatment of any renal cancer is surgical removal of the kidney (*nephrectomy*). No other treatment is effective because the malignancy does not respond to radiation or chemotherapy. Because these cancers are commonly found in the elderly, patients and families often express concern over the risk involved in surgery. Since current anesthetic and surgical techniques have decreased the mortality rate for kidney surgery to less than one percent, age is rarely a sufficient reason to defer surgical treatment.

While kidney stones and infections (*pyelonephritis*) sometimes appear for the first time in individuals fifty years of age or older, these disorders actually occur more often in the younger age group. Treatment is often medical and surgery is not needed. For most people, if the kidneys have functioned normally the first fifty years, few problems may be expected in the remaining years.

Ureters

The ureters (one for each kidney) are smooth tubes that propel urine from the kidneys to the bladder by a wave-like sequence of muscular contractions (*peristalsis*). A valve prevents urine from reversing its flow when the bladder empties. Blockage of the bladder outlet, if persistent, can enlarge the ureter and cause a backflow of infected urine to the kidneys.

The same stones, infections, and malignancies that can afflict the kidneys can also appear in the ureters. Although aging does not specifically change ureteral function, diseases may spread to the ureters from the kidneys above or the bladder below.

Bladder

The bladder is a hollow sac composed of an inner lining of mucous membrane, a middle layer of muscle, and an external covering membrane. It is located in the pelvis behind the pubic area, in front of the vagina in women.

Controlling nerves extending from the spinal cord permit the bladder to relax while urine enters. When the capacity of 350–500 cc (about one-third to just over one-half quart) is reached, there is a sensation of fullness. Voluntary control then takes over and the urine is retained until an appropriate time for expulsion. A signal from the brain then relaxes the ring-shaped muscles around the urethra (outlet tube) and simultaneously contracts the bladder muscles. This normally generates a smooth urine flow until the bladder is empty.

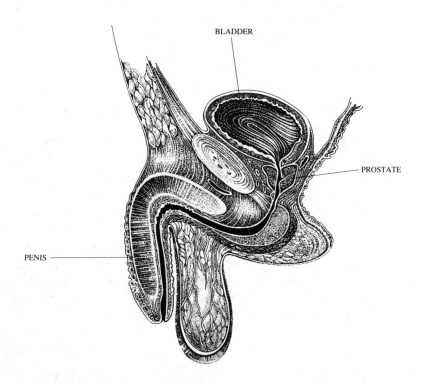

Figure 2. Male bladder and genitals.

Aging may bring problems with urination to both sexes, but with some anatomical differences of cause and effect. As men age, the prostate glands (Figure 2) surrounding the urethra may swell as a result of benign growths or cancer and tend to compress the urethra. Then, just as more pressure is required to force water through a squeezed garden hose, the bladder muscles must work harder to expel urine. If the obstruction grows greater, the bladder muscle may deteriorate, causing the wall to thicken or allowing the inner lining to protrude between muscle fibers and form pouches (*diverticuli*) in the outer covering. Inability to pass urine may develop gradually or come suddenly, accompanied by the risk that stagnant urine may lead to bladder infection. The various symptoms of bladder infection include:

- Burning during urination
- Increased frequency of urination
- Waking at night to urinate
- Double voiding (urge to repeat within minutes after previous urination)
- Dribbling stream
- Decrease in width and force of urinary stream
- Blood in urine (visible or microscopic)

Physical examination for diagnosis of a bladder outlet obstruction or infection may reveal a mass in the lower abdomen. Palpation of the prostate by the physician's probing finger inserted in the rectum will often find it enlarged, tender, or both. A urine specimen may contain white blood cells, bacteria, or blood. An intravenous pyelogram will frequently show an enlarged bladder with thickening walls and possibly diverticuli. An X ray taken after urination may show retained urine. The physician examining the bladder interior through a cystoscope inserted through the urethra (Figure 3) may view bladder abnormalities directly, and the inner lining may appear inflamed. After thorough inspection and assessment, the obstruction or infection may be treated medically with antibiotics, drugs (chemotherapy), or female sex hormones (estrogens), or more aggressively by surgery or radiation.

Following menopause, women may experience episodes of bladder infection, often after sexual intercourse. The urethra may become stiffer and constricted and susceptible to small outpouching of the mucous lining. With slackening of the pelvic muscles, the bladder may sag and protrude into the vaginal entrance (*cystocele*), causing protrusion and shortening of the urethra (*urethrocele*) and leading to a condition (*cystourethrocele*) which may permit bacteria from the rectum and vagina to escape into the bladder. A secondary infection can result from stagnant urine in the relaxed bladder. However, the most distressing problem stemming from pelvic relaxation can be loss of urine upon coughing, sudden movement, or laughter (*stress incontinence*).

Diagnosis of cystitis (bladder inflammation) and cystourethrocele requires thorough pelvic examination. Urinalysis will disclose white

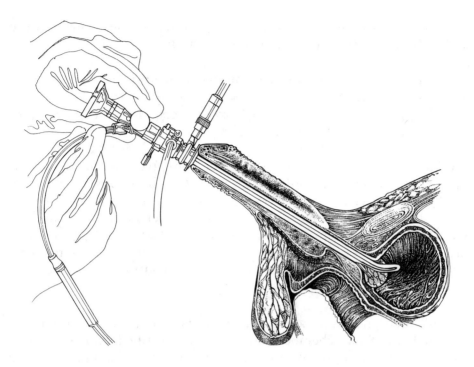

Figure 3. Cystoscope inserted through the penis to examine bladder.

blood cells and possibly red blood cells and bacteria. Special X rays taken as the bladder empties will show the extent of bladder descent and fore-shortening of the urethra and changes in the angle at which the urethra joins the bladder. Direct viewing by cystoscopy will confirm the diagnosis.

A *cystometrogram* is a study of the bladder nerve function and muscle tone. Water or gas (carbon dioxide) is introduced into the bladder through a narrow tube, and a graph of bladder pressure then shows if bladder function is abnormal. Abnormal nerve stimulation of bladder muscle (*neurogenic bladder*) may cause incontinence by involuntary bladder contraction—a condition which should be ruled out before a firm diagnosis of stress incontinence is made.

Bladder relaxation—with or without cystis and stress incontinence—can be treated with antibiotics, drugs to increase urethral tone, or surgery. Surgery may be done through the vagina or lower abdomen. The method chosen depends on the degree of relaxation and accompanying pelvis or bladder disease. The operation normally relieves incontinence and markedly lessens the likelihood of infection.

Bladder cancer occurs three times as often in males as in females, and whites are afflicted four times as often as non-whites. The most vulnerable group ranges in age from 75 to 84 years. However, recent statistics show that 60 percent of those patients properly treated survice at least five years. The causes of this type of cancer include industrial compounds, breakdown products of metabolism in the body, parasites that invade the bladder, and viruses. In addition, several studies have shown that the risk of bladder cancer for cigarette smokers is twice that for non-smokers. While the cancer-causing mechanism has not yet been clearly defined, the disease probably involves the production of cancerous agents in the urine. A diagnosis of cancer may be suspected on the IVP or cystogram X rays, but only cystoscopic examination can confirm the presence of malignancy.

Bladder cancer is usually treated by surgery, radiation, or a combination of both. Some chemotherapeutic drugs instilled into the bladder have been useful in cases of superficial cancer, but oral administration of similar agents has not proved successful to date.

Surgery for superficial bladder cancer is performed by means of a special type of cystoscope. An electric knife permits the surgeon to simultaneously excise cancerous growths and seal off bleeding vessels. While this technique is effective with superficial cancer, periodic cystoscopic examinations following surgery are essential because the cancer tends to recur in other areas of the bladder. It is important also to avoid further exposure to cancer-causing agents such as cigarettes.

Advanced cancer of the bladder requires a total *cystectomy* in which the bladder, prostate, seminal vesicles and sometimes the urethra are removed. Urinary drainage is effected by placing the ureters in a segment of small bowel. The bowel is then brought to an opening made in the abdominal wall where urine is collected in a bag appliance. In some cases, the ureters are attached to the intact large bowel and urine is then retained in the rectum and expelled through the anus with feces.

The stage the cancer has reached determines the type and extent of required surgery. Because early diagnosis favors conservative surgical therapy, medical attention should be sought promptly when blood appears in the urine. Periodic physical examination and urinalysis are strongly recommended for everyone 50 years of age or older.

Prostate and Seminal Vesicles

As men age, the prostate may enlarge—a condition known as *benign prostatic hyperplasia* (BPH). The cause of enlargement is unknown, but some evidence indicates involvement of an imbalance in sex hormones. The development and maintenance of the prostate gland requires normal amounts of male hormones.

Generally, prostatism (signs of prostate problems) does not appear until after age 55, and is most prevalent from 60 to 80. On physical examination, the bladder may be felt as an abdominal mass; rectal examination will reveal an increase in prostatic size or stiffness or both. Urinalysis may disclose bacteria and white or red blood cells. The IVP X ray will frequently show incomplete emptying of the bladder, increased prostatic size, and in severe cases, widening of the ureters. Cystoscopy will reveal the size of the prostate and the condition of the bladder, and a biopsy of the gland may confirm the presence of cancer.

The treatment of prostatism will vary with the severity of the symptoms, the presence or absence of infection, and evidence of deterioration of the upper urinary tract. The possibility of malignancy and the age and medical condition of the patient will also be significant factors.

In cases of mild prostatism—*prostatitis*—infection rather than the size of the gland is likely to be the source of the symptoms, and these will disappear under treatment with appropriate antibiotics. Urologists will usually try this therapy when treating the younger age group.

Surgery is required in advanced cases of prostatism when the enlarged prostate, benign or malignant, more severely obstructs the bladder. The surgical technique depends on the size of the gland, the training of the surgeon, and the medical condition of the patient. The length of convalescence following surgery varies from two to six weeks depending on the size of the gland and the surgical procedure utilized.

Cancer of the prostate is second only to lung cancer as a cause of death in males. Twenty percent of men over sixty will develop prostatic cancer, the likelihood increasing as they grow older. The malignancy may be present undetected for long periods, manifesting itself only when it spreads to other areas of the body. The earliest and most reliable method of detection is periodic rectal examinations in which the prostate is palpated. Malignancy, if present, will be felt as a hard area within the gland.

The symptoms of prostate cancer can be similar to those of more benign prostatism. Pain may develop and spread to bones, accompanied by nerve compression. There may also be anemia, weakness, lethargy, and fatigue. Treatment here too is determined by the stage and extent of the malignancy and the person's age and medical condition.

If the cancer patient is passing urine adequately, surgery may be unnecessary. However, if surgery is indicated and the cancer is localized to the prostate, with no evidence of spread to other structures, a radical prostatectomy may be performed. In this procedure, the prostate and seminal vesicles are entirely removed. The lymph nodes draining the prostate are also removed and examined to make sure the cancer is not spreading. The procedure often cures the malignancy, but unfortunately only 10 to 15 percent of all men with prostate cancer are suitable candidates for this surgery. Undesirable side effects can include sexual impotence, urinary incontinence, and the possibility of later narrowing of the urethra.

Radiation, either from an external source or from radioactive isotopes inserted in the prostate, has successfully cured cancer confined to the prostate. However, radiation can have debilitating side effects on surrounding tissues, and impotence may occur in up to 40 percent of all patients. A combination of surgical removal only of the lymph nodes draining the prostate (*pelvic lymphadenectomy*) and insertion of radioactive gold or iodine in the prostate is now employed in many medical centers. This method has the advantage of confining radiation to the prostate with little effect on surrounding structures. While the amount of radiation is greater and is applied over a long period, the incidence of post-radiation impotence is much lower.

Hormonal treatment may be beneficial when prostatic cancer has spread to other parts of the body. Female sex hormones (estrogens) decrease the rate of growth of cancer cells and relieve symptoms. Similarly, elimination of the male hormone, (testosterone), by removal of the testicles (*orchiectomy*) often proves effective. A combination of orchiectomy and estrogens gives maximum results.

Chemotherapy is being tried in many places and is promising. However, it remains a hard truth that the outlook for prostate cancer depends heavily on the stage of the disease at the time of diagnosis, the patient's age, and the response of the tumor to treatment. Proper therapy at the right time can mean survival for twenty years or more.

Urethra

The urethra is not only a tube through which the bladder empties but also serves men as a conduit for semen. In both women and men, aging causes no significant changes in the urethra, and cancer is rare.

Injury to the male urethra at an early age may cause a gradual narrowing (*urethral stricture*). Such injury may result from a blow to the area between the scrotum and rectum (*perineum*), pelvic fracture, gonorrheal infection, the use of catheters, or prior surgery. A narrowed urethra may obstruct the bladder outlet. Diagnosis of urethral strictures is made by cystoscopy or X ray, and urinalysis can detect infection.

Where the stricture is not severe, treatment can be conservative, consisting of periodic widening of the bladder with metal rods which stretch the scar tissue to a normal inside diameter. In severe cases, or if the stricture recurs rapidly, surgery (*urethroplasty*) may be required to cut away diseased or narrowed tissue and to restore a normal structure.

Penis

The penis undergoes no specific changes with aging, although uncircumcised men are more susceptible to cancer in this area. The incidence of this cancer is low—up to 3 percent of all genitourinary malignancies—but the condition is debilitating. If the foreskin cannot easily be drawn back to permit cleaning and inspection of the top of the penis, circumcision should be performed. While many men feel they are too old for this, it involves little risk and minimal post-operative discomfort.

When cancer of the penis has been substantiated by a biopsy, surgery is commonly performed to remove the malignancy, and radiation may also be used. As with cancer elsewhere in the body, the choice of technique will depend on the size and state of the malignancy and whether it has spread to nearby lymph nodes.

Scrotum, Testicles, Epididymides, and Vas Deferens

The scrotum contains the testicles which produce sperm and sex hormones. The *epididymides* conduct the sperm to the *vas deferens,* a tube which carries the sperm to the ejaculatory ducts in the prostatic urethra. Aging produces no specific change in these structures. While the menopause ends female fertility, the testicles continue to produce active sperm to an advanced age. Testosterone levels usually remain normal through old age, but occasionally levels drop and symptoms similar to female menopause may develop. These can be alleviated by testosterone taken by mouth or injection.

Sexual Capacity in Males Over 55

Sexual capacity peaks in adolescence and gradually declines thereafter. In the aging man, the frequency of erections slowly declines, they take longer to attain, ejaculation is delayed, and the amount of semen discharged decreases. Repetition of a climax shortly after a first one is more difficult after the age of 40 and the average frequency of intercourse falls from two or three times a week in early adulthood to once a week at age 65. An end to all sexual activity is experienced by only five percent of those under 65, but half of all men are affected by age 75.

Erectile impotence is a condition where erection cannot be achieved or maintained; ejaculatory impotence is either failure to ejaculate or premature ejaculation. The predominant problem among the aging is erectile impotence, an affliction which has a disturbing affect on interpersonal relationships no matter when it occurs. It had been believed that 90 percent of all cases of impotence were functional or emotional in origin, but medical authorities now find that the proportion of true organic impotence may range as high as 50 percent.

Erection is effected by a flow of blood into two bodies of tissue in the penis called the *corpora cavernosa.* The flow is regulated by nerve impulses that allow more blood into than out of the penis. Poor erections can be caused by infection in various organs such as the prostate, seminal vesicles, or bladder. While antibiotics often bring improvement, inflammation of arteries or nerves supplying the penis may linger and prolong impotence. *Peyronie's disease* is a condition of uncertain origin in which fibrous patches of tissue grow over the corpora cavernosa, preventing normal expansion. It often causes an erect penis to bend at an angle that prevents insertion into the vagina. In severe cases, the penis may become totally limp.

Various endocrine diseases such as diabetes mellitus, hyperthyroidism, and adrenal failure (Addison's disease) can disturb blood flow, nerves, or hormones in ways that may lead to impotence. Insufficient blood supply to the penis as a result of aging can bring total impotence.

Diseases that cause kidney or liver failure can also disturb hormone levels and have sexual side effects. Any disease or injury involving the central nervous system can interfere with normal erection. Erections can also be adversely affected by accidental damage to any of the pelvic structures and by surgery on the rectum, colon, bladder, or prostate.

Vascular diseases which narrow the blood vessels and decrease blood flow to the penis will limit the firmness of erection and also the ability to maintain it. Probably the most common cause of impotence in the aging is hardening of the arteries (*atherosclerosis*). Malignancies such as cancer of the penis, prostate, or bladder are especially damaging in their tendency to affect the complex hormonal and neurological systems responsible for normal sexual activity.

Drugs that can hinder erection include estrogens, morphine, barbiturates, medications to control blood pressure, tranquilizers, antihistamines, alcohol, dilantin, and bromides. The widespread belief that a few drinks bring relaxation while increasing sexual sensitivity and capability is quite false. The two-martini lunch not only adversely affects efficiency at work, but also puts a crimp in the night's efforts in bed. The ability to metabolize alcohol also diminishes with age so that side effects last longer when you are older. However, this problem usually abates when drinking is reduced.

Impotence in men over 55 may be insidious, appearing as a gradual decrease in the strength, duration, and number of erections. The first perceived symptom may be the absence of morning erection on awakening with a full bladder. Ejaculation may be attained only with a semierect penis, and the period between erections will lengthen.

Diagnosis of impotence includes a physical examination and a study of the patient's history. The pulse in the groin and legs may be weaker, indicating diminished blood supply to the lower half of the body. A malignancy in a pelvic structure may be discovered. Laboratory tests may disclose high blood sugar or subnormal blood hormone levels. Psychological tests and psychiatric evaluation can be employed to rule out emotional causes, and X-ray studies will reveal diseases of the sex organs or arteries. A special test to monitor erections during sleep—nocturnal penile tumescence test—can distinguish between organic and emotionally caused impotence.

Treatment of impotence depends on the cause. Medical treatment may suffice with antibiotics to eliminate infection, hormones to correct low serum testosterone levels, or modification of blood pressure medication to reduce its side effects. In severe cases, or failure to respond to medical or psychiatric treatment, surgery may be necessary. Fortunately, within the past decade significant advances in surgical techniques have alleviated impotence. They include the development of the penile prosthesis, an artifical erection device which has revolutionized treatment of sexual dysfunction in the aging male.

There are two basic types of penile prostheses. The first, the semi-rigid rod, consists of a pair of rods made of silicone rubber or plastic which are inserted in the corpora cavernosa. These maintain the penis in a semi-erect state which permits its insertion into the vagina. While this type of prosthesis has the advantage of having no mechanical parts to malfunction, the presence of a constant erection can be a source of embarrassment in public places. The most popular models of the semi-rigid prosthesis are the Small-Carrion and Finney types, which have achieved success rates up to 93 percent in several series of treatments.

In 1973, Scott, Bradley, and Timm introduced the inflatable penile prosthesis, a pair of hollow silicone-rubber cylinders that are inserted in the corpora cavernosa (Figure 4). They are connected by tubing to an inflate-deflate mechanism placed under the skin of the scrotum, which in turn connects to a fluid-filled reservoir located under the muscles of the pelvis. When the patient squeezes the skin of the scrotum over the inflate mechanism, fluid is pumped from the reservoir into the cylinders to produce a full erection. When sexual activity has ended, pressure on a deflate valve releases the fluid, permitting it to return to the reservoir and the penis to revert to a flaccid state.

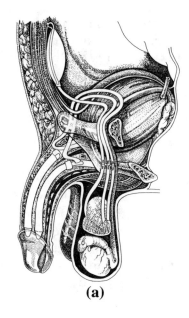

(a)

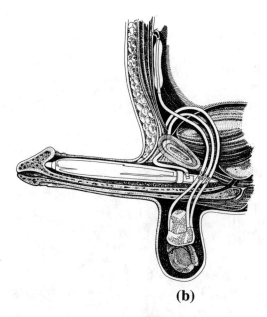

(b)

Figure 4. Prosthesis for impotent males. Fluid stored in reservoir under pelvis muscles above penis (**a.** Top) is released by pressure on valve mechanism in scrotum (shown above testicle) and inflates pair of silicone rubber tubes implanted in penis to produce erection (**b**).

The inflatable penile prosthesis has a number of advantages. It produces a full erection without concealment problems. Also, the length, diameter, and hardness of the penis can be varied, and erosions of the device through the penis are rare. A particular advantage may be the fact that the sexual partner need not be aware of the prosthesis. Disadvantages include a reported failure rate of up to 35 percent in some test groups, and the fact that the prosthesis is expensive because it requires lengthy hospitalization and special surgical skill for successful placement.

Nevertheless, several medical centers have reported success rates of 82 to 95 percent with the inflatable prothesis. One of the authors has achieved a long term success rate of 93 percent, and further experience and improvements in the device can be expected to bring even better results and greater satisfaction to impotent men. Thus, men need no longer submit to impotence as an inevitable consequence of advancing age; men in their eighties have enjoyed renewed sexual pleasure with the device.

Causes of Organic Erectile Impotence

Inflammatory
  Prostatitis
  Seminal vesiculitis
  Urethritis
  Cystitis
  Neuritis
  Arteritis
  Peyronie's disease

Endocrinologic
  Diabetes mellitus
  Hypogonadism
  Hypothyroidism
  Hyperthyroidism
  Addison's disease
  Cushing's syndrome
  Acromegaly

Metabolic
  Renal failure
  Hepatic cirrhosis

(continued)

Neurologic
Multiple sclerosis
Tabes dorsalis (syphilis)
Spinal cord compression
Epilepsy
Pernicious anemia

Traumatic
Castration
Pelvic fracture
Urethral rupture
Prostatectomy
Cystectomy
Removal of rectum
Sympathectomy
Lymphadenectomy
Vascular surgery
Spinal cord trauma
Brain damage
Pelvic radiation
Perineal biopsies

Vascular
Atherosclerosis to pelvic vessels
Arterial obstruction
Aneurysms
Priapism
Senility

Neoplastic-Malignancies
Pituitary tumors
Hypothalamic tumors
Adrenal tumors
Spinal cord tumors
Prostatic cancer
Bladder cancer

Medications
Estrogens
Morphine
Barbiturates *(continued)*

Medications to control blood pressure
Tranquilizers
Antihistamines
Alcohol
Dilantin
Bromides

DIABETES

Theodore G. Duncan, M.D.

Assistant Professor of Clinical Medicine,
University of Pennsylvania School of Medicine
Head, Section of Diabetes Mellitus and Metabolism,
Pennsylvania Hospital
President, Garfield G. Duncan Research Foundation, Inc.

Diabetes is a disease marked by an inability to metabolize sugar due either to failure by the pancreas to secrete enough insulin or to the body's inefficient use of the hormone. As a result, sugar in the blood may rise to harmful levels. It is rapidly becoming a serious threat to the nation's health, ranking with heart disease and cancer as a major cause of serious complications and premature death. New cases of diabetes have multiplied six hundred times in the same period that our population has doubled. Diabetics now number about 5,000,000, and another 4,000,000 to 5,000,000 without overt symptoms have undetected diabetes.

Types of Diabetes

The two types of diabetes are called maturity-onset and juvenile. They differ in their beginning, clinical course, treatment, and sometimes in physical characteristics.

Maturity Onset

Ninety percent of all diabetics have the maturity-onset type. This milder form of the disease usually appears after the age of 30 and about 80 percent of its victims are over 40. The chance of getting diabetes doubles with each additional decade of life. Now that one of every nine Americans is at least 65, diabetes can be expected to afflict a greater number of people. Maturity-onset diabetes also has a hereditary component. It tends to recur in families, and about 50 percent of diabetics can name a blood relative who also has the disease.

Maturity-onset diabetes develops gradually. The symptoms are insidious because high blood-sugar levels may exist for as long as ten years before more overt indications of the uncontrolled disease appear. Familiarity with subtle clues can help early diagnosis. Because the pancreas does continue to produce insulin in maturity-onset diabetes (insulin levels may actually be above normal but peripheral muscle and fat cells do not use the hormone effectively), the devastating effects of *ketoacidosis* (a form of excessively acid blood) and diabetic coma are rare.

Juvenile

Juvenile diabetes, although it normally occurs before age 30, is not limited mainly to the young, despite its name. The pancreas simply stops producing insulin and may do so at any age. Since the 10 percent of diabetics afflicted with this form of the disease produce no insulin of their own, they must receive sustaining insulin dosages or risk the acute symptoms of ketoacidosis which can rapidly progress to diabetic coma and then death.

Suspecting Diabetes

When the blood sugar exceeds 185 (milligrams per milliliter, or mg/ml), it spills over into the urine. A test for urine sugar becomes positive, indicating the condition called *glycosuria*. If the problem persists, a large amount of sugar leaves the body in an increasing volume of urine and the patient becomes thirsty and loses weight. Initially, the appetite increases to compensate for the loss of calories with the sugar, but if the disease progresses without treatment, *acidosis* (excessively acid blood) develops, leading to nausea and vomiting and then diabetic coma. Increased thirst, frequent urination, awakening at night to urinate, weight loss, all herald the onset of diabetes.

Long before acute signs become evident, subtle changes may suggest the disease, especially if the patient is obese or has a family history of diabetes. A number of ailments should be regarded as indicating the desirability of a test for diabetes. These include:

Recurrent skin infections, such as boils, carbuncles, and furuncles which are more frequent in undetected or poorly treated diabetics (Figure 1)

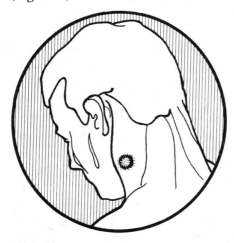

Figure 1. A boil or carbuncle can be a warning sign of diabetes.

"Shin spots," clearly defined pigmented areas, round or irregular and usually about the size of a dime, which appear on the front of the leg over the shinbone (more often in men than in women)

Itching "down below," a common warning signal in women and caused by a fungal infection that irritates and inflames the vaginal and vulvar areas (high blood-sugar levels create a good culture medium for fungus, but control of the diabetes and administration of antifungal medication make the symptoms vanish quickly)

Functional *hypoglycemia*, or low-blood-sugar symptoms, occurring three to four hours after a meal, can be a sign of mild maturity-onset diabetes. The condition can co-exist with diabetes or, in some individuals, precede it by many years. The symptoms of hypoglycemia include nervousness, tremors, frontal headaches, weakness, fatigue, anger, rage reactions, sweating, and sometimes a feeling of being all washed out. Unconsciousness occurs, but is rare. Eating candy or drinking orange juice or a coke usually relieves the symptoms within 15 to 20 minutes. The diagnosis is confirmed with a five-to six-hour glucose-tolerance test. If at least one blood sugar value in this period is below 45, and is associated with the symptoms, hypoglycemia exists.

Obesity, a major form of malnutrition—actually overnutrition—is directly related to the number of diabetics in the population. The most obese individuals are more likely to have diabetes. The disease was rare in American Indians and Eskimos before 1945, but now that these groups have adopted western civilization's habits of eating and diminished activity, the rate of new cases has increased. Our modern way of life demands little exercise, and junk foods—ice cream, soft drinks, beer, pretzels, cookies—provide excess calories that are converted into fat cells. During the second World War, the rate of new cases of diabetes fell in England, Germany, and Japan because the food supply was limited and physical activity increased. When the war ended, food again became plentiful, activity lessened, and the rate of new cases rose to the previous level.

When a diabetic patient loses weight through a proper dietary regimen, blood sugar levels drop toward normal, occasionally reducing or eliminating requirements for oral hypoglycemic drugs and insulin therapy. In all cases, the adjustment of these medications must be made by a physician.

Sometimes the signs and symptoms of diabetes complications precede the acute symptoms such as thirst, frequent urination, and weight loss. A patient with nerve damage secondary to diabetes can feel numbness and tingling in the feet without being aware of having the disease. Fifty percent of male diabetics over age 50 are impotent. Because of this, when a patient brings this symptom to the attention of a urologist, a glucose-tolerance test is usually done to determine if diabetes is the cause.

Since impaired vision in one or both eyes can occur in the mildest type of diabetes, it may be an early warning sign of the disease. A doctor examining the eyes with an ophthalmoscope looks for damage to the retinal blood vessels in the back of the eye (*diabetic retinopathy*). Early detection and prompt treatment reduce the likelihood of blindness.

Peripheral vascular disease—hardening of the arteries—is more common and occurs at an earlier age in diabetics than in the normal population (see earlier section on *Peripheral Vascular Disease*). A cramping pain in the calf muscles while walking is a cardinal sign of impaired circulation of the lower extremities caused by narrowing of the arteries. Pain is rarely noted while walking in the home, but is felt after sustained walking outside. Resting for a moment, for example, while waiting for a traffic light to change, permits the pain to subside. Patients usually describe the pain as "a charley horse," but it is technically known as intermittent claudication. When the symptoms are first noted, they should be brought to a physician's attention so an appropriate evaluation of the blood supply can be made. Cramping of the calf muscles while at rest in bed is not usually due to arterial disease.

Diagnosing Diabetes

When a warning sign or obvious acute symptom of diabetes appears, certain tests are indicated to establish the diagnosis. Sustained high blood-sugar values over 200 confirm diabetes without the need for further testing. If randomly taken values are borderline, a three-hour glucose-tolerance test gives helpful additional information.

In this test, a patient fasts for at least eight hours and is then given 50 to 100 grams of glucose (*glucose load*) orally. The blood sugar is measured just before administration of the glucose and again 30, 60, 90, 120, and 180 minutes afterward. No eating or exercise is permitted during the test which is performed early in the day (blood-sugar values change from morning to afternoon). Normal blood-sugar values would fall below 110 after fasting, 160 one hour after the glucose is taken, 120 an hour later, and 110 an hour after that. If two or more of the measured values are high, the patient is said to have diabetes.

Since there is a correlation between blood-sugar values and age, the reference blood-sugar level can be increased 10 units for each decade of life beyond 50. For example, the fasting blood sugar of a 70-year-old patient can be 130 and still be considered normal.

If a functional or reactive hypoglycemic reaction to eating a carbohydrate like glucose is suspected, a glucose-tolerance test is extended for an additional two to three hours. Blood-sugar values below 45 associated with the other symptoms of hypoglycemia establish the diagnosis of reactive or functional hypoglycemia. The symptoms usually occur three or four hours after the glucose is given. Blood-sugar values in the 50–60 range are frequently seen in normal people and do not indicate hypo-glycemia.

Treatment—Diet and Oral Medication

General

Teamwork is essential for diabetes therapy. It is started by the physician and then supported by a dietitian and a nurse educator. Since diabetes is a lifelong disease, the patient must learn the basic habits of good health and when to change the medication dosage and diet as directed by the physician. Some patients prefer not to make the changes themselves, but those who do so enjoy the freedom of a flexible medical regimen.

While mild maturity-onset diabetes without complications can usually be treated by diet alone, patients' compliance, unfortunately, is frequently unsatisfactory, making additional therapy necessary. Either oral hypoglycemic medication or insulin can be used at this point to lower the blood-sugar value, the choice being made by the physician. Good control is maintained by a proper balance of activity, diet, and hypoglycemic medication (Figure 2).

Diet

The calories eaten each day are adjusted to attain or maintain ideal weight. They are decreased if the patient is obese, increased if the patient is underweight. Slender, active diabetics have a much better chance of achieving control with less medication than do inactive patients with the most common U.S. disease: overconsumption and overweight.

The number of calories needed varies with body build, sex, and activity. First, the ideal body weight is estimated. For a female of average build, allow 100 pounds for 5 feet of height and 5 pounds more for each additional inch. For an average male, allow 106 pounds for 5 feet and 6 pounds for each additional inch. Subtract 10 percent for a smaller-than-average frame; add 10 percent for a large one.

As an example, a 58-year-old woman with a medium frame who is 5 feet 5 inches tall would have an ideal weight of 125 pounds (100 for the 5 feet, 5 × 5 = 25 for the extra 5 inches). A 60-year-old man with a large frame who is 6 feet tall would have an ideal weight of 196 pounds (106

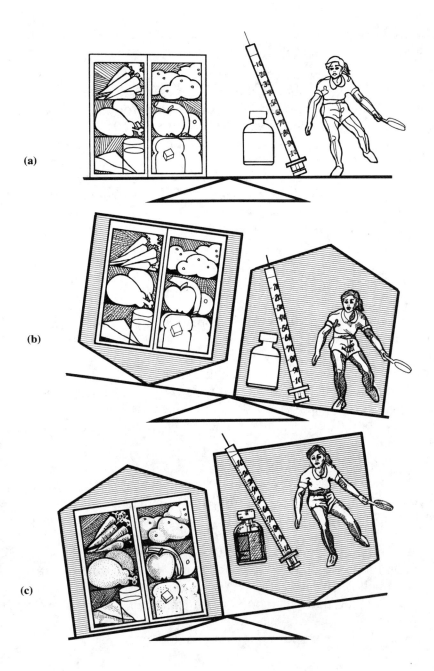

Figure 2. Blood sugar levels are influenced by diet, insulin, and exercise: **(a)** A proper balance of the three factors keeps blood sugar normal. **(b)** Less eating, more insulin, or more exercise lower blood suger. **(c)** More eating, less insulin, or less exercise increase the sugar level.

for the 5 feet, 6 × 12 = for the extra 12 inches, totaling 178, and 10 percent more for his big frame).

The basal number of daily dietary calories (the number that does not take into account extra nutritional requirements for physical activity) is simply the estimated ideal weight multiplied by 10. The basal calorie count for the woman in the example would be 125 (ideal weight) × 10 = 1250 calories. If she did light work (housework and shopping), add 30 percent to bring the total to about 1600 calories per day. The man whose ideal weight is 196 pounds would have a basal calorie count of 1960. If he is a construction worker, we add 40–50 percent for heavy physical activity, bringing the total to about 3000–4000 calories.

An obese or portly diabetic patient should consume fewer calories to reduce weight, about 500–1000 calories less than the number calculated for the ideal weight, to insure an effective weight loss of 1 to 2 pounds per week. For example, suppose the woman whose maintenance diet (for ideal weight) contained about 1600 calories actually weighed 225 pounds. Her prescribed diet would be about 600–1100 calories per day. (A patient who eats less than 1000 calories needs one multivitamin tablet as a daily supplement.) If the woman weighs only 87 pounds, she should increase her diet to 2000–2500 calories per day until she reached her 125-pound ideal body weight, then decrease her intake to the 1600-calorie level.

The times of day that meals and snacks are eaten are of paramount importance for the patient taking insulin. Delaying a meal or overlooking a snack can drop the blood sugar precipitously, causing hypoglycemia. Food helps to prevent this. Six feedings—three meals and snacks at midmorning, midafternoon, and before bed—give protection six times daily against low-blood-sugar reactions. The amount and timing of eating can do more to help maintain good control of diabetes than any other single factor, making the patient's cooperation essential. When the physician prescribes medications and diet, the patient must follow through rigorously to receive the maximum benefits of therapy.

After the physician calculates the number of calories needed, the dietitian reviews the specific diet with the patient to make sure the foods prescribed by the exchange list are compatible with the patient's normal needs and tastes. A patient once complained, "Doctor, your diet is no good. You gave me a low calorie WASP diet, and you know I like mostly bagels and lox.''

The American Diabetes Association (600 Fifth Avenue, New York, NY 10020) and American Dietetic Association (430 North Michigan Avenue, Chicago, Illinois 60611) have compiled an easily understood diet plan called the Exchange System which lists similar foods together. Foods on one list can be exchanged for others on the same list, permitting variety in the diabetic's diet.

Oral Hypoglycemic Drugs

When diet alone does not return the blood sugar to normal values, insulin or oral hypoglycemic therapy is indicated. The physician makes the determination. Given a choice, most patients elect an oral hypoglycemic drug in preference to a daily insulin injection. The maturity-onset diabetic who does not require insulin can usually be treated effectively with one of the oral hypoglycemic drugs called *sulfonylureas*. However, it is unwise to treat with medications if blood-sugar values can be controlled by diet alone.

The oral drugs have a good safety record. Fewer than four percent of patients taking them report side effects. A study called the University Group Diabetes Program (UGDP) has suggested that one of the sulfonylurea drugs might increase the risk of fatal heart attacks, but its findings are the subject of considerable criticism and controversy and are still open to question.

Patients receiving oral drugs must observe the same precautions as those prescribed insulin therapy. These medications can decrease the blood sugar to below-normal values if activity is increased or calories are decreased. Since the dosage will vary, safety precautions of routine visits to the doctor and urine-sugar testing are necessary. When practical, patients are asked to test urine sugar at least once daily, either at bedtime or before breakfast. If the results remain relatively negative, control is good. If glycosuria (sugar in the urine) persists for a few days, the patient should have the physician determine appropriate changes in drug therapy or diet. Because more medication is needed to gain control than to maintain it, periodic adjustments of oral drug therapy are necessary. At first, the patient should see the doctor every few weeks, then monthly, and, when good control is established, about once every three months.

Oral hypoglycemic drugs should not be taken if the patient has kidney damage or liver disease, since these drugs are either metabolized in the liver or excreted by the kidneys. Your doctor will know if kidney or liver problems exist.

Abnormal accumulations of these medications in the body can cause severe hypoglycemia that may last for several days. The patient who is unconscious due to low sugar caused by oral hypoglycemic medication requires hospitalization since the effect may linger. Temporary treatment for the unconscious patient at home may consist of candy, orange juice, or a cola drink, until the physician can take over. Loss of consciousness due to hypoglycemia can be life-threatening. The unconscious patient should never be force-fed because fluid may get into the lungs and cause aspiration pneumonia.

Once control has been achieved by diet and the proper oral hypoglycemic medication, the therapeutic regimen can be effective for many years. At times of stress, such as an accident or surgery, increased oral medication or insulin may be necessary.

Occasionally, the blood sugar levels cannot be controlled solely by oral hypoglycemic drugs and diet, leading to a condition called secondary failure. Strict diet should be maintained to insure that poor control is not caused by dietary indiscretions, but when blood sugar stays high despite good diet control, insulin is the only choice. The patient may enter a hospital to determine the type and dosage of insulin, and also to participate in a structured education program about diabetes. The knowledge acquired during hospitalization will serve for a lifetime to prevent subsequent complications and further hospitalization.

Insulin Therapy

The normal pancreas automatically releases the correct amount of insulin to regulate blood sugar, increasing the output when food is eaten and decreasing it during fasting periods. Since diabetics do not have this built-in regulating mechanism, insulin must be injected once or twice a day at a dosage that depends on food intake and exercise.

Because these three factors interact, they must always be considered together when adjustments are anticipated. Insulin and activity decrease the blood sugar, while food and inactivity increase it. Thus, activity cannot be changed without a corresponding change in the insulin dosage or diet, nor can diet be altered at a given exercise level without an adjustment of insulin dosage. This may seem complicated, but when a patient has received instruction in a diabetes education program and has gained practical experience, the adjustments become second nature.

Insulin Types

The ability of insulin to lower the blood sugar depends upon the dosage and type of insulin used. There are three general types: short-acting, regular (R), and semi-lente (S). Intermediate-acting insulins include lente (L) and NPH (N), and long-acting ones are PZI (P) and ultra-lente (U).

Short-acting insulins taken before breakfast have a major blood-sugar-lowering effect in the period between breakfast and lunch. Hypoglycemic reactions may occur before lunch if too much insulin is injected or if the patient has either forgotten the mid-morning snack or delayed lunch. If a reaction occurs that is not due to increased exercise or decreased activity, the insulin dosage can be decreased the following day by four units to prevent repeated hypoglycemic reactions. But if the blood-sugar values are high between breakfast and lunch, the regular or semi-lente dosage can be increased in the morning by two units. Patients should consult their physician before making changes.

Intermediate-acting insulins lower blood sugars in the afternoon and evening. Lente has somewhat longer lasting effects than NPH. If urine sugar is elevated before supper or bedtime, or before breakfast the next day, the dosage can be increased by about two units. If a hypoglycemic reaction occurs before supper or during the night, the dosage of insulin may be decreased by about four units to prevent recurrences. Insulin may be necessary twice during the day to maintain good control through the night, so an additional intermediate type of insulin can be added before supper. A mixture of intermediate and short-acting insulins can be given together in one syringe before breakfast to combine both a.m. and p.m. control.

Preparation for Insulin Injection

Insulin is usually stored in the refrigerator, but a bottle in current use can be kept at room temperature without the insulin's losing strength. An adept diabetic can routinely inject the appropriate amount of insulin into the fatty tissue under the skin of the thighs, abdomen, buttocks, or upper arms with little difficulty. However, some with poor vision, diminished mental capacity, or complications may have problems. A magnifier attached to the barrel of the syringe (Figure 3) can help the visually handicapped by making the numbers and markings larger and easier to see. For the totally blind, an Insulgage (Figure 4) attached to the plunger measures the exact dosage of insulin drawn into the syringe. Two gauges can be used when a mixture of insulins is required. If this technique is too cumbersome, a visiting nurse or a relative can prefill the syringes once a week so that a week's supply can be kept on hand.

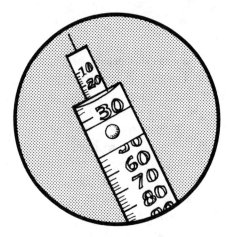

Figure 3. A magnifier attached to a syringe makes numbers easier to read.

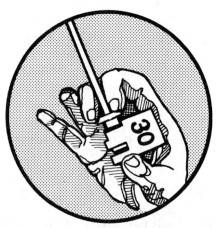

Figure 4. An Insulgage allows the blind to draw a proper insulin dosage into the syringe.

Diabetics with hand tremors or weakness resulting from strokes or other causes sometimes find it difficult to hold the bottle in one hand while drawing insulin into the syringe with the other hand. For such a problem, a portable insulin bottle holder with a magnetic back (Figure 5) can be placed temporarily against a metal door or refrigerator. It holds the bottle in an upside-down position so that the insulin can be withdrawn correctly, in effect providing an additional hand.

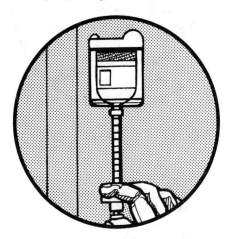

Figure 5. The Insulin Aid bottle holder provides a steady "third hand" for diabetics with hand tremors or weakness.

Insulin Therapy Hypoglycemia

When a diabetic exercises more than usual, additional food should be eaten to compensate for the additional calories used by the body. For example, if one who is normally sedentary plans to play 18 holes of golf during the day, more food can be eaten at breakfast and the size of the snack can be doubled. Also, drinking orange juice or a cola beverage before teeing off will provide sugar. This extra sugar will be burned up during the activity with no adverse effect on the blood-sugar level. If more calories are not eaten, hypoglycemia may result.

A hypoglycemic diabetic may become unconscious. An unconscious person should not be given liquids by mouth (Figure 6) because they may be inhaled into the lungs where they can impair respiration and cause aspiration pneumonia. Instead, a member of the family can inject Glucagon the way insulin is injected, and the diabetic will awaken within 20 minutes. Sometimes, a physician will give glucose intravenously in a hospital emergency room to restore the blood sugar to a normal value.

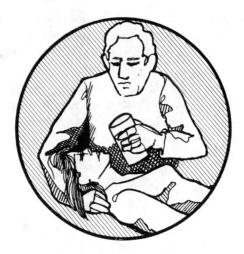

Figure 6. Don't force fluids into an unconscious person's mouth.

To avoid hypoglycemia, diabetics should follow these rules:

- Never begin driving a car when hypoglycemia threatens. If it occurs while you are driving, pull over, stop the car, and take sugar.

- Before driving, test yourself by doing mental arithmetic such as subtracting 7 from 100. Continue through several further subtractions to make sure you are alert and do not have hypoglycemia.

- Keep Lifesavers or similar candy in the glove compartment or pocketbook to use when hypoglycemia starts. Eat half a roll of Lifesavers and allow 15–20 minutes for them to take effect.

- Never omit a snack or delay a meal.

- Eat additional food for increased activity.

- Eat a package of peanut butter crackers to avoid a reaction if you must delay a meal.

- Teach a spouse, friend, or family member to recognize hypoglycemia because the diabetic is often unaware of it. Sugar in the form of juice, candy, or cola will correct the condition.

Education

Since diabetes is a life-long disease, patients must learn to manage and control it. A good diabetes education program for teaching the basics about the disease usually requires about 10 hours of instruction, whether done in a classroom or individually. Important topics include:

Diet Management	Oral hypoglycemic agents
Insulin therapy	Hypoglycemia
Poor Control	High blood sugar
Ketoacidosis	Urine sugar testing
Record keeping	Adjustments of insulin dosage
Foot Care	Special care of minor injuries
Sick day routine	When to call the physician
Daily living	Emotional considerations
Community programs	Diabetic emergencies
Travel provisions	Diabetes identification card

A team of professionals, including nurse educators, physicians, podiatrists, dietitians, pharmacists, social service personnel, psychiatrists, and psychologists, provides both teaching and treatment. Before the course begins, a simple test is given to determine the patient's previous knowledge about diabetes. The results of the test are used to shore up weak areas of understanding, so that when the course is completed, all necessary topics will have been adequately covered.

In addition, a profile outlining socioeconomic factors, dietary history, medical history, diabetes education background, mental acuity, home situation and handicaps is completed. A blind patient will need special training in the use of the insulin gauge and syringes. The patient with limited vision can be taught to use the magnifying attachment on the syringe. Patients with mental impairment due to strokes, Parkinson's disease, or other causes, may have to be cared for by a relative. In such cases, family attendance at the course is encouraged.

A visiting nurse and a home-care coordinator are enlisted to see that the program instituted in the hospital is carried forward at home. A "diabetes hotline" (Figure 7) can be used to call a nurse or physician in a medical center for help with adjustment of the insulin dosage or to review problems before they become major difficulties.

The patient and family should have an up-to-date diabetes instruction manual at home for quick reference, for example, the Joslin Diabetes Manual, 11th Edition, published by Lea & Febiger, Philadelphia, Pennsylvania. The manual is a source of information on questions that

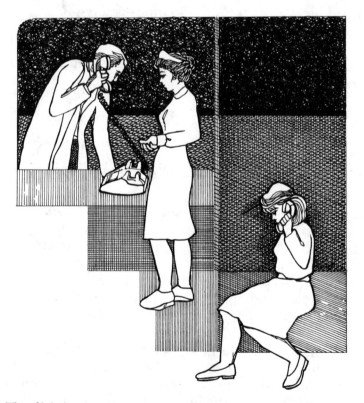

Figure 7. The diabetes hot line is a ready source of advice about diabetes problems and treatment.

may arise infrequently so that answers tend to be forgotten. Current information on research, foods, and other important topics can be gleaned from the American Diabetes Association magazine, *Diabetes Forecast*. Other suggested reading is *The Good Life with Diabetes*, available at the Diabetes Information Center, 829 Spruce Street, Suite 302, Philadelphia, Pennsylvania 19107, and *Diabetes in the News*, issued by the Ames Company division of Miles Laboratories, Inc., Elkhart, Indiana 46514.

Urine-Sugar Testing

Patients with either maturity-onset or juvenile diabetes can judge their degree of control by testing their urine for sugar. High urine sugars usually reflect high levels of blood sugar. The juvenile diabetic is asked to test urine sugar four times daily, before meals and the bedtime snack. If sugar value is high before lunchtime in a diabetic receiving insulin, the short-acting insulin dosage is increased by a small amount. If the urine sugars are elevated in the evening, the intermediate or long-acting insulins are increased.

A small amount of sugar in the urine is advisable since no sugar—*aglycosuria*—may indicate blood sugar low enough to cause a hypoglycemic reaction. If the urine is totally free of sugar, the usual insulin dosage should be reduced. Patients with maturity-onset diabetes receiving oral hypoglycemic agents have less difficulty controlling the level of blood sugar and can tolerate less sugar in the urine without concern about reactions.

Periodic visits to the doctor will further document the degree of control maintained by the patient. Blood and urine sugar values measured in the office will help to determine whether they are too high, just right, or too low, and medication can be adjusted accordingly. The interval between visits is determined by the ease of control and presence or absence of complications.

Blood-Sugar Testing

Some patients now use a "finger-stick" method to test blood sugar (Figure 8). A drop of blood is obtained by piercing the finger painlessly with a simple device (Autolet), the drop is placed on the end of a specially prepared stick (Dextrostix), and the stick is inserted in the portable apparatus (Dextrometer) to measure the blood-sugar value. By testing several times a day, the diabetic is able to monitor accurately the adequacy of control and to determine the amount of insulin needed. Centers are now being established throughout the United States at existing diabetic education facilities to teach patients to use this equipment.

Blood sugar can now also be monitored at less expense with Chemstrip BG made by the Bio-Dynamics company. It provides clinically significant accuracy and does not require a costly instrument and daily calibration.

Travel

While diabetics need not limit activity or travel because of their disease, certain precautions are advisable. If treatment is by diet alone and/

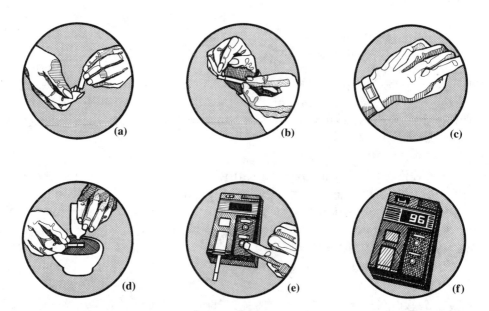

Figure 8. Measuring blood sugar with a Dextrometer: (a) Prick finger to draw blood. (b) Place drop of blood on test strip. (c) Wait one minute. (d) Wash off blood with water. (e) Insert test strip in Dextrometer. (f) Read blood-sugar value on meter display.

or hypoglycemic medication, maintaining good control will entail little or no difficulty. Oral hypoglycemic agents lower blood sugar just as insulin does, so a regular eating pattern should be maintained and overeating avoided to prevent a rise in blood sugar and weight gain.

Insulin-dependent diabetics must be more careful. Before starting a trip, they should obtain from their physician the name of the doctor in the new location in case of emergency. If traveling by plane, they should inform the ticket agent of their condition since a special diet is available on some airlines. They should take along an extra set of prescriptions to insure an uninterrupted supply of insulin, syringes, and other medications, and should also keep enough supplies in carry-on luggage for immediate use.

Diabetics should discuss a possible change in insulin dosage with their physician before starting the trip. The dosage will usually be lowered on the day of departure to compensate for the exercise involved in packing and other activities. Extra food can also compensate for this activity.

Wearing an identification bracelet or necklace can be helpful in case of emergency when special medical care is needed. A card in a wallet or pocketbook identifying the carrier as a diabetic who must carry insulin and syringes will help with customs officials. Syringes are regarded with suspicion and the card will prevent embarrassment.

On any kind of trip, it is best to travel with a companion who will detect developing hypoglycemia before the diabetic does. If the diabetic must travel alone, it is advisable to inform the hotel desk clerk or host at a private home of the guest's condition. If the host is unaware of the problem, prompt therapy may be delayed in an emergency with possibly dangerous consequences. If alone in a room, the diabetic should ask for a wake-up call, informing the operator of the need for immediate medical attention if the call is unanswered. These simple routine precautions will insure safe and pleasant journeys for diabetic travelers.

Complications

Life insurance studies indicate that mortality is greatest among younger diabetics and decreases progressively with advancing age. Most who develop diabetic complications do so within 15 years after the onset of the disease. Those who survive this early period have a better chance of a more normal lifespan. Factors that reduce life expectancy are obesity, hypertension, impaired circulation, and kidney and heart disease.

Coronary artery disease is the major cause of death of diabetics over 55 years old. Strokes, or cerebral vascular disease, are also more prevalent among older diabetics while younger ones are more likely to die of kidney problems secondary to diabetes. Major complications of diabetes include eye, nerve tissue, urinary tract, and peripheral vascular disease.

Diabetic Eye Problems

Diabetic retinopathy is a disease of the small blood vessels in the back of the eye which causes most new cases of blindness in the United States. It is rare in the first years of diabetes, but increases in frequency with time. After ten years, diabetics have a 50 percent chance of developing diabetic retinopathy, and by the 25th year the incidence is 95 percent. The incidence of glaucoma and cataracts also increases.

There are two types of diabetic retinopathy: background retinopathy and the more serious proliferative retinopathy. Background retinopathy produces small leakages of fluid from the blood vessels, aneurysms (bulges in the vessel walls), and hemorrhages, which usually cause little vision loss. Proliferative retinopathy forms new weak small blood vessels which hemorrhage and impair vision. Fortunately, laser beam treatment of proliferative retinopathy can diminish the likelihood of blindness by

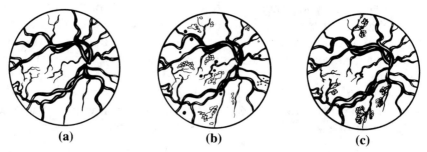

(a)   **(b)**   **(c)**

Figure 9. Diabetes can damage blood vessels in the retina: **(a)** Vessels are normally smooth and leak no blood or other fluid. **(b)** Mild diabetic retinopathy produces "background" changes, including small hemorrhages, aneurysms, and some fluid leakage. **(c)** More severe diabetes proliferation retinopathy produces clusters of weak new vessels.

60 percent. Patients should have an annual examination to determine the degree of diabetic effect on the eyes.

An operation (*vitrectomy*) is now performed when blindness secondary to bleeding into the fluid portion of the eye is not alleviated naturally in six to twelve months by reabsorption of the blood. An instrument is inserted into the chamber of the eye to wash out coagulated blood and cut away scar tissue, partially clearing the area and restoring some vision. Restoration of enough vision to enable a previously totally blind patient to walk about freely helps to reduce dependency on others.

Diabetic Neuropathy

A "pins-and-needles" sensation or numbness in the feet is a symptom of *diabetic neuropathy* (nerve disease), probably the most common of all the chronic diabetic complications. It is due to the fact that nerves in the feet do not transmit the proper sensations to the brain. Pain in the lower extremities can be severe, particularly in bed at night. Symptoms may last for months and then diminish after a waxing and waning course.

Such problems of sensation are usually caused by an abnormality of the peripheral nerve. Occasionally there are weakness and wasting of the muscles of the lower extremity related to motor nerves. This may also develop in the hands but less frequently than in the legs and feet. When the nerves of the gastrointestinal tract are affected, the stomach empties more slowly. Involvement of the small bowel results in nighttime diarrhea, frequently with no warning of an impending bowel movement.

A disorder of the internal genitourinary nervous system causes impotence in 50 percent of diabetic males over 50. Impotence due to diabetic neuropathy has a slow, gradual onset and is characterized by an absence of erections on morning awakening and persistence with all partners. In contrast, the patient whose impotence stems from psychologic factors usually has only intermittent difficulty, sometimes wakes up with an erection, and may have normal intercourse with certain partners but difficulty with others. Diabetics who are impotent have a normal desire for sex (*libido*) and can experience orgasms, but are unable to have an erection.

A sophisticated internal prosthesis has been developed which enables the impotent diabetic to achieve an erection with fluid forced into the apparatus by means of a small pump implanted in the scrotum. Following intercourse, a release button in the scrotum is pressed to relieve the pressure in the implant, and the penis again becomes limp. The operation to implant the pump has had a 90-percent success rate.

Kidney Disorders

Kidney disease caused by diabetes is more prevalent in young patients but is also found in older age groups, together with other kidney problems. *Proteinuria*—protein in the urine—seldom occurs in younger diabetic patients before their tenth year, but is seen in 10 percent of patients over 60. A small amount of albumin in the urine is not necessarily related to advanced kidney disease, but a large amount (over 5 grams per day) is, which can be demonstrated by kidney function tests. Routine kidney function tests should be performed annually.

Pyelonephritis—infection in the urinary tract—is more frequent in diabetics than in normal individuals. Signs and symptoms of the disease include fever, back pain on one side, frequent urination, a burning sensation during urination, and a need to urinate at night (*nocturia*), but one or all may be present. The infection is detected by urinalysis. A urine culture is done to identify the bacteria causing the infection and the appropriate antibiotic to be administered. A urologist should evaluate the patient with recurrent urinary tract difficulty. An *intravenous pyelogram*—X ray of the kidney—will outline the anatomy of the urinary tract system. If necessary, a cystoscope is inserted to examine the bladder and lower urinary tract.

Older diabetics may develop a *neurogenic bladder*, a disorder that may cause urinary retention, a frequent urge to urinate, nighttime urination, and sometimes distention of the bladder without a normal sensation of fullness. The patient has difficulty emptying the bladder completely and may also have difficulty starting the urine flow, produce a weak stream, and sometimes be incontinent. Massive urinary retention in the bladder requires catheterization and drainage. Persistent urinary tract distention can lead to kidney failure and frequent infections and must be treated promptly.

Peripheral Vascular Disease

Diabetics have an increased risk of a reduced blood supply to the lower extremities due to narrowing of both the large and small vessels.

Early in the disease, this can cause cramps in the calf muscles when walking. This symptom, known as *intermittent claudication*, usually arises from walking some distance in the street and is relieved by a short rest. Cramping of the legs at night in bed does not necessarily stem from vascular disease. A physical examination will disclose the decrease or absence of blood vessels in the legs and feet, and the extent of the problem can be measured by various peripheral vascular tests. An X ray of the arteries (arteriogram) in the involved extremity will reveal blockages or narrowing of the blood vessels. If the disease is severe, the patient may develop constant pain, gangrene, and ulcerations. (See separate section on *Peripheral Vascular Disease*)

Diabetic Aids

Medic Alert emblems –Necklaces and bracelets are provided by the Medic Alert Foundation engraved with the medical difficulty, the telephone of the Medic Alert central file, and the file number of the wearer. The address of the Medic Alert Foundation International is P. O. 1009, Tuckahoe, California 95380. Phone 209-632-2371.

Cemco syringe magnifier –This stainless steel and plastic clip-on magnifier attaches to the syringe to enable a diabetic with poor vision to read the calibrations. It is available from Cemco, P. O. Box 21, Scandia, New Mexico 50073.

Insulgage –This instrument helps the handicapped diabetic to prepare an accurate insulin dose for injection. Dosage is varied by using different gauges. Gauges are available with Braille markings. Two gauges are required to draw a mixture of insulins into the syringe. Medicaid, Inc., 9485 E. Orchard Drive, Englewood, Colorado.

Insulin-Aid –This is an insulin bottle holder with a magnetic back that clings to any metallic surface. It holds the bottle firmly so insulin can be drawn into the syringe with only one hand. It is particularly helpful for diabetics weakened by strokes.

NEUROLOGIC DISEASES

Gunter R. Haase, M.D.

Professor of Neurology, Pennsylvania Hospital

It has been remarked that, whatever may be claimed in its favor, old age is a losing proposition. Taken literally, the comment contains some truth. There is a progressive loss of cells—especially in the nervous system—as we age. This results in some loss of functional capabilities with normal aging, independent of any disease process, which is experienced by most aging individuals. The resultant disabilities frequently trouble the aging individual and family members who question whether the failings are "normal" or "abnormal."

The following is a survey of normal neurologic disturbances that are part of the aging process, and of several diseases that are more or less specific to the older age group. It will be seen that indicators of disease in a young individual often fall within the range of average in later life, when they are then defined as normal.

Normal Neurologic Signs In Aging Individuals

Impairment of memory is a common complaint of the elderly, often expressed as, "I just can't remember anything anymore," or even, "I must be losing my mind." Close inquiry usually reveals that memory loss is greatest for the names of people, places, and things. However, while ready access to names has failed, such people frequently have little difficulty describing in detail what they are unable to name. This is in no way abnormal. Only rarely does such memory loss progress to more general intellectual deterioration.

Memory impairment is usually most troublesome when recent events are forgotten while experiences of the more distant past are remembered vividly. Such lapses can be especially annoying to family members suspected of having taken missing articles such as money or glasses which had simply been put down in forgotten locations. The physician is often asked by the patient or family for medication to improve memory. Unfortunately, none has yet been found. Other changes in the nervous system as we age include visual and hearing losses and dulling of the senses of smell and taste. These may stem from a variety of causes.

Normal elderly individuals frequently have a reduction of muscle bulk. While this may be most prominent in the shoulder girdle and buttocks, the muscles of the temples, neck, hands, and feet may also become smaller. Muscle tissue loss may be severe enough to justify the comment, usually made by a family member, that "his bones stick out." Muscle strength normally lessens only slightly, but reflexes, as tested with a reflex hammer, diminish significantly in both degree and swiftness. These changes are often accompanied by a mild impairment of coordination.

Minor tremors are common in advanced age, most frequently involving the hands, head, lips, or voice. Tremors can be evidence of disease, especially Parkinson's disease, but are more often isolated events known as *senile tremor*. Although tremors only occasionally respond to treatment, people who have them are usually relieved by firm assurance that they do not reflect serious disease.

Postural changes in normal elderly individuals commonly include a bending forward of the body and head. The gait usually loses some of its natural spring, the stride shortens, and walking may become shuffling. All muscular movements may become stiffer and slower.

Dementia

Occasionally, the normal mild forgetfulness of the elderly progresses to a more general mental loss, including disorders in thinking, confusion, poor judgment, careless personal hygiene, and frequent changes of emotional expression. Family members often remark, "He is not himself anymore." This condition is known as *dementia*. The disorder usually progresses slowly, and care of the one undergoing personality changes may be quite difficult for relatives.

There is a tendency to ascribe these changes to "hardening of the arteries," but scientific findings indicate that arteriosclerosis is rarely the cause. The brains of individuals with dementia more often show extensive cell loss and other widespread microscopic changes, rather than arteriosclerosis. Because Alois Alzheimer, a German neurologist, was the first to describe these changes, the disorder is also known as Alzheimer's disease. The shrinkage of brain substance can now be detected with a CAT-scanner, a computer-assisted X-ray instrument of great diagnostic value for brain diseases. It displays a cross section of the brain (or other part of the body) that can also reveal such evidence inside the skull as blood clots and brain tumors.

The specific cause of dementia remains unknown, but immune factors, viruses, and hereditary predisposition have been variously suspected. Unfortunately, although various vitamins, blood-vessel dilators, lecithin, and other drugs have been tried, no drug or other treatment has yet proved successful in arresting the progress of the mental changes.

Dementia is sometimes due to various medical conditions, rather than an unknown source associated with aging, and may then possibly be halted or reversed. In some instances, symptoms may be brought on by severe depression or the excessive use of sedative or tranquilizing drugs. In others, they may be due to reversible causes such as inadequate thyroid function, certain blood disorders, brain tumors, and kidney and liver diseases. Dementia should always receive careful medical investigation to determine if treatment can be helpful.

Stroke

The brain receives its nourishing blood by way of three large arteries which branch into smaller and smaller vessels. *Carotid* arteries in the right and left sides of the neck supply the front of the brain, and the *basilar* artery deep in the back of the neck supplies the rear of the brain. Disorders of the brain's blood supply account for a large percentage of all deaths and an even larger percentage of disabilities in older people. Medically classified as cerebrovascular disease, these disorders are commonly called "strokes," especially if their onset is sudden.

The nervous system functions through the activities of nerve cells called *neurons*. Projections called *axons* connect neurons with other nerve cells in the brain and spinal cord to form networks, or circuits. A neuron must have an adequate supply of oxygen and glucose to perform its task. If oxygen supplied in the blood falls below a critical level (*hypoxia*), for example, because heart or lung action temporarily stops, tissue may be damaged. Neurons in the outer layer (*cortex*) of the brain are especially vulnerable. A person with damaged cortical neurons may continue simple reflex activity such as breathing and chewing, and may appear alert, but may not be able to speak, recognize, recall, or think.

If oxygen deprivation lasts less than about 3—4 minutes, recovery is usually complete. However, longer periods without oxygen usually cause permanent brain damage and the condition known as "a human vegetable." The person may breathe without assistance and move the eyes, but cannot respond to the external world. With good nursing care and control of infection, such patients may survive for years, but are very unlikely to recover sufficiently to resume the ordinary activities of daily living. In cases of even more severe hypoxia, all brain function ceases, including breathing, and only the heartbeat and blood pressure are maintained. This state is brain death from which there is no recovery.

The above conditions involve the entire brain. If only one of the vessels supplying the brain becomes obstructed or otherwise disabled, only part of the brain will lose its blood supply and only the activities associated with that part will be affected.

The effects of stroke thus depend on the site and degree of brain damage. The left side (*hemisphere*) of the brain controls the right side of the body, and vice versa. In each hemisphere, one part, the motor area, is concerned with muscle movements, while a nearby part, the sensory area, interprets information such as the nature of surfaces and shapes and the location of body parts. The back part of the brain (*posterior* or *occipital cortex*) receives and interprets visual information. Speech, both speaking and listening, is associated with the left hemisphere (Figure 1) in all righthanded people and in about half of those who are lefthanded, and with the right hemisphere in other lefthanders.

Ischemic Infarction

The most common cause of stroke is reduced blood flow due to an obstructed artery. A deficient blood supply is known as *ischemia,* and the resulting damage to tissue served by the obstructed vessel is termed *ischemic infarction.* When the blockage is caused by arteriosclerosis

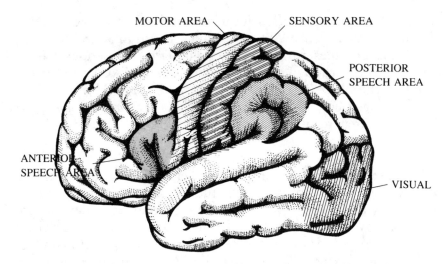

Figure 1. Left side of brain, showing areas associated with different functions.

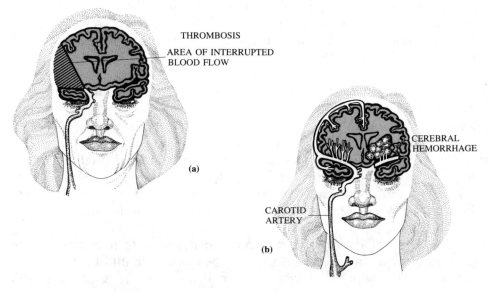

Figure 2. Stroke: **(a)** Thrombosis blocks brain artery. **(b)** Cerebral hemorrhage diverts blood from brain tissues.

(thickening of the wall and narrowing of the opening) of a brain artery, resulting in formation of a blood clot (*thrombus*), the disease is referred to as *cerebral thrombosis (Figure 2),* and the affected artery may be named specifically (middle, anterior, or posterior). In other instances, the obstruction may be due to a loose piece of matter (*embolus*) formed in the heart valves or broken off a clot in an arteriosclerotic artery leading to the brain, and then delivered by the blood stream to a cerebral artery. If the embolus becomes firmly wedged in place and seriously impedes blood flow, it can cause a permanent neurologic disorder (ischemic infarction). If the blockage is only temporary, the trouble may last only a few minutes or several hours. It is then called a *transient ischemic attack,* or TIA. TIA's may recur repeatedly and may be followed by a full-scale stroke.

The onset of neurologic problems in cerebral embolus and thrombosis is usually very sudden, although thrombosis symptoms may develop over hours or days (*stroke-in-evolution*). External signs depend on the blood vessel involved. For example, ischemic infarction in the right middle cerebral artery causes weakness or paralysis of the left arm and leg and the left side of the face. The head and eyes may be turned to the right and sensation may be disturbed on the body's left side, described as numbness, tingling, "pins and needles," or simply "strange." The right eye may become temporarily blind and, if the posterior cerebral artery is involved, both eyes may lose some vision on the side of the visual field opposite the blocked artery.

A thrombosis of the left middle cerebral artery involves the right side of the body in a similar pattern, and may also affect speech. The stroke patient may have difficulty finding a right word (*expressive aphasia*), forming a sentence (*motor aphasia*), and comprehending statements (*receptive* or *sensory aphasia*). Less common are difficulty in reading (*dyslexia*) and solving mathematics problems (*dyscalculia*), confusion of right and left, and poor muscular coordination in tasks involving limbs on both the paralyzed and normal sides of the body (*apraxia*).

Ischemic infarction of either cerebral hemisphere does not usually produce a coma, but consciousness may be lost as a result of infarction of the brain stem which connects the spinal cord and the brain. Impulses originating in the cerebral hemispheres travel through fibers in the brain stem to their destinations in various parts of the body, as do signals from the body destined for the brain. The brain stem also contains nerve tissue essential for maintaining consciousness and control of eye movements, blood pressure, and respiration. Thus, infarction of the brain stem is a devastating and often fatal event.

A typical stroke case involved a 70-year-old woman driver who side-swiped several parked cars on her right side. Examination revealed complete loss of vision to the right of the midline in each eye (she simply had not seen the parked cars), and X-ray tests showed infarction in the rear of the left cerebral hemisphere.

Another patient, aged 59, was hospitalized with marked weakness in his right arm and leg, first noted when he collapsed on getting out of bed. He was unable to form words and could not understand what was said to him. His family reported that he had experienced four episodes of

difficulty in forming words in the three weeks preceding his attack, none lasting more than five minutes. On two of these occasions he had dropped objects held in his right hand. A clinical diagnosis of thrombosis of the left middle artery, preceded by ischemic attacks involving the same vessel, was confirmed by X-ray studies.

Complete recovery can be expected after each transient ischemic attack and some recovery after ischemic infarction (depending on the patient and the therapy). The extent of recovery will be greater if the patient tries to exercise affected muscles relatively soon after the onset of stroke. Especially when accompanied by supportive measures, physical therapy is an important component in stroke treatment. Transient ischemic attacks are treated with drugs such as aspirin and anticoagulants to reduce the chance of blood clots. Anticoagulant drugs are used cautiously because they increase the risk of internal bleeding. Surgery may be necessary to restore free blood flow to carotid arteries choked by arteriosclerosis.

Cerebral Hemorrhage

Ischemic infarction causes about 80 percent of all strokes. The other 20 percent are caused by hemorrhages, which also rob the tissues of their blood supply because they divert the blood flow from useful to harmful paths (Figure 2). Cerebral hemorrhage tends to occur most often in people who have a long history of high blood pressure. They are less often due to injury, congenital abnormalities, inflammatory diseases of the blood vessels, and blood clotting deficiencies.

Cerebral hemorrhage is typically sudden and may be related to physical exertion. The victim may abruptly lose consciousness, or initial drowsiness may progress to coma. Paralysis develops quickly in limbs on the side opposite that of the hemorrhage, and a conscious patient may complain of a severe headache. Convulsive seizures occasionally occur during the early stages. Cerebral hemorrhage is often fatal, and survivors may recover slowly and incompletely.

Treatment of hemorrhagic stroke includes general supportive measures and physical therapy. Surgical removal of the blood clot is rarely useful.

Parkinson's Disease

Parkinson's disease usually occurs after the age of 50. Symptoms develop gradually: a tremor in the limbs when at rest, slowness of move-

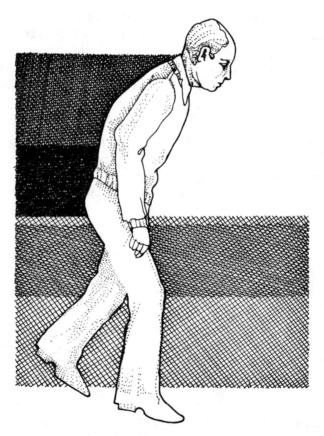

Figure 3. Typical walking posture in Parkinson's disease.

ment, or rigidity in groups of muscles. Initial symptoms may be so slight, only the person with the disease is aware of them: handwriting may grow smaller, dressing and undressing may take more time, and tasks requiring close muscle coordination may become more difficult. Others may sometimes notice that movements are slower, the hands tremble, the facial expression has become wooden, and steps are shorter during walking and the normal arm swing is absent (Figure 3). Certain groups of muscles may ache, and arms and legs may feel sore and tight. Frequently, saliva drools from the mouth and the voice becomes feeble and monotonous. The disease may become increasingly disabling for many years if not treated.

The cause of Parkinson's disease is generally unknown. In a few cases, the cause has been traced to viral encephalitis contracted at an earlier age. In some others, the cause appears to have been prolonged use of tranquilizing drugs.

Treatment of Parkinson's disease has consisted of anticholinergic drugs such as Artane (*trihexyphenidyl*), Congentin (*benztropine mesylate*), and several others. These are still used, especially for early treatment in mild cases. Their possible side effects include dryness of the mouth, blurred vision, constipation, and sometimes confusion or hallucination.

The recognition that Parkinson's disease reflects the lack of a substance, *dopamine,* in certain parts of the nervous system has, in recent years, led to treatment with *levodopa* (L-dopa) which converts to dopamine in the brain. L-dopa is usually given with *carbidopa* to prevent rapid chemical breakdown. L-dopa benefits most patients, but its effectiveness depends on regular administration, whether alone or in combination with carbidopa. Side effects may include nausea and vomiting, lowering of blood pressure, and involuntary movements such as facial grimaces and twisting or jerking of the arms and legs. Because the side effects can sometimes be related to the dosage and timing of medication, the treatment requires close supervision by an experienced physician. Drug treatment is combined with physical activity such as walking, swimming, or stationary bicycling. Patients with Parkinson's disease often become depressed, which may need special attention.

GASTROINTESTINAL DISEASES

Scott H. Wright, M.D.

Assistant Professor of Medicine,
University of Pennsylvania
Section Gastroenterology, Pennsylvania Hospital

William H. Lipshutz, M.D.

Associate Professor of Medicine,
University of Pennsylvania
Head, Section of Gastroenterology, Pennsylvania Hospital

Gastrointestinal complaints are common among men and women of all ages, but tend to be especially prevalent in the elderly. This is partly due to the aging process itself and partly to diseases associated with aging that have gastrointestinal symptoms. The following are among the most widespread disorders of the gastrointestinal tract.

Swallowing Difficulty and Heartburn

Swallowing difficulties can indicate various disorders and should not be ignored either by the sufferer or the doctor. Diagnostic evaluation, including consideration of the history of the complaint, usually discloses a cause and indicates the most effective treatment. An understanding of the anatomy between the mouth and the stomach and what happens when we swallow is helpful as background to a discussion of the disorders that can make swallowing difficult.

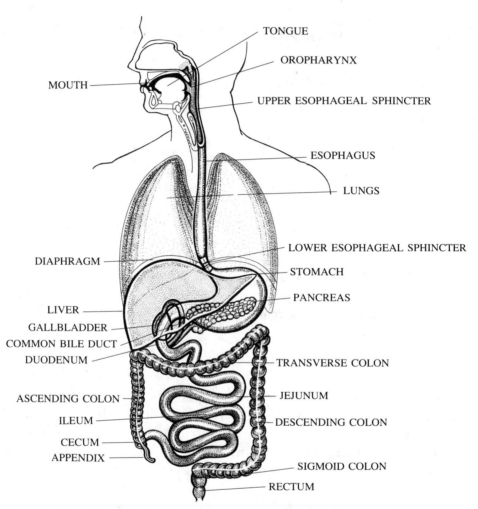

Figure 1. Gastrointestinal tract.

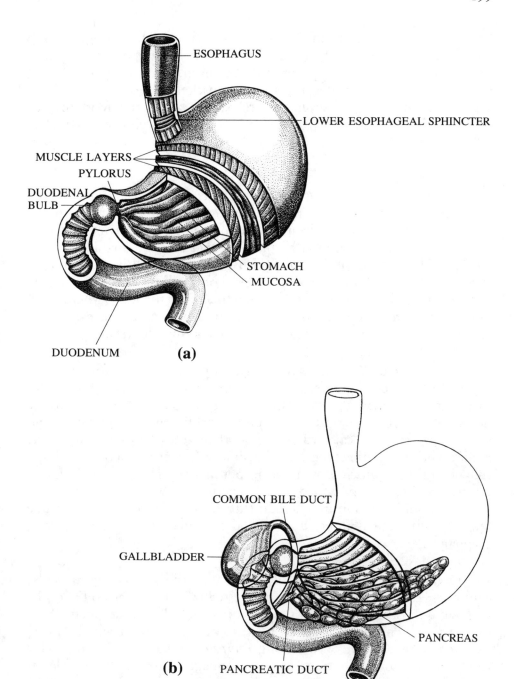

Figure 2. Stomach and neighboring organs, showing (a) details of stomach and esophageal muscles, and (b) gallbladder and pancreas.

When we place food in the mouth, a combination of tongue action and sudden contraction of throat muscles propels the food to the top of the *esophagus,* the tube leading to the stomach. The airway to the lung automatically closes while a ring-shaped muscle (*sphincter*), that guards the upper end of the esophagus, relaxes to allow the food to pass through. This first step of swallowing is normally a well coordinated act of nerves and muscles. It can be disrupted by neural or muscular disorders.

Patients with such diseases as multiple sclerosis, Parkinson's disease, tissue damage (*infarction*) in the swallowing center in the brainstem due to an inadequate local blood supply, poliomyelitis, myasthenia gravis, or muscular dystrophy, will usually complain that they are unable to start a swallow. They will have difficulty with both solids and liquids, in contrast to the effect of a tumor which blocks only solids. They may also regurgitate food through the nose and breathe it into the lungs where it can cause pneumonia requiring hospitalization. Problems at this early stage of swallowing require neurologic evaluation and muscle tests.

Motion pictures of the swallowing action slowed down for study can provide a limited diagnosis, also disclosing tumors or tissue formations such as webs and bands that restrict the esophagus. If further steps are necessary, an ear, nose, and throat specialist will examine the mouth and throat down to the vocal cords, using local anesthesia to check for tissue abnormalities, whether vocal cords come together properly, or if the tongue or throat muscle is weak or uncoordinated. This may be followed by *pharyngoscopy* and *esophagoscopy*, performed with a local anesthetic spray and mild sedation in less than fifteen minutes, in which a flexible optical instrument is inserted for visual examination of the throat and esophagus.

Occasionally, the cause is still not found, and swallowing difficulty continues. Esophageal motility is then tested. Motility is the ability of the esophagus muscles to perform properly: first, to relax the sphincter muscle at the top end to let food in; next, to contract certain muscles in sequence to create a wave of squeezing (*peristalsis*) that drives food quickly from the top to the bottom of the esophagus; then to relax a lower sphincter to let the food into the stomach. Peristalsis can be a primary response triggered by swallowing or a secondary response triggered by esophageal distention after food has passed through the upper sphincter. The motility test involves insertion of a tube that senses the pressure at various points along the esophagus so that the dynamics of swallowing can be measured and aberrations detected.

Swallowing disorders caused by a lack of normal esophageal peristalsis, such as esophageal spasm, *achalasia* (failure of the lower sphincter to relax at the right time), and *scleroderma* (hardening and shrinking of the esophageal tissue), usually cause difficulty with both solids and liquids. A general spasm of the esophagus causes chest pain during swallowing and occasionally regurgitation of undigested food. Swallowing very hot or very cold liquids often brings on the chest pain. Fear of a possible heart attack often causes the sufferer to seek medical attention. A *barium swallow* (X-ray inspection as an opaque liquid is swallowed) and an *esophageal pressure test* (similar to the motility test) are used to confirm the diagnosis of spasm. A physical examination and resting and stress electrocardiograms are also routine since one of the main objects of treatment is to reassure the patient that the pain is not caused by coronary artery disease. Muscle relaxants are given to reduce the spasm.

The lower esophageal sphincter normally contracts to prevent acid stomach contents from rising into the esophagus, but must relax to pass swallowed food before contracting again. Failure of the sphincter to relax causes a buildup of pressure and resistance to further swallowing.

Gastroesophageal Reflux Disease

Symptoms: Heartburn, regurgitation, pain at night, pain when swallowing, swallowing difficulty, esophageal bleeding

Cause: Lower sphincter (valve muscle) fails to prevent acid stomach contents from rising to esophagus (not related to hiatus hernia)

Treatment: *Drugs*—Antacids, Tagamet (Cimetidine) to decrease acid production, Urecholine to increase sphincter pressure. Avoid atropine and Isuprel which decrease sphincter pressure. *Foods*—Avoid chocolate, alcohol, fats, and coffee which all decrease sphincter pressure, and orange and tomato juices which burn. *General*—Raise head of bed; don't eat shortly before bedtime; don't lie down soon after eating; don't wear clothes that bind the abdomen.

The lower sphincter may also weaken and fail to keep stomach contents from entering the esophagus. This may cause severe heartburn, a burning in the chest that travels upward and is associated with the rising of sour material from the stomach to the mouth. Heartburn due to an ineffective lower esophageal sphincter is often confused with *hiatus hernia,* a displacement of the junction between the stomach and esophagus from its normal position. Recent studies have shown the disorder to be unrelated to hiatus hernia.

It was also recently discovered that various foods and drugs used to treat other disorders can weaken the lower esophageal sphincter and cause heartburn. The reflux (backward flow) of stomach acids can seriously inflame the esophagus (*esophagitis*) which may ulcerate and produce severe bleeding, or heal so that scar tissue narrows the esophagus and causes increasing difficulty in swallowing solids.

Therapy consists of neutralizing stomach acids with liquid antacids; lessening acid production with drugs such as cimetidine; avoiding irritants such as aspirin, coffee, tobacco, and alcohol; and physical precautions, including raising the head of the bed so that gravity assists a downward flow, making sure clothing (for example, girdles) is not tight, and refraining from eating just before bedtime or lying down after a heavy meal. If such therapy fails, or if severe complications develop, surgical correction of the weak sphincter is usually successful.

Cancer of the esophagus invariably causes swallowing difficulty. It is readily diagnosed with X rays (barium swallow), biopsy, and microscopic examination of tissue cells. Because people tend to disregard minor difficulties in swallowing, however, detection is sometimes too late for good therapeutic results. Many other disorders can also produce swallowing difficulty. With these, too, proper and prompt attention and early diagnosis and treatment have the best chance of success.

Jaundice

The term "jaundice" refers to yellowing, most easily seen in the eyes or at the base of the tongue, but occasionally visible throughout the skin. It is caused by an abnormally high blood content of *bilirubin,* a residue of old red blood cells normally removed from the bloodstream by the liver. The liver converts the bilirubin into bile which may be stored temporarily in the gall bladder but ultimately empties into the upper end of the small bowel where it aids in food digestion.

A small amount of bilirubin is normally present in the blood. Yellowness first becomes apparent when the level rises to two or three times normal and increases as the level becomes higher.

A high bilirubin content in the blood may result from three different abnormalities. First, excess bilirubin may be produced beyond the ability of the liver to process it. Second, liver cells may be disabled by drugs or disease so that bilirubin backs up into the blood. Third, the common bile duct, into which the liver normally discharges the converted bilirubin, may be mechanically blocked so that bilirubin backs up into the liver (a long-lasting duct block can cause liver damage).

These three conditions are common in the elderly. For example, the blood released during surgery breaks down after the operation and increases the load of bilirubin delivered to the liver. Liver disease such as hepatitis due to infection or drugs may partially incapacitate the liver cells. Alcohol is a very common drug that can cause liver damage and jaundice. (Although jaundice may be related to some types of liver disease, it is not always the most sensitive indicator.) The common bile duct can be blocked by cancer of the pancreas through which the duct passes, by cancer of the bile duct itself, or by gallstones lodged in the duct. Occasionally, surgery in the area of the gallbladder or common bile duct may result in inadvertent damage that narrows the bile duct and leads to jaundice.

Diagnosis involves not only a physical examination but also a medical history. The doctor will ask about medications being taken, alcohol consumption, previous episodes of hepatitis or personal contact with people who have had hepatitis or jaundice, and symptoms that might suggest present hepatitis or gallstones. (Hepatitis usually produces a tired feeling and weakness before the onset of jaundice. Gallstones often bring severe pain to the upper right abdomen frequently accompanied by fever and chills.) A recent weight loss may suggest cancer since pain and other effects often reduce appetite. The physical examination probes for signs of cancer, tenderness over the liver which may indicate disease of the liver cells, and an apparent mass in the abdomen which might indicate a blocked bile duct, especially if the patient also has fever and chills.

Initial testing is oriented toward distinguishing between a blocked bile duct and liver disease as the cause of the jaundice. This is essential because a blocked duct is often surgically correctable, whereas medical treatment is preferred for liver disease and surgery is usually avoided. Blood tests may show a characteristic pattern. X rays of the liver and gall-bladder are often helpful and may be supplemented by ultrasound tests, similar in principle to sonar detection of submarines, which use reflections of sound waves to display a picture of internal organs such as the pancreas and common bile duct. The ultrasonic scan can show if the common bile duct is dilated suggestive of mechanical blockage, if stones are present in the gallbladder, and sometimes if a tumor exists in the pancreas or liver. If the duct is dilated, it can be filled with an opaque dye and X-rayed to give more details about the possible blockage.

If the duct is blocked by cancer or a nonmalignant obstacle such as a gallstone, surgery is usually necessary. If the duct is not dilated, the likely cause of jaundice is liver disease, but a liver biopsy may be performed to confirm the diagnosis. This involves use of a local anesthetic such as Novocain and the insertion of a needle to obtain a small sample of liver tissue for microscopic examination.

The tests determine if medication is indicated to treat liver inflammation. Occasionally, liver disease requires only improved nutrition and observation. The patient is usually advised to avoid alcohol and other medications known to affect the liver until the inflammation heals.

Rectal Bleeding

Rectal bleeding is a common problem in the general population, but in those over 50, it is more likely than in younger people to be due to cancer or blood vessel disorders in the bowel. The blood may be bright red or, if it is totally mixed with the stool, invisible (occult). Slow bleeding can be detected only by a chemical test of the stool. Chronic bleeding may cause anemia or a low blood cell count.

Discovery of the source is not as urgent when the bleeding is slow as when it is fast. The sudden loss of a large amount of red blood through the rectum is a medical emergency which requires immediate hospitalization and evaluation. Excessive loss can cause anemia, fatigue, headache, malaise, and sometimes psychiatric disturbances. Replacement of lost blood by transfusion helps to relieve the symptoms, but the cause of the bleeding must be found to prevent further loss.

Previous heartburn, indigestion, or ulcers would suggest that the bleeding originated in the stomach or esophagus. A recent change in bowel habits or red blood on toilet tissue would indicate a lower source such as the rectum or colon. Black tarry stools, if not related to taking of iron or other medications such as Pepto-Bismol that can darken the stool, suggest bleeding from the stomach. The doctor will study the skin, lips, and abdomen for clues to the source of the bleeding, and will also ask about a family history of blood-clotting abnormalities and previous bleeding problems.

The blood is tested for proper clotting, anemia, and signs of disease that might cause bleeding. The first step to localize the source of the bleeding is insertion of a tube through the nose or mouth into the stomach to sample the area for blood. If no blood is detected, and the medical history does not suggest ulcers, the focus of the search shifts to the lower bowel or colon.

The last several inches of the bowel are visually examined with a *sigmoidoscope* inserted though the rectum. This reveals cancers, *colitis* (inflammation), hemorrhoids, and other possible causes of bleeding in the anal region. If this examination is negative, the bleeding is assumed to originate higher in the bowel, and a barium enema is given. The lower gastrointestinal tract is filled with opaque liquid and X-rayed to disclose the condition of the bowel beyond the reach of the sigmoidoscope. The X rays can disclose cancer, *polyps* (small growths on the intestine wall), colitis, blood vessel malformation, *diverticulosis* (ballooning of weak spots in the colon wall into pockets called *diverticuli*), and other rarer causes of lower bowel bleeding. If the search is still not fruitful, the upper gastrointestinal tract may be X-rayed.

Early Warning Signs of
Cancer of the Colon

- Change in bowel habits
- Change in size of stool
- Rectal bleeding
- Blood in stool (visible or occult)
- Previous colon cancer
- Family history of colon cancer
- Polyps

- Family history of polyps
- Ulcerative colitis for at least 8 years

If the bleeding source is not found and bleeding continues, but not at a rate that requires immediate surgery, more specialized tests will be performed. The inner surface of the bowel can be visually examined with a *colonoscope,* a long, flexible, optical tube that is inserted in the rectum and threaded through the entire colon. The colonoscope is especially effective for finding certain sources of bleeding, but requires more time and skill than a barium enema does. Also, the patient is given a sedative so that preparation and observation may have to be done in a hospital. An instrument similar to a colonoscope may be inserted through the mouth into the stomach after the patient is mildly sedated and given a local anesthetic in the throat to prevent gagging. This allows the doctor to visually inspect the lining of the esophagus and the stomach and the upper portions of the *duodenum* and *jejunum* (beginning portions of the small intestine).

If none of these measures discovers the source of bleeding, *arteriography* may be recommended. In this procedure, a dye is injected into the blood vessels that supply the gut so that they are clearly seen in X rays. Bleeding sites are revealed by leakage of the dye.

After the patient's condition has been stabilized, treatment focuses on preventing the bleeding from recurring. Hemorrhoids are treated with stool softeners and the application of soothing agents to the anal area to relieve discomfort. Colitis may be treated by medication or, if necessary, surgery. A tumor will be surgically removed or treated with medication or X rays. Life-threatening bleeding from diverticulosis or blood vessel malformations may require surgical removal of the affected part of the intestine; less severe bleeding may be treated medically. Ulcers usually respond to medication, but may also sometimes require surgery. In general, emergency surgery is reserved for bleeding that is so heavy it cannot be stopped long enough to permit satisfactory evaluation.

Most rectal bleeding has a nonmalignant cause. However, since the chance of a malignancy increases with age, people over 50 should have even minor bleeding promptly and thoroughly checked. Since colon tumors grow slowly, early detection usually allows a complete cure. It is also important to correct anemia due to bleeding from any source because the older person's heart is especially sensitive to the harmful effects of a low blood cell count. When bleeding is stopped and anemia is corrected, the long-term outlook for patients with rectal bleeding is usually good.

Change in Bowel Habits: Diarrhea or Constipation

Changes in bowel habits and discomfort in having bowel movements are fairly common among the elderly. Since the susceptibility to both bowel cancer and nonmalignant causes of such changes increases with age, sufferers should seek early medical attention. Diarrhea, constipation, and any change in the frequency or consistency of stools may signal health problems that can worsen if left untreated.

In evaluating a change in bowel habits, the doctor first considers common, easily corrected disorders. For example, many medications other than laxatives and anti-diarrhea drugs affect the stool. Some of these may be unnecessary or replaceable by less harmful substitutes. A dietary history is important because water, milk, beans, cabbage, and certain other foods can affect bowel movements. Stresses and emotional upsets can cause certain fluctuations in bowel habits known as the *irritable bowel syndrome,* characterized by alternating constipation and diarrhea. A medical history may be informative, since the aftermath of previous surgery may also affect bowel flow.

If the preliminary investigation is not conclusive, the doctor then considers such possible causes as viral or bacterial infection in the colon, other illnesses such as hyperthyroidism or infection elsewhere in the body that can affect colonic activity, and blood circulation to the bowels, since poor circulation can also change bowel habits and occasionally cause pain. The doctor may request a stool specimen for culturing and microscopic identification of parasites or their eggs.

The search then turns to possible narrowing of the colon by mechanical obstructions. Blood in the stool, detected by sensitive chemical tests (the blood is often invisible), strongly suggests a tumor or colitis. Obstruction and a change in bowel habits may be due to diverticulosis or *diverticulitis,* infection of the diverticular pockets. A sigmoidoscope inserted in the rectum permits direct inspection of the lining of the lower bowel for tumor or colitis. With a barium enema, the entire colon can be examined in X rays, including parts beyond the reach of the sigmoidoscope.

Occasionally, disease in the stomach or small bowel may cause diarrhea. If examination of the lower gastrointestinal tract proves unrevealing, the upper tract is X-rayed. These X rays and stool tests help to rule out rare disorders such as diseases of the lining of the upper bowel that prevent it from absorbing food, diseases of the pancreas and other organs that secrete digestive juices, cancers of the upper gastrointestinal tract, and scarring, adhesions, or other abnormalities from previous surgery.

If these investigations fail to yield a diagnosis, it is quite likely that no serious disease is present. However, if the symptoms are severe or the stool contains blood, further tests may be performed, including arteriography (X rays after a dye is injected into the arteries), colonoscopy, or upper gastrointestinal endoscopy (inspection of the upper tract through a tube inserted in the mouth).

Treatment of diarrhea or constipation depends on cause. Often, only a change of diet or medication is necessary. For diverticulosis or irritable bowel syndrome, bulk may be added to the diet and muscle-relaxing drugs given to relieve cramps. Infections respond to appropriate antibiotics or anti-parasite drugs. Diverticulosis and diverticulitis are usually treated with antibiotics and resting of the bowel, but surgery is sometimes necessary.

A tumor usually requires hospitalization for tests to determine its extent. Surgery can often cure a localized tumor, but if the tumor has spread from its initial site, chemotherapy or radiation may be judged to be more effective.

Although changes in bowel habits are not usually the sign of serious disease, they should be brought to the attention of a physician. Early diagnosis and treatment greatly increase the chances for a complete cure of any disease, and undue delay may be fatal. The medical tests usually cause little discomfort and may give peace of mind.

Intestinal Gas

Excessive intestinal gas is another frequent complaint of older people, appearing as abdominal distention, bloating, cramps, belching, and passage of gas through the rectum. Some common causes are air swallowing, intolerance to milk sugar, and a spastic colon.

Excessive Intestinal Gas

Cause 1. *Air Swallowing*
Treatment: Learn to eat slowly and quietly; abstain from liquids at meals; avoid cigarette smoking and gum chewing; keep a piece of hard candy in the mouth or a small wooden stick between the teeth.

Cause 2. *Irritable colon*
Treatment: More bulk such as bran cereal in diet; bulk-type laxative; smooth-muscle relaxant (prescribed by physician)

Cause 3. *Intolerance to milk sugar (lactose)*
Treatment: Avoid milk, cheese, and ice cream.

Cause 4. *Abnormal bacteria in colon*
Treatment: Restrict carbohydrates in diet; identify and eliminate offending foods.

Belching and a bloated feeling can be due to overindulgence in carbonated beverages. Air swallowed (often unknowingly) during hurried eating or under emotional stress inflates the stomach and can cause discomfort. Drinking more carbonated drinks, Alka-Seltzer, or bicarbonate of soda for relief merely increases the distention and the belching.

A simple remedy is to swallow less air by learning to eat slowly and quietly, to abstain from liquids at meals, and to avoid cigarette smoking and gum chewing. Simethicone-containing prescriptions such as Mylicon help to absorb internal gas. Keeping a piece of hard candy in the mouth or a small piece of wood between the teeth can help to break the habit of swallowing air.

Lactose (milk sugar) intolerance can cause gas, cramps, and occasional diarrhea. It is due to an enzyme deficiency widespread in the United States, especially among Orientals, blacks, and people of Mediterranean origin, such as Jews, Armenians, and Italians. Excessive amounts of milk, hard cheese, or ice cream can trigger the distress. Unabsorbed milk sugar passes on to the lower intestine where bacteria ferment it and produce gases such as hydrogen and methane. The gases distend the colon and cause diarrhea and abdominal cramps. A history of recurrences of the disorder and a physical examination to rule out other possibilities are usually sufficient to diagnose the deficiency, but a special lactose-tolerance test may sometimes be required. Restricted eating of milk products usually brings lasting relief.

The spastic colon syndrome includes intestinal gas and cramps and alternating constipation and diarrhea. Victims are found to have abnormal muscle activity in their gastrointestinal tracts that cause normal amounts of gas to produce cramps and pain. Treatment consists of adding bulk in the form of bran cereal and Metamucil to the diet and administering an anti-spasmodic or smooth (involuntary) muscle relaxant such as Bentyl or Librax.

A rare cause of excessive intestinal gas is an abnormal variety of bacteria in the colon. These bacteria produce gas as they metabolize certain carbohydrates found on the skins of prunes, apples, and other foods which do not bother most people. The remedy is a diet with severe restrictions on carbohydrates and a trial-and-error elimination of gas-producing foods.

Weight Loss

Weight loss, especially in the elderly, may be due to depression (poor appetite), lack of help in preparing food, swallowing difficulties, pain, or a tumor or other disease that alters either the need for or ability to absorb nutrition. Normally, if the diet contains enough calories, weight is maintained.

Hyperthyroidism may increase the metabolism so that a normal intake of food is not enough. Certain diseases of the pancreas or the lining of the small bowel, or deforming gastrointestinal surgery may impair the transferring of nutrients from the bowel to the blood stream so that nutrition is deficient in spite of a normally adequate diet.

To find the cause of weight loss, the physician first investigates dietary intake and eating habits. Hospitalization may sometimes be necessary to determine if a controlled and adequate diet succeeds in maintaining weight. Pain or other symptoms are noted that may suggest gastrointestinal or other disease. The blood is tested for evidence of poor nutrition and to rule out thyroid disease. A physical examination discloses abdominal or other abnormalities that may indicate serious chronic disease or cancer. If necessary, X rays are taken of internal organs.

A chest X ray and electrocardiogram provide clues to possible heart disease, lung tumors, chronic lung disease, and bone disease in the chest. If an abnormality is found, further X rays may be taken of the colon, esophagus, stomach, liver, pancreas, and bones. To minimize discomfort and expense, tests are limited to those necessary to arrive at a specific diagnosis.

Treatment of weight loss due to inadequate diet is simple improvement of the diet. For some elderly people, the family may need help from a social work agency. A metabolic problem such as thyroid disease is treated with medication or radiation to normalize the metabolism. Infection or chronic disease is treated with appropriate antibiotics and pain relievers. Tumor of the gastrointestinal tract requires surgery, radiation, or chemotherapy. Chances for complete recovery are good if cancer is treated at an early stage. Treatment of incurable cancer may still permit a more or less normal life for an extended period of time. If the weight loss is related to intestinal deformation by previous surgery, therapy consists of corrective surgery, where feasible, or dietary supplements.

Abdominal Pain

Occasional abdominal pain is commonplace and simply tolerated, but continuous pain should receive medical attention. A history of the pain and its relation to eating, bowel activity, and physical exercise will usually locate the source and indicate appropriate tests and therapy.

Peptic ulcers are a common source of abdominal pain. Non-malignant types, usually *gastric* (stomach) or *duodenal* (end of the small intestine near the stomach), create pain between meals when the stomach is empty. Generally described as a burning discomfort in the middle of the abdomen, the pain is usually relieved by eating food, drinking milk, or taking an antacid. Particular foods or drugs bring abdominal distress, including caffeine drinks such as coffee and cola, salicylate drugs such as aspirin, and, sometimes, spicy foods. The discomfort may be interrupted by several pain-free months before recurrence brings a visit to a physician. Diagnosis is usually confirmed with a series of X rays of the upper gastrointestinal tract which show the location of the ulcer.

The pain of gallstones can be excruciating. It characteristically occurs in the upper right abdomen under the lower ribs and sometimes makes its victim double over and sweat heavily before it spreads under the right shoulder blade. The pain may come at any time, but most often appears after a heavy meal.

After the pain is first felt, the urine may darken and the stool lighten, indicating jaundice as a result of passge of the stone from the gallbladder into the common bile duct. The diagnosis of gallstones is confirmed by X ray or ultrasonic scanning.

Disease of the pancreas can cause abdominal pain of vague origin. The pancreas is difficult to investigate because its location at the back of the upper abdomen shields it from probing fingers, and it doesn't show up on routine X rays. It can be studied only with sophisticated techniques such as ultrasonic scanning, computerized axial tomography (CAT-scan), and endoscopy (insertion of a long optical tube for visual inspection) of the upper gastrointestinal tract. These tests require expertise that may not always be available in community hospitals.

Pancreatic pain normally starts two or three hours after a meal and is located deep in the upper abdomen. It usually seems to be associated with the back, and bending the upper part of the body often eases the pain by relieving the pressure on the pancreas where it lies across the spine. Although less intense than that due to gallstones, pancreatic pain can be severe and make it impossible to find a comfortable position.

Inflammation of the pancreas due to excessive alcohol consumption, previous nearby surgery, drugs, or infection can produce the pain. Such inflammation is not usually accompanied by significant weight loss. However, the cause of the pain is often cancer of the pancreas which is associated with significant weight loss and fear of eating because it increases the pain.

The pain of colonic disease usually occurs below the *umbilicus* (belly button) on both sides. It feels like a cramp that may or may not ease with a bowel movement or passage of gas. The pain is common in constipated people.

Diverticulitis (inflammation of bulging sacs in the colon wall) or rupture of a sac usually causes severe pain and tenderness to touch in the lower left abdomen. It signals the onset of acute disease and requires hospitalization, antibiotic treatment, and bowel rest.

Appendicitis causes pain and tenderness in the lower right abdomen. It is easy to diagnose in the young but is frequently overlooked in the elderly. A pain in the critical area should be investigated regardless of the age of the sufferer.

A leaking or ruptured *aneurysm* in an abdominal blood vessel (ballooning of a diseased segment) is usually a catastrophic event characterized by severe abdominal pain and a lapse by the victim into a shock-like state from loss of blood. However, it is usually preceded by warning symptoms of intestinal pain that tend to occur immediately after a meal. The pain is due to a decrease in the intestinal blood supply required for digestion and absorption of food. The disorder is called *intestinal angina* because it resembles *angina pectoris,* the chest pain caused by diseased and narrowed coronary arteries that diminish nourishment to the heart.

The pain of *peritonitis* is usually part of an intense reaction to the perforation of an abdominal organ and the spilling of its contents into the peritoneal cavity (space in the abdomen between the organs). It is frequently so severe and aggravated by any body movement that the victim cannot even shift position from side to side. The abdomen is rigid to the touch and no bowel sounds are heard through a stethoscope. Often, the physician's hand can feel free air over the liver, indicating the escape of air from an internal organ. Peritonitis can be caused by rupture of a peptic ulcer, the gallbladder, a diverticulum in the colon, or a cancer. It requires emergency care and hospitalization. The perforated organ is located and surgery performed to drain the peritoneal cavity, rid it of infection, and close the perforation.

Obstruction of the small intestine may cause a colicky abdominal pain which starts mild, builds to a maximum, and then subsides. The rhythmic pain pattern is caused when the intestinal channel is constricted by attached tissue that squeezes the intestine or prevents it from expanding, or by growths or inflammation inside the intestines. The cause is usually determined by X ray (barium series) and corrected or relieved by surgery or medication.

CANCER

Harvey Lerner, M.D.

*Head, Section on Surgical Oncology
and Cancer Chemotherapy
Pennsylvania Hospital*

Cancer may be the most dreaded six-letter word in the English language. Because of widespread ignorance about this disease, the word can cause panic when mentioned in a diagnosis. Such fear discourages people from becoming informed about the nature of the disease and doing what they can to help guard against it.

Cancer is truly an equal opportunity disease. It doesn't discriminate against anyone regardless of age, sex, race, or social status. In the United States, it is estimated that one of every four in the general population will develop some form of cancer, one of every seven will eventually die from the disease, approximately 675,000 new cases of cancer will be reported in 1981, and 365,000 of these new patients will die during the year.

What is Cancer

It is not a specific disease, but most likely a group of different malignant diseases gathered under a common name. To describe its nature requires consideration of how the body normally works.

The human body consists of many organs or organ systems such as the heart, lung, bone, gastrointestinal tract, and so on. These are in turn made up of billions of tiny living cells which perform different, and often very specific functions for their particular organ. Each cell reproduces itself by repeatedly dividing in two, thus providing growth and repair of body tissues. The entire process of cell division, growth, and tissue repair is normally regulated by a body control mechanism. When this control is lost, a group of cells may begin to multiply at an abnormally rapid rate. The uncontrolled growth becomes a tumor. Tumors may be benign or malignant (cancerous). Benign tumors may continue to enlarge but do not invade neighboring tissue or spread to remote areas of the body. Malignant tumors have this ability, and the spreading of the disease is known as *metastasis*.

A malignant growth can metastasize to other areas of the body in two ways. One way leads to nearby or regional lymph nodes through the lymphatic, a system of vessels that carry lymph somewhat like the system that circulates the blood. The second way is by invasion of small local blood vessels. Malignant cells that break away from the parent tumor can then travel with the blood stream to distant areas where they are nourished, multiply rapidly, and destroy their new home.

Early detection and treatment is the surest means of combating and curing cancer. The longer tumors are permitted to grow without treatment, the more likely they are to have time to metastasize.

What Causes Cancer

The true cause of uncontrolled cell growth leading to cancer is unknown. However, a great deal is known about the development of some cancers. It is generally agreed that people develop cancer mainly through repeated or long-term contact with one or more cancer-causing substances known as carcinogens. There are many sources of cancer. The few examples that follow are now widely recognized:

1. Cigarette smokers are ten times more likely to develop lung cancer than are non-smokers. They also run a higher risk of developing other types of cancers.

2. There is a direct relationship between alcohol consumption and cancer, especially when drinking is combined with heavy smoking.

3. Exposure to radiation can cause cancer, whether the radiation is from machines (for example, X rays), radioactive

substances, or the sun. A sun worshiper may pay a penalty years after exposure when heavily sunburned areas develop skin cancer.

4.   Certain chemicals are specifically known to cause cancer and may create occupational hazards. For example, an asbestos worker without a face mask risks lung cancer by breathing asbestos particles over a long period of time.

5.   Viruses are suspected of causing one or more forms of cancer.

There is no evidence to support the claim that repeated injury can cause cancer. Most physicians agree that tumors found under such conditions probably existed prior to the injuries. There is also no evidence that a cancer can be developed by contact with another person who already has the disease.

It is known, however, that cancer is a long-term process which may develop slowly over a period of 15 to 30 years. The earliest phase of the disease—the induction phase—may result from repeated contact with one or more carcinogens. Local growth, the pre-invasion phase, then follows and may last from five to ten years before the next, invasion, stage of growth appears. Dissemination, or metastasis, may follow the invasion phase after one to five years, and normally also lasts about one to five years.

Cancer Treatment

At present, there are three standard treatments for cancer: surgery, radiation, and chemotherapy, which may also be used in combination with one another. In planning treatment, it is important to gather as much information as possible on the extent of the disease, using all available diagnostic means. If technically feasible, a biopsy should be performed so that the type of tumor can be determined by microscopic examination. This may be the single most important factor in helping to decide the best treatment.

Treatment may be curative or palliative. Cure implies that all of the cancer, including its extension and metastases, has been eliminated from the body. No matter how long the patient lives, this particular tumor will not recur. Palliative treatment implies that no cure is possible. The therapeutic goal is then maximum possible comfort for the patient.

Surgery

Surgery is the oldest method of treating cancer and has been the mainstay of curative therapy. It can cure only disease which is still localized in the tissue of origin and in regional draining lymph nodes, with no metastases beyond this region.

Radiation

Radiation therapy (X rays, radium, and cobalt) is highly specialized and is administered by a physician specifically educated and trained in this field. Radiation therapy, like surgery, can be used for cure or palliation, depending on the type and extent of the tumor. In addition, radiation therapy may be adjunctive, that is, used to destroy any residual tumor cells after surgical removal of all the gross tumor.

Chemotherapy

Chemotherapy is the treatment of cancer with drugs and has become one of the major modalities available. Certain types of tumors are now treated almost exclusively with anti-cancer drugs with relatively high long-term survival rates. *Adjuvant* chemotherapy may be used after the local disease has first been eradicated by surgery or radiation when there is still a high risk of distant spread of the disease. However, anti-cancer drugs are most effective when only a small number of tumor cells remain. Adjuvant chemotherapy is usually employed over an extended period of time.

Nutritional Problems

The most common nutritional problem in cancer patients is weight loss due to a variety of causes. It may be secondary to the cancer or a side effect of treatment. The tumor may block the intestine and interfere with passage of food. Some tumors produce a substance that decreases the appetite. A tumor may cause pain that diminishes interest in food, and the very diagnosis of cancer can kill the appetite. Sometimes the patient's sense of taste is altered and some foods become unpleasant. The effects of surgery, chemotherapy, and radiation can create nutritional problems.

Whatever the cause of the decreased appetite, the end result is the same. When food is lacking, the body consumes reserves of fat and protein, loses weight, and eventually depletes its reserves. Because a well-nourished body is more able to withstand the stress of cancer and its aggressive treatment, it is very important that the cancer patient accept regular nourishment. Adequate nutrition helps the patient to withstand major surgery as well as higher doses and more prolonged periods of chemotherapy and radiation. Malnutrition depletes the body's natural defense mechanisms and renders the patient much more susceptible to infection. In most clinical cancer centers, a patient will receive nutritional support throughout the course of therapy.

Rehabilitation

Rehabilitation has been one of the most neglected aspects of cancer treatment. Physical restoration is very important, but the patient's social, psychological, vocational, and economic problems are also significant and should not be overlooked. Most hospitals now have rehabilitation departments for the cancer patient.

Head and neck surgery or a major amputation may require physical rehabilitation, including prostheses, or speech training may be needed after a laryngectomy (removal of the voice box). Breast surgery is usually followed by special training, and instruction is necessary for management of difficulties after the various ostomies such as *colostomy, ileostomy,* and *ureterostomy.*

Psychosocial or vocational problems can be debilitating. Anxiety is generated by the fear of prolonged suffering, mutilation, loss of sexual capability, employment difficulties, and possible death. The problem involves not only the patient but also family and friends. The patient may anticipate being unwanted and alienated, which can lead to complete withdrawal. Most hospitals have social service departments to assist in individual or group counseling. In addition, the American Cancer Society has helped to establish many ostomy, laryngectomy, and mastectomy clubs. Through these groups, patients and families contact others with similar problems whose previous experience provides helpful support.

Follow-up

The physician's responsibility for the cancer patient does not end when surgery is over, radiation treatment completed, or the last drug given. After primary treatment, a follow-up schedule should be carefully planned. This will often require appointments every three months for three years, then every six months for five years, and yearly thereafter. In addition to the usual physical examination, there will frequently be follow-up testing appropriate to the type of primary cancer that was treated.

Common Types of Cancer

Lung Cancer

Lung cancer is the number one cancer killer in the world and continues to rise in epidemic proportions. Cigarette smoking is reported to be responsible for 90 percent of all lung cancers, and the rest may be attributed to exposure to industrial carcinogens or other air pollutants. Despite repeated warnings from the American Cancer Society and the Surgeon General, people continue to smoke. Lung cancer appeared to be restricted to males as long as most smokers were men. Now, the rate for females is rising sharply as more and more women smoke.

The symptoms of lung cancer are usually connected with obstruction of a bronchus (one of the larger air pasages in the lung) caused by the tumor, and include a cough, with or without blood, the development of pneumonia behind the obstructing tumor, and chest pain. The diagnosis is usually established by chest X ray and bronchoscopic examination (an optical instrument is inserted through the mouth into the major air passages of the lung). A piece of tissue may also be removed and examined. Appropriate treatment may be surgery, radiation therapy, or chemotherapy, alone or in combination.

The prognosis for lung cancer patients is extremely poor. Eighty percent die within one year of the initial diagnosis. For this reason, countermeasures are mainly preventive. The recognition of industrial carcinogens, for example, has stimulated the use of proper protective equipment. However, cigarette smoking remains widespread, guaranteeing that lung cancer will be with us for many years to come.

Breast Cancer

Over 80 percent of all lumps found in the female breast are not malignant. The vast majority are cysts or other benign lumps which are not a serious health hazard but should not be ignored. Pain in the breast is most often due to hormonal changes during the menstrual cycle and only rarely to breast cancer. Also, breast cancer is not caused by a blow or repeated blows to the breast, by caresses, by nursing or not nursing a baby, by sexual contact, or by contagion. Nonetheless, more than 90,000 new cases of breast cancer will be reported this year in the United States.

One out of every 13 women will develop breast cancer at some time during her life, making this the most common form of cancer and leading cause of cancer death in women today. The chances for recovery and cure are significantly greater when the disease is detected at an early localized stage. Frequent self-examination (Figures 1, 2, and 3) of the breast is essential. If a woman is menstruating regularly, the examination should be performed after her period; otherwise, it should be done routinely at the same time each month. The purpose of the examination is to detect changes in the size and shape of the breast or nipple, any discharge, dimpling, or puckering of the skin, or any other unusual feature.

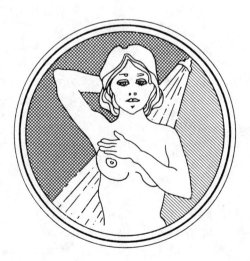

Figure 1. In the shower (hands glide more easily over wet skin). Holding fingers flat, move hand gently over entire breast to check for any lump, hard knot, or thickening. Repeat with other breast.

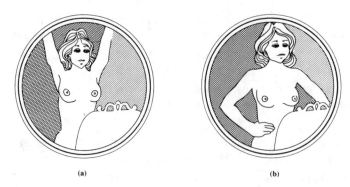

Figure 2. Before a mirror, look for any changes in breast shape such as a swelling, dimpling of skin, or change in the nipples, first with arms at your sides, then **(a)** with arms up, and then **(b)** with hands on hips pressing down firmly to flex chest muscles.

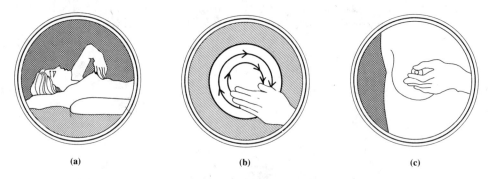

Figure 3. Lying on back. **(a)** Place pillow under right shoulder and right hand behind head to examine right breast with left hand. Holding fingers flat, press gently in small circular motions **(b)**, starting at top of breast (12 o'clock) and proceeding clockwise to 1 o'clock then full circle back to starting point. Repeat in smaller circles (at least three), ending at nipple. A ridge of firm tissue in lower curve of breast is normal. **(c)** Squeeze nipple between thumb and forefinger. Any discharge should be reported to your doctor. Repeat with left breast and pillow under left shoulder.

Mammography (breast X ray) is an important diagnostic technique performed by radiologists with highly sophisticated equipment. It can often reveal a developing breast cancer long before it can be felt by the physician's fingers. If a lump or suspicious area on a mammogram is found, a biopsy is performed. The tissue is examined by a pathologist, a physician who interprets the changes caused by disease in body tissues.

Before any surgery is performed, the patient must sign a consent form outlining the type of surgery for which she is giving permission. She has the choice of having the biopsy performed and then waiting for a definitive diagnosis and a discussion of available options if she does have breast cancer. On the other hand, she may decide to have a mastectomy at the time of the biopsy if the biopsy shows the presence of cancer.

Clearly, when a diagnosis of cancer is confirmed, it is best to begin treatment in a hospital that has the staff and resources necessary to apply all forms of effective treatment. Before treatment is begun, the patient has the right to request opinions from other physicians to confirm both the diagnosis and the recommended treatment.

Several types of mastectomy (breast removal) are performed in American hospitals today.

1. Radical mastectomy is removal of the entire breast, the muscles of the chest wall, and the lymph nodes in the *axilla* (armpit).

2. Modified radical mastectomy is removal of the entire breast and the lymph nodes in the axilla, but not the muscles in the chest wall.

3. Simple or total mastectomy is removal of the breast but not the lymph nodes or the muscles in the chest wall.

4. Partial, or segmental, mastectomy is removal of only a portion of the breast. The tumor is removed along with a margin of normal tissue in all directions, and the breast is cosmetically reconstructed. In addition, some lymph nodes usually are removed from the armpit, and radiation therapy may or may not be given. Partial mastectomy is usually performed on a very select group of women in whom the cancer is relatively small, particularly in comparison with the size of the breast. This procedure is usually reserved for women who volunteer to participate in an important clinical trial being conducted by the National Surgical Adjuvant Breast and Bowel Project in an effort to determine whether a partial mastectomy is as effective as a more extensive procedure.

Regardless of the procedure, if the excised cancer is smaller than 0.5 cm (about 0.2 inches), the patient has greater than a 10-to-1 chance of surviving for 10 years.

If the lymph glands beneath the arm are involved with the tumor, or if there is evidence of remote spreading, the physician will probably elect to administer chemotherapy. Clinical trials have demonstrated that women who receive chemotherapy appear to remain free of cancer much longer than those who don't. Radiation therapy may be used in special cases, for example, to reduce the tumor size before surgery, or to destroy secondary tumors resulting from spreading, especially if the spread has been to bone, which causes pain, or to the chest wall.

Some breast cancers depend on hormones such as estrogen for growth and may be treated with other hormones or specific anti-hormones. If the patient responds to hormone therapy, and the tumor seems to depend on estrogen, further surgery may be performed to remove sources of growth-stimulating hormones, such as the ovaries, the adrenal glands (situated above the kidneys), or the pituitary gland (at the base of the brain).

The American Cancer Society's *Reach to Recovery Program* has been very helpful to breast cancer patients. It is staffed by American Cancer Society volunteers, each of whom has had a mastectomy. These volunteers assist patients in such ways as exercises, the use of prosthetic breast forms, and in answering their questions.

Some women who undergo mastectomy may wish to consider breast reconstruction in which a suitable prosthesis is placed underneath the skin to form a realistic breast mound. However, reconstruction is normally not considered until at least six months after the mastectomy.

It is essential that the breast cancer patient undergo careful and long-term follow up. Women who have had cancer in one breast have about one chance in ten of developing a cancer in the other. The risk is greater if there is a family history of breast cancer. There is also an increased risk for women who began menstruating very early and for those who either had their first child after age 30 or never had children.

Cancer of the Colon and Rectum

Almost 100,000 Americans will develop cancer of the colon and rectum this year and nearly half will die from the disease. Only breast cancer kills more women; only lung cancer kills more men. As in all cancers, early diagnosis and treatment are the key to higher cure rates. Unlike many cancers which are secret until the disease is beyond cure, cancer of the colon is detectable and easily localized at a very early, asymptomatic stage.

The colon (large bowel) is the lower five or six feet of the intestine. The last five or six inches of the colon form the rectum, which ends at the anus through which the body eliminates its waste as bowel movements. The most common symptoms of colorectal cancer are abdominal discomfort or pain, blood in or on the stools, and change in bowel habits. If any of these symptoms last for more than two weeks, a physician should be consulted. Blood in the stool is always a serious symptom which should be brought to the attention of your physician.

The examining physician will feel the abdomen and probe the rectum with a gloved finger. A more extensive visual examination may be done with a proctosigmoidoscope inserted into the rectum to permit the physician to see the lower ten or twelve inches of the colon and rectum. A large number of tumors develop in this area. If a tumor is evident, a biopsy may be performed so that the specimen can be examined under the microscope and identified. A flexible instrument called a colonoscope may be used for further examination. It is about as thick as a finger, maneuverable around bends and curves to explore the entire colon, and permits taking of tiny tissue samples for biopsy. The colon may also be filled with opaque material (barium enema) and X-rayed.

The type and location of a malignant bowel tumor are among the factors that determine the best treatment, usually surgical removal. After surgery, the physician may suggest radiation therapy to help prevent recurrence of the cancer. Chemotherapy may also be recommended to combat both local recurrence and distant spread of the tumor.

A colostomy is sometimes necessary after surgery. It consists of an opening of the colon placed on the front abdominal wall to allow the passage of bowel movements and thus substitutes for the rectum. A colostomy may be permanent, particularly if the lower portion of the colon is removed, or temporary, to allow other surgery to proceed or to permit some other part of the bowel to rest and heal. Since bowel function is not impaired, the patient can live a normal active life but will usually wear a colostomy bag to receive waste material.

Patients with colostomies are often eligible for assistance from the American Cancer Society or the United Ostomy Association, a group whose members have all undergone colonic or rectal surgery. Information about local chapters may be obtained from the United Ostomy Association, 1111 Wilshire boulevard, Los Angeles, CA 90017.

With more advanced bowel cancers, radiation treatment may be given for several weeks before surgery to shrink the cancer and relieve pain. Chemotherapy and radiation may also be used in combination at different times to destroy or control the cancer.

Cancer of the Cervix

Cancer of the uterine cervix (neck of the womb) is the second most common form of cancer in women. Its symptoms may be minimal, such as a slight vaginal discharge or bleeding, irregularities in menstruation, or bleeding following sexual intercourse. Diagnosis is usually easy and quick, and the disease can be readily cured. However routine laboratory tests (Pap smears) and gynecologic examinations are essential, followed by a biopsy if the test result is abnormal. The diagnosis can usually be made before the disease invades nearby tissue. Even if there are early signs of invasion, the cure rate can be very high, but falls dramatically if the cancer is allowed to advance without being treated. Effective treatment may combine radiation therapy and surgery.

Malignant Lymphomas

Malignant lymphomas are cancers of the lymphatic system (lymph nodes). This system is part of the general circulation and is related to the ability to resist infection. Malignant lymphomas can be divided into two main groups—Hodgkin's and non-Hodgkin's.

The disease usually begins as a painless enlargement of one of the lymph glands. If left untreated, it may spread through the lymphatic system and to other organs. Other symptoms that may develop are fatigue, weight loss, and occasionally itchy skin and night sweats. When the disease has become widespread, the body's resistance to infection is markedly reduced. Because the symptoms are vague, they are often incorrectly associated with other diseases.

An accurate diagnosis is established by biopsy of a lymph node, including a microscopic examination to determine the lymphoma type.

The physician then tries to determine the extent of the disease, a procedure known as staging which includes a clinical examination, X rays to reveal the possible spread to other lymph nodes, and biopsies. Biopsies may cover not only the lymph nodes, but also the liver and especially the bone marrow to see if the disease involves blood-making tissues. Treatment and prognosis depend on whether the cancer is still localized or has already advanced. Therapy may consist of radiation, chemotherapy, or a combination of both.

Unproven Cancer Treatments

Home remedies do not cure cancer, and unproven treatments are as much a part of the cancer problem as the disease itself. Fear of cancer is universal. Fear of surgery, radiation, and chemotherapy tempts many to seek unorthodox alternatives that promise to be easier, faster, and surer.

Cancer quackery is big business in the United States. Patients and their families are often unfortunate prey for schemes that exploit anxiety and ignorance. One such scheme is the sale of diets or pills "specifically designed" to destroy cancers. These have never been shown to help any patient and usually waste valuable time while the tumor grows until the patient finally seeks medical attention when the disease is no longer curable.

Can Cancer Be Cured

The answer to this question is an emphatic yes. However, the key is early detection. The American Cancer Society has prepared a booklet which stresses the warning symptoms of cancer known as "The Seven Key Signals:"

1. Any unusual bleeding or discharge through the mouth, nose, vagina, penis, bowel, or bladder.

2. A sore or an ulcer that does not heal normally.

3. Indigestion or difficulty in swallowing.

4. Much hoarseness or a persistent cough.

5. Changes in bowel or bladder habits.

6.   Hardening or lump in the breast or any other part of the body.

7.   Changes in color or size of a wart or mole.
            Figure 4 from an American Cancer Society publication on

GYNECOLOGICAL PROBLEMS

Frank Gaudiano, M.D.

Assistant Professor of Obstetrics and Gynecology
Pennsylvania Hospital

In 1979, new cases of breast cancer in women exceeded 100,000. In the same year new cases of uterine and ovarian cancer reached 70,000, and many of these were fatal. This lamentable statistic and the fact that increasing age brings women a greater risk of breast and other types of cancer, make regular breast and pelvic examinations essential. Early detection of these disorders assures the older woman the best chance for complete cure.

Ideally, every woman should have continuity of care from one gynecologist through the menstrual and childbearing years and into old age. However, for obvious reasons, this is not practical for most women. The older woman especially is likely to avoid a pelvic examination because it has become increasingly uncomfortable, or simply because she is no longer in touch with her former gynecologist. A good relationship with their gynecologists is very important for most women, for even in the best circumstances they often find many matters, for example, sexual problems, difficult to discuss with other professionals, however sympathetic.

Finding a gynecologist with whom you can be at ease may not be easy, but here are guidelines to test if the one you have is satisfactory (from *Our Bodies Ourselves* by the Boston Women's Health Collective, published by Simon & Schuster, New York, 1973). If your physician does not do the following, you have failed to communicate your wants or it is time to find a new physician:

1. Give an accurate diagnosis of your condition, healthy or otherwise, at your request.

2. Obtain results and meanings of any tests or examinations done by him or by others at his direction as soon as they are available.

3. Clearly explain indications for treatment, varieties and alternatives; pros and cons of particular treatment; and the opinions of other experts, as well as the doctor's own preference and the reasons for it.

4. Offer answers to your questions about any examination or procedure he may perform in advance of, or at any time during the performance of it.

5. Stop any examination or procedure at any moment at your request.

6. Offer complete information about purpose, content and known effects of all drugs prescribed or administered, including possible risks, side effects, contraindications, especially of combination drugs.

7. Show willingness to accept and wait for a second medical opinion before performing any elective surgery which involves alteration or removal of any organ or body parts.

8. Give answers to your questions about your body or about your general health and functions, in addition to any particular conditions or encouragement to seek these answers from other sources.

The Older Woman

A woman's life may be divided into three separate periods: childhood, childbearing, and post-childbearing. The changes that take place after the childbearing years are hormonal, physical, and psychological, and affect both her own life and the lives of her husband and family.

Preceding ovulation in each menstrual cycle, the ovary produces estrogen, a hormone which has an effect on the female genital organs—the breasts, the lining of the uterus, and the mucus at the neck of the uterus (cervix). During the second half of the menstrual cycle, following ovulation, the ovary produces progesterone, a hormone which prepares the uterine lining to accept a fertilized egg, should conception take place. With menopause, these cycles end, menstruation ceases, and organs such as the vagina and breasts no longer receive estrogen stimulation. The effects of low estrogen can be disturbing. Figures 1 and 2 illustrate the parts of the female urogenital tract.

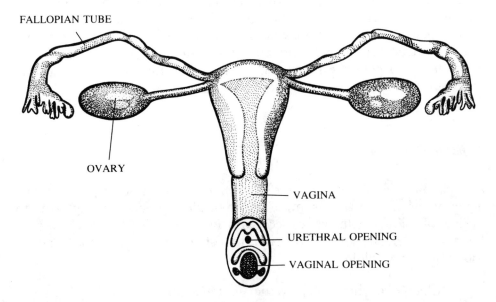

Figure 1. Female urogenital tract.

Psychological changes and the intensity with which they are felt vary with the individual. Some women are relieved when they can no longer bear children, while other become depressed. However, the absence of the need for contraception often makes the mature woman's sexual relations more pleasurable.

The "empty nest syndrome" is a common sad reaction when children leave home to pursue their own lives and careers. However, for many women this becomes a time to regain or restore a sense of purpose. Release of the pressures of raising a family is a positive influence that leaves them free to carry on activities and interests previously put aside. The inability to make a successful adjustment to this freedom is appropriate for discussion with a gynecologist, who will often suggest sources for further assistance or advice.

Following menopause, physical changes related to a decrease in estrogen will often justify a visit to a physician. Problems that may need medical attention include diminished genital response to sexual stimulation, pain on intercourse or urination, loss of urine with coughing or straining, and, frequently, "hot flashes." However, it should be noted that a decrease in estrogen may not be the cause of a particular problem. Many life changes, such as the stresses of aging and the strangeness of new roles, can generate pressures which make professional help a welcome surce of comfort.

What to Watch For

While it would be unwise for a woman to diagnose or treat her own gynecologic problems, it is important to be alert to bodily changes and to seek professional help when necessary. Prevention is the watchword in medicine. Here are some of the signs that should be brought to the attention of the gynecologist:

1. Changes of the vulva (external genital area)

- Any dark spot, especially one which is new, has changed in color or size, or bleeds

- Any lump

- Any red or red-and-white area that is crusted or bleeds

- Persistent itching or scaling of the skin

- Thinning or thickening of the vulvar skin

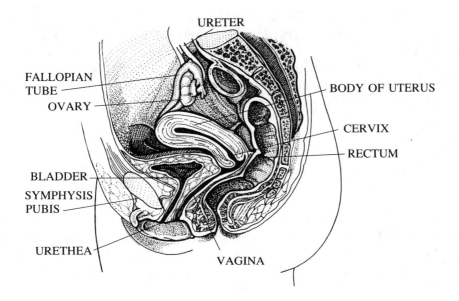

Figure 2. Pelvic organs.

2. Changes of the vagina

- Any bleeding, spotting, or red or brown staining

- Any discharge, with or without itching, especially with an unpleasant odor

- Any protruding growth

- Any problems encountered during sexual intercourse because of dryness, tightness, or poor muscle tone in the walls of the vagina

- Any protrusion of normal body structures through the vaginal opening

3. Changes in body function

- Loss of urine on coughing, straining, or lifting

- Any change in bowel habits such as inability to pass stool, chronic constipation, dependence on laxatives, or the need to press the vagina to eject stool

- Blood in stool or urine

The gynecologist will advise you as to their meaning and suggest a course of action or treatment. In some instances, a second medical opinion may be sought. The findings described are not cause for alarm, for most reflect benign conditions. Some are long-term results of childbearing and loss of muscle tone and hormones, and may occasionally warrant surgery. Others will benefit from treatment with estrogens.

Certain conditions will require excision of a small piece of tissue (biopsy) for laboratory study to determine whether it is benign or malignant. In-hospital diagnostic tests may be needed before or after the initial biopsy.

Occasionally patients reject biopsy out of their fear of pain or the suspected presence of cancer. It is unwise to balk when the physician suggests a tissue sampling. When you are in doubt, a second opinion can be reassuring, but the issue should never be evaded, for early diagnosis invariably offers the best chance of cure if cancer is found.

Breasts

Concern for their breasts is a lifelong preoccupation for most women. As an adolescent, the young woman fears that her breasts will not be large enough to make her attractive; in the childbearing years she may be concerned that the milk produced will be insufficient to feed the baby properly.

In the later stages of life, it is very important that the breasts be examined by a physician twice a year, and equally important that self-examinations be made once a month. Regular attention to breast examinations is necessary to detect and diagnose any abnormality. However, a lump in the breast is *not* a sure sign of cancer; most such lumps are benign.

The breast is the site of 28 percent of all cancer in females. The incidence of the disease increases with age, making the risk of its appearance at age 70 six times that at age 40. Unfortunately, despite substantial advances in therapy, breast cancer proves fatal to as many women today as it did 40 years ago. Nonetheless, detection of a cancerous lump at an early stage greatly improves the odds of living five or more years following surgery. Breast cancer is diagnosed too late for cure in about one-third of all cases, and for this reason regular breast examination is essential. Because nine out of ten breast cancers are detected by the woman rather than by her physician, conscientious personal medical care is the best insurance against cancer hazards.

On discovery of a lump, the physician may suggest a soft-tissue X-ray. If the lump appears to be a cyst, however, the doctor may elect to drain it while the patient is in the office. This procedure is only slightly uncomfortable, much like taking a blood sample from the arm.

A firm diagnosis of breast cancer can be made only by performing a laboratory examination of a sample of tissue removed from the breast under anesthesia. Anesthesia may be local or general, depending on the preference of the surgeon. Following laboratory examination of the tissue, the physician will confer with the patient to determine the appropriate therapy. If no cancer has been found, close follow-up will be recommended for added assurance.

The risk of developing cancer is higher for some women than for others. Any of the following factors will place a woman in the high risk group:

- A history of previous breast cancer
- Presence of a dominant lump, localized pain, or nipple discharge
- A family history of breast cancer
- No record of childbearing, or birth of a first child after age 40
- First menstrual period before age 11, or late menopause

Sex and the Older Woman

It is often assumed that a woman's ability to respond sexually diminishes with advancing age and her interest in sexual activity declines. Neither assumption is true. As Masters and Johnson have noted, "There is no time limit drawn by the advancing years to female sexuality." Masters and Johnson also assert that women reach their erotic peak in middle age, and that sexual capacity does not decline until very late in life, with orgasmic response continuing into the eighties.

Exposure to regular and effective sexual stimulation is an important factor in a woman's ability to respond. Effective sexual stimulation is not easily defined, but it can be said that it depends on communicating to the partner whatever is found pleasing or exciting. Sexual patterns which were pleasurable early in life will remain pleasurable in later years; it is essential to maintain the response with regular sexual relations. When this condition is met, a woman in her eighties is able to respond with the intensity of a young woman.

Apart from the physiological ability to respond, a number of factors can affect the maintenance of a satisfactory sexual relationship. Discomfort during intercourse because of dryness or tightness of the vagina may detract from enjoyment, leading to avoidance of intercourse. Estrogen cream prescribed by a gynecologist for local application will provide relief from such symptoms. A partner's inability to establish or maintain an erection because of chronic disease or other infirmity can foreclose the opportunity for sexual intercourse. The potential for closeness and pleasure in touching will remain unaffected, and this kind of intimacy will often provide much satisfaction for the older person who is denied the enjoyment of intercourse.

A satisfactory sexual relationship will have a salutary effect on psychological well-being as well as on physical health. Whether the relationship is nurtured by touching and closeness or by sexual intercourse, its purpose is the realization of the special contentment generated by the warmth and closeness of a loved one.

The Estrogen Controversy

In July of 1977, the Food and Drug Administration issued regulations concerning the proper labeling of estrogens prescribed for female patients. Since that time there has been a continuous debate as to the effects of estrogen use. It might be argued that estrogens should be prescribed when, in the physician's opinion, the patient is likely to benefit from their use. However, their use should extend over the shortest period of time consistent with the alleviation of menopausal symptoms, and dosage should be no larger than needed to effect relief.

Studies suggesting a link between the use of estrogens and cancer of the uterus are indeed cause for concern. This is especially so in light of the possibility that, in some women, estrogens may affect an abnormality in the lining of the uterus in a manner that can progress to cancer. However, the issue remains ill-defined. It is clear that there is significant benefit to a large number of women, and that when there is no contraindication, use of the drug under appropriate medical supervision is justified. Such supervision is best performed by a gynecologist, who will make periodic examinations to ascertain that there is no ill-effect.

Questions Often Asked by Older Women

Is it possible for a woman over 50 or postmenopausal to become pregnant?

While 98 percent of all women over 55 have passed through menopause, a few will continue to menstruate. Though fertility is greatly diminished, pregnancy is possible as long as ovulation and menstruation persist. Contraception in this age group is therefore advisable. A safe precaution is to continue to use some form of contraception for one year after the last period. Either condoms and foam or diaphragms are suitable. Intrauterine devices (IUD) or oral contraceptives should be avoided since irregular bleeding associated with either may necessitate diagnostic tests to exclude a serious disorder.

I've heard that cancer of the ovary is hard to detect. How can I be sure I don't have this form of cancer?

It is true that cancer of the ovary is difficult to detect without actually checking the ovaries or taking a tissue sample. However, as with breast examinations, frequent pelvic examinations by a gynecologist will reduce the possibility that an undetected ovarian cancer will develop to an advanced stage.

My period stopped a few years ago. I had some bleeding since then, and my gynecologist wants me to have a D & C. The bleeding has stopped, but he still wants to operate. Is this necessary?

The problem of postmenopausal bleeding involves the question as to whether the bleeding indicates cancer of the lining of the uterus. Such bleeding is most often not due to cancer, but a sample of the uterus lining must be taken to be certain of the true cause. Bleeding may be caused by a number of benign conditions, such as polyps of the uterus or cervix, uterine fibroids, vaginal infections, and benign growths of the vagina.

My gynecologist told me I have fibroids and recommends a hysterectomy. What are fibroids—and is surgery required?

Fibroids are benign muscle tumors of the uterus which can grow to quite large size. When they become large enough to generate symptoms such as backache, frequent urination, and difficulty in passing stools, or when they make thorough examination of the ovaries difficult, they should be removed. Hysterectomy is therefore indicated.

My husband and I enjoy a good sexual relationship. I'm concerned about what the future may bring.

This is an important concern common to many aging women. Sexual response and enjoyment develop over the years. If a couple continue to share a desire for sexual activity, the female can enjoy intercourse well into her seventies and eighties. One researcher reported a woman who still experienced orgasms in her nineties. It should be kept in mind that regular sexual contact is essential. Because sex drive declines over the years and is difficult to renew if allowed to lapse, the best way to keep a sexual relationship functioning is to continue to have sex as often as desired by both partners. Loss of desire for sex can pose a serious problem for the older woman, but it can often be overcome by mutual caring communication between partners, and patience.

We want to have sex but my vagina is tight, and it hurts each time we try. What can I do?

As the ovaries decrease their production of estrogen, those parts of the body which depend on it for their function are affected. The uterus no longer bleeds (no menstruation), the breasts become smaller, and the vagina may become dry and tight. If there are no other symptoms, the gynecologist may prescribe an estrogen cream to be inserted in the vagina a few times a week. This will often solve the problem. However, the decision as to whether estrogen is likely to be helpful should be made by a physician.

My period stopped three years ago and I still have severe hot flashes several times a day. This interferes with my work. What can I do?

Many women experience these symptoms, complaining that their daily lives are adversely affected. We recommend estrogen tablets taken by mouth to relieve such symptoms, accompanied by careful monitoring. Because the question of the possible involvement of estrogen in cancer of the uterus remains unresolved, caution is advised. An appropriate procedure is to sample the lining of the uterus before starting estrogen and every six to nine months thereafter. Further diagnostic procedures may be indicated if bleeding occurs.

I am 68 years old and I lose may urine when I cough, lift a laundry basket, or even when I climb stairs. My gynecologist tells me my bladder has dropped and he wants to operate. Am I too old for such surgery?

Your gynecologist and internist are well qualified to judge the state of your health. If both clear you for surgery, it is well to proceed. It is not necessary to suffer the discomfort and embarrassment of spontaneous loss of urine. The recommended surgery involves little risk and normally corrects the condition.

It burns when I urinate and I lose urine when I cough or lift anything heavy. My doctor recently examined me and said everything seemed normal. What can I do?

The urinary bladder and urethra are affected by estrogen. As estrogen levels decrease, the bladder and urethra are more easily injured, making them more vulnerable to infection. An infection in the bladder is a possible cause of your condition. See your physician for a re-examination.

INFECTIOUS DISEASES

Stephen J. Gluckman, M.D.

Assistant Professor of Medicine, University of Pennsylvania School of Medicine, Chief, Infectious Disease Section, Pennsylvania Hospital

What Causes Infection?

Infectious diseases are caused by microorganisms that vary widely but can be grouped into four classes: parasites, fungi, bacteria, and viruses.

Parasites live on or in another organism from which they get nourishment to survive. Many parasites, such as lice, ticks, and various intestinal worms, are large enough to see with the unaided eye. Some others, such as the amoeba, are composed of single cells visible only under a microscope.

Fungi are microscopic plants that occasionally cause infections in humans. Such skin infections as athlete's foot and ringworm are common fungal infections. Only rarely do fungi infect our internal organs and cause more serious illnesses.

Bacteria are simple one-celled organisms that can infect any part of our bodies. *Streptococci,* the source of some sore throats, and *pneumococci,* the cause of some pneumonias, are examples.

Viruses are the smallest of the infecting microorganisms. They are little more than packets of genes that can be made visible only with extremely powerful electron microscopes. Influenza and the common cold are caused by viruses.

Each of the four classes of infectious agents is composed of thousands of different specific types. Antibiotics are effective in treating most parasites, fungi, and bacteria, but are completely ineffective against viruses. At present, there is little specific therapy for viral infections.

However, it should be noted that microorganisms are not necessarily harmful. Our bodies and our environment have myriads of microorganisms, and many of these are not only harmless but distinctly helpful.

Diseases caused by microorganisms vary in severity. Thus, one person with pneumonia (a lung infection) may have a low-grade fever and a mild cough, requiring only moderate care at home, while another with the same disease will be seriously ill and need prolonged hospitalization. Similarly, many persons have such mild hepatitis that they are completely unaware of it, while less fortunate victims are incapacitated for weeks or months. The explanation for this variability is that most illnesses can be caused by many different microorganisms, some more virulent than others. Also, different individuals can get diseases of different severity from the same infecting agent, depending on their resistance to infection at the time of exposure.

Fever and Chills

Fever is normally the primary symptom of an infectious disease. However, some infectious diseases are not necessarily associated with fever, and some non-infectious diseases may occasionally cause fever. Fever is an above-normal body temperature. But what is normal body temperature? Actually, there is no single "normal" temperature, but rather a normal range, because the body's temperature varies throughout the day. An oral temperature may be 97°F (36.1°C) in the morning, rise steadily during the day, peak at about 99°F (37.2°C) in early evening, then decrease to a low of 96°F (35.8°C) between 2:00 and 4:00 a.m. An oral temperature above 99°F is generally considered to be elevated. Since rectal temperatures are about one degree higher than oral, a rectal reading must exceed 100°F (37.8°C) to be considered abnormally high. This daily cycle is important to remember, because most illnesses that generate fever tend to follow the same pattern of a lower temperature in the morning and a higher one in the evening. Thus, when you are ill, a relatively low morning temperature may not necessarily signal improvement, and a relatively high evening temperature may not indicate a relapse.

Fever is often accompanied by chills. These are of two types, each with a different significance. Less serious is the common "sick" feeling described as "chills up and down my spine," or "I just can't warm up." On the other hand, a severe chill involving teeth-chattering and uncontrollable shaking of the entire body is less common and generally implies a graver illness. It can often be artificially induced by improper use of antipyretics (fever-reducing medicines).

What should be done about fever? First, it is important to recognize that fever in adults usually does little harm unless it is exceptionally high, at least 104°F (40°C). Fevers are generally treated only to relieve discomfort. There is usually no need to reduce the temperature to normal during an illness. It should merely be brought down to a level at which the patient is more comfortable.

Aspirin-containing compounds are standard temperature-reducing medications, usually in quantities of one or two 325-mg pills every four hours. Abrupt lowering of fever is often accompanied by much sweating; this is normal. As the antipyretic effect wears off, and the temperature starts to rise again, a chill may be felt. Unpleasant cycles of fever, sweats, chills, and then more fevers can be avoided by taking the antipyretic more frequently. It is also important to increase fluid intake because the fever accelerates fluid loss.

Respiratory Tract Infection

Infections of the respiratory tract can be grouped under several headings: (sore throat) *pharyngitis,* upper respiratory tract infections (the common cold), bronchitis, pneumonia, and influenza. These categories are not mutually exclusive, since their various symptoms may coexist.

Sore Throat

In adults, most sore throats are caused by viruses for which there is no specific treatment. Often in children, but only rarely in adults, the cause is streptococcal bacteria—the "strep throat." It's usually impossible to distinguish between a viral and a bacterial sore throat solely on the basis of the sufferer's complaints or a doctor's visual examination. A distinction can be made only by taking a sample from the throat for culture and analysis, a process that takes 24 to 48 hours. Strep throats are treated with an antibiotic. Penicillin is preferred, but if the patient is allergic to penicillin, erythromycin is often used.

Physicians may disagree concerning the treatment of a patient with a sore throat. Should all be cultured to identify the few who have strep throats? Or should all be treated with antibiotics without culturing? Culturing a sample from every sore throat adds to the cost of medical care, and giving antibiotics in every case needlessly exposes some individuals to potential side effects. If culturing can be done inexpensively, it is probably the better approach.

Very little can be done to relieve the throat soreness. Sucking lozenges and gargling with warm salt water may help (an atomizer is probably more effective than gargling), and medications such as aspirin may ease the pain.

Upper Respiratory Tract Infection

Upper respiratory tract infections are among the most common illnesses in the United States. The average adult catches about four per year. They primarily involve the nose, the throat, or both, and symptoms usually include low-grade fever, mild sore throat, sneezing, runny nose, stuffy head, and a mild-to-moderate cough. However, the symptoms may vary greatly in different individuals and in successive infections in the same person. These infections are commonly caused by viruses. Although special techniques can identify the specific virus, no specific treatment is available, so that such diagnostic tests are rarely performed.

Treatment is essentially symptomatic: aspirin for fever, extra fluid for dehydration, and antihistamine/decongestant medication for the stuffed head and runny nose. (It should be noted that antihistamines make some people feel tired.) There are many such cold remedies and the milder ones can be obtained without a prescription. Despite advertising claims, differences are minor. Though these medicines help to a degree, they do not cure. The disease will run its course, and the victim must be prepared for several uncomfortable days.

Besides the discomfort and time lost from work, colds can present an additional difficulty, bacterial superinfection. Tissues weakened by a virus can develop a bacterial infection, leading to sinusitis, *otitis media* (middle ear infection), bronchitis, or bacterial pneumonia. Fortunately, superinfection is not common, but a cold sufferer who also has a chronic respiratory problem such as emphysema is more susceptible to superinfection. Warning signs include failure of a viral upper respiratory infection to improve after four or five days, a viral infection that does improve but then worsens, and an increase in the quantity of sputum or nasal discharge and its change to a yellow-green color.

Antibiotics can be used to treat bacterial superinfection, but probably cannot prevent it. In fact, they can be harmful if used for prevention because they may kill normal protective bacteria and thus allow more dangerous, antibiotic-resistant bacteria to increase. People with viral colds should be warned to report the signs of bacterial superinfection as soon as they appear so that it can be treated early with antibiotics.

The use of vitamin C in the treatment and prevention of colds has aroused a good deal of interest in recent years. This question remains controversial; there is little evidence to date that this medication is as helpful as claimed by its advocates.

Bronchitis

Bronchitis may be either acute or chronic. Acute bronchitis occurs in generally healthy persons. Its main symptom is a deep, persistent cough, commonly accompanied by a burning pain that spreads outward from the center of the chest and lasts for several seconds. There is often sputum, and there may or may not be fever. Acute bronchitis may occur alone or as part of a more general respiratory infection. Therapy includes antibiotics, expectorants, and fluids to help loosen the mucus. Judicious use of a cough suppressant may be helpful when the coughing is intolerable. However, since coughing is a normal mechanism for clearing out the infection, it should not be unnecessarily suppressed.

Chronic bronchitis occurs most often in people who have other underlying lung problems. In the United States, the most common predisposing condition is cigarette smoking. The disease is characterized by a habitual cough, often accompanied by large amounts of sputum, which is typically more severe when a sleeper awakes in the morning. Most victims have periods when the disease worsens, frequently during winter months. They may then need antibiotics and other medication to help clear the lungs for easier breathing.

Pneumonia

Pneumonia is infection in the lung itself. It can be caused by organisms of any type, but is most often due to a virus. Bacterial pneumonias are also important because they occur fairly frequently, and, unlike viral pneumonia, are treatable with antibiotics.

The symptoms of pneumonia vary widely depending upon the causative organisms. They include cough, breathing difficulty, fever, malaise, chills, exhaustion, and chest pain that increases with deep breathing or coughing. Persons with viral pneumonias tend to feel less ill than those with bacterial pneumonias, and their coughing typically produces little if any sputum. The cough of bacterial pneumonia yields large quantities of grey-green-brown sputum and may contain streaks of blood.

Treatment of pneumonia does not necessarily require hospitalization. The decision is based on several factors, including severity of the illness, age, other medical problems, and the availability of family and friends to help care for the patient at home. Aspirin or acetaminophen is given to reduce fever. A dry, non-productive cough can be eased with a cough suppressant. If the cough produces sputum it is usually best to withhold suppressants in favor of expectorants and large quantities of fluid to help clear the lungs.

Antibiotics are helpful in the treatment of bacterial pneumonias but useless for viral types. However, certain unusual bacteria, such as mycoplasma and the bacterium responsible for Legionnaires' disease, may cause an illness similar to viral pneumonia. Since these bacteria respond to treatment with erythromycin, misdiagnosis of such pneumonias as viral may deprive a patient of lifesaving therapy. Because such unusual bacterial pneumonias are often difficult to distinguish from viral types, many physicians treat all apparently ''non-bacterial'' pneumonias with erythromycin.

Influenza

Influenza is also a viral respiratory infection. The influenza virus is one of the most serious and difficult challenges to modern medicine because of its unique ability to periodically change its ''outer coat,'' thus evading recognition by the defenses our bodies' systems developed during a previous siege. Small changes allow the virus to generate a new wave of influenza every few years. After most of the people in an area have been infected, the number of new infections drops until the virus again changes its coat, once more slips through our defenses, and begins a new cycle of illness.

In addition to the small changes every two or three years, much larger shifts occur every ten to twenty years. A new wave of influenza then sweeps over the entire world, resulting in many illnesses and fatalities. This happened in 1918 with the Swine flu, in 1957 with the Asian flu, and in 1968 with the Hong Kong flu. Such pandemics of influenza have been recorded for over 400 years. Man has yet to develop a method for predicting the shifts and the resulting pandemics, or for slowing the spread of the disease after it begins.

Influenza is mostly a disease of the winter months. The virus is spread by coughing and sneezing, and the spread is probably facilitated by increased indoor living. Influenza has distinctive symptoms and should not be confused with the common cold. After a short 48-hour incubation period (the time between exposure and the development of illness), the patient usually notices a rather abrupt onset of fever, *myalgia* (muscle ache), headache, a dry cough, and general malaise. If present, runny nose, watery eyes, and sore throat are mild. Diarrhea and vomiting may also occur.

In most cases, the fever is gone in three or four days, and all other symptoms disappear within a week except for a persistent cough and fatigue which may last a few weeks longer. While it lasts, influenza causes considerable discomfort and can occasionally be extremely severe especially in elderly persons with lung or heart problems or diabetes.

Because it is a viral disease, there is no specific cure. Treatment aims to control symptoms and includes rest, aspirin for the fever and aches, and cough suppressants for an intractable cough. Vaccination has successfully prevented the disease for many years, and should be given each year during the fall. The vaccine is most strongly recommended for those such as the elderly who are most likely to contract a severe infection (see *Immunization* below).

Since the ill-fated Swine flu vaccination program in 1977, there has been much concern about side effects. Of those who receive the vaccine, about one-third will have some local discomfort, such as swelling and redness; one or two percent will experience 12 to 20 hours of fever, usually mild to moderate; and about one in 1,000,000 will develop the serious complication, the Guillain-Barre syndrome. This complication, for which influenza vaccine is only one of several causes, produces varying degrees of paralysis which usually resolves itself but may take several months to do so. This syndrome created the controversy surrounding the Swine flu vaccine.

Legionnaires' Disease

In the summer of 1976, national attention focused on Philadelphia when a mysterious illness affected almost 200 people who had attended an American Legion convention. More than 15 percent of the cases were fatal. Since then, it has been learned that the disease is caused by a bacterium which has been responsible for many epidemics during the past several decades, as well as for illness not associated with epidemics. In most cases, the victim is unable to distinguish this disease from other respiratory ailments with similar symptoms, but several clues alert the physician who can now administer effective antibiotics. Although this bacterium usually causes respiratory illness, it can also cause disease in other organs such as the intestine, liver, kidneys, brain, and muscle. Its effects have been felt throughout the United States and in several foreign countries.

Despite the advances in knowledge, much about this illness is unknown or uncertain. Where does it live in nature, by what mechanism does it cause disease, and exactly how does it spread?

Tuberculosis

Tuberculosis (TB) has been known since antiquity. Most characteristically, it is a chronic illness for which the main symptoms are cough, weight loss, fever, malaise, and drenching sweats at night. It is a variable disease that can range from having no apparent symptoms to extensive involvement of several organs.

The disease is spread when TB bacteria are coughed into the air by an ill individual and inhaled by other people. The bacteria taken into the lungs may exist there for years without causing illness. Individuals harboring the bacteria will register positive on a tuberculin skin test, indicating that they have TB bacteria in their bodies although they are otherwise completely well. The bacteria remain in a quiescent state until, for some reason, the balance between the bacteria and the body's control changes to favor the bacteria, causing them to multiply rapidly with resultant illness.

Tuberculosis is no longer prevalent in this country. It is now seen mostly in elderly persons who contracted it years earlier when the disease was more widespread. Though a detailed description of tuberculosis is beyond the present scope, the following facts should be noted:

- Before effective medications for treating tuberculosis were developed, infected patients were often hospitalized for long periods. This is no longer necessary.

- If medication is being taken regularly, treatment does not require special environments, diets, or prescribed periods of rest. Medications for active disease should be taken daily for a period ranging from months to years.

- Individuals with active tuberculosis who are taking proper medication are no longer contagious and need not avoid contact with others. They can resume normal daily activities as soon as they feel well enough.

- A positive tuberculin skin test is not a cause for alarm. It affirms exposure to tuberculosis and often requires additional diagnostic tests to determine the extent of the disease. There is rarely a need to repeat the test.

- A person who has had close contact with a patient with known active tuberculosis should be evaluated by a physician.

Urinary Tract Infections

Urinary tract infections are classified according to the area involved. *Cystitis* is an infection in the urinary bladder; *pyelonephritis* is an infection in the kidney. They can occur independently or together. The symptoms, severity, and treatment of bladder or kidney infections differ.

Microorganisms usually gain entrance to the urinary system by ascending the *urethra,* the tube through which the bladder excretes urine.

Until relatively late in life, urinary tract infections are predominantly a problem of females, probably because their shorter urethras make it easier for bacteria to reach the bladder. It has been estimated that 15 to 20 percent of all women will have urinary tract infections at some time in their lives.

As we age, other factors may interfere with urine flow and contribute to the development of urinary tract infections. Neurological problems associated with aging, and enlargement of the prostate gland in males, may make it more difficult to empty the bladder completely so that urination no longer adequately flushes out bacteria that have managed to make their way up the urethra to the bladder. Also, for various reasons, older people are more likely to require insertion of a urinary catheter (a thin tube threaded through the urethra to ease passage of urine) which provides more opportunity for bacteria to be carried into the bladder. Even with the most careful sterile technique, persistent *bacteruria* (bacteria in the urine) develops in a small number of patients after only a single urinary catheterization. If the catheter must be left in place, bacteruria is unavoidable. Although bacteria in the urine do not invariably produce disease, they may cause cystitis or pyelonephritis.

Typical cystitis symptoms are a strong, sometimes uncontrollable, urge to urinate; increasingly frequent urination, sometimes hourly, typically passing little urine and often with a feeling that the bladder is never empty even just after voiding; and burning with urination. Other characteristics are lower-abdomen discomfort and dark, occasionally bloody and foul-smelling urine. Although cystitis brings much discomfort to its victims, it is not serious and rarely necessitates hospitalization.

Pyelonephritis usually produces a sudden onset of fever, chills, and aching pain in the lower side. These symptoms may be accompanied by those of cystitis if the bladder is also involved. Occasionally, pronounced gastrointestinal symptoms such as nausea and vomiting appear and can be somewhat misleading to the physician. Pyelonephritis can be extremely serious and often requires hospitalization.

Ultimately, proper diagnosis of a urinary tract infection, whether cystitis or pyelonephritis, is made by microscopic examination of the urine and, if needed, culturing the urine for bacteria. Collecting women's urine specimens for bacterial studies involves two common problems.

First, as women urinate, the stream often picks up vaginal material. Since vaginas normally contain bacteria, examination of such a urine specimen may give misleading results. This necessitates ''clean-catch'' midstream collections. The region of the urethral opening is first cleaned while the *labia* (vaginal lips) are held apart. Then, when urination starts, some urine is allowed to flow into the toilet before a sample is collected from the continuing stream in a sterile container which is taken to the laboratory for examination. Although this procedure is somewhat awkward, it is necessary to obtain a reliable specimen for evaluation.

The second problem relates to the fact that bacteria can multiply rapidly in the urine. Unless the specimen is examined and cultured promptly, an insignificant initial number of bacteria may rapidly increase, giving the urine a false appearance of infection. If the examination cannot be made immediately, the specimen must be refrigerated to inhibit bacterial growth until the test can be performed.

Often, the expense of a urine culture can be avoided if early microscopic analysis clearly shows the presence of infection. Need for a urine culture, or for investigation by *cystoscopy* (visual examination of the urinary tract with an optical tube) or *intravenous pyelography* (series of X rays of the urinary system), is a decision of the attending physician who weighs various factors, including the severity of the illness, history of urinary tract infections, recently taken antibiotics, and known urinary tract abnormalities. Generally, recurrent urinary tract infections in women or one such infection in men will warrant these diagnostic studies.

Many antimicrobial agents combat urinary tract infections effectively. Those commonly used include sulfonamides, ampicillin, tetracycline, and cephalosporins. Patients with cystitis and mild pyelonephritis can be treated as outpatients. Patients with more severe pyelonephritis should be admitted to the hospital and treated with more potent, and potentially more toxic, antibiotics until the antibiotic sensitivities of the infecting microorganisms can be determined by laboratory studies. With this information, an effective drug with relatively low toxicity can often be selected. Duration of treatment will vary, ranging from a single dose to several months of medication, but typically one to two weeks. An increase in fluid consumption is often recommended to promote urine flow, but probably has minimal effect on the outcome.

In cases of recurrent urinary tract infections, it is important to un-
cover and treat correctable predisposing problems, such as an enlarged
prostate or a kidney stone. When these conditions are treated, the infection usually clears up. If nothing correctable is found, regular use of antimicrobial drugs over a period of time will often eliminate the disease or
decrease the frequency of recurrence.

Gastroenteritis

The symptoms of gastroenteritis include nausea, diarrhea, and abdominal cramps. Fever may or may not be present. Several conditions
other than infectious agents, for example, ulcers, gall bladder disease,
and appendicitis, may also produce some or all of these symptoms. A
physician can distinguish between "food poisoning" and these conditions by history, physical examination, and, when necessary, laboratory
tests.

"Food poisoning" is not a medical term, but is generally used when
gastroenteritis symptoms seem to be related to the eating of contaminated food. The symptoms can be caused by a variety of agents, including
many types of bacteria, viruses, and parasites, and toxic substances such
as lead and arsenic. When a patient complains of apparently food-related
nausea, diarrhea, vomiting, and abdominal cramps, the physician's initial goal is to decide whether the disease is self-limiting and manageable
with symptomatic therapy, or more serious so that it requires specific
treatment and may have public-health implications. Warning signs of a
more serious disease include extreme toxicity, a high fever of 102°F
(38.9°C) or more, and mucus or blood in the stool.

The degree of patient discomfort is not a reliable indicator of the
severity of the disease. One of the most common types of food poisoning
produces several truly miserable hours of agonizing abdominal cramps
and frequent vomiting. However, it causes neither fever nor blood stools,
and recovery is usually complete within 12 to 24 hours without special
treatment.

Before treating gastroenteritis, the physician will study the patient's
history and determine what foods have been eaten recently. Certain illnesses are associated with specific foods. Contaminated food often looks,
smells, and tastes entirely normal, with no indication that it is
"spoiled." Also, because many infections take several days to develop

after harmful organisms are ingested, it is important to consider food consumed for days preceding the onset of the illness. Recent travel may give a significant clue to the involvement of unusual microogranisms. A similar illness in the patient's family or associates may also help to identify the source.

Therapy for gastroenteritis requires consideration of the patient's need for fluids and the choice of the most effective antibiotic or other medication. Extra fluid replaces losses due to persistent vomiting and diarrhea and so prevents dehydration, potentially one of the most serious complications of gastroenteritis.

Appropriate fluids include broths, tea, fruit juices, and soda that contain easy-to-digest sugar and electrolytes. Heavy liquids and solid foods should be avoided at first, but may be added gradually later as the patient recovers. Milk and milk products should not be given until recovery is complete. If vomiting is intractable so that fluids cannot be retained, hospitalization may be required for intravenous fluid replacement.

The many medications for gastroenteritis vary both in efficacy and in side effects. Antibiotics are helpful only if the gastroenteritis is caused by *Shigella, Yersinia, cholera,* certain types of *E. coli,* and some parasites. In the majority of cases, antibiotics are ineffective and may even be harmful. In some more severe forms of infectious gastroenteritis, the use of medications to treat diarrhea and abdominal cramps may interfere with the body's natural means of clearing the disease microorganisms out of the system. For these reasons, treatment is sometimes limited solely to fluid replacement until the disease resolves itself, usually within a few days.

If a social event or restaurant appears to be implicated in an outbreak of gastroenteritis, the public health department has the responsibility and authority to investigate and make specific recommendations. Most states have laws restricting the occupations where known carriers of gastroenteritis-causing microorganisms, such as *Salmonella,* can be employed.

Traveler's Diarrhea

Travelers to foreign countries have long been familiar with the distress of diarrhea after their arrival, giving it such whimsical names as Montezuma's Revenge and Delhi-Belly. Its causes and possible means of treatment and prevention have only recently been discovered.

Seventy-five percent of all cases appear to be caused by a normal bacterium of the intestine, *E. coli,* that has acquired the ability to make toxins. Because of natives' long exposure to the altered bacterium in the area visited by the traveler, they are no longer susceptible to these toxins; hence the name Traveler's diarrhea.

Since the infection is spread by contaminated food and water, prevention includes drinking only bottled beverages or boiled water and avoiding salads, ice, and unpeeled fruit. Also preventive is a daily dose of doxycycline, a tetracycline-type antibiotic, or 60 cc of Pepto-Bismol liquid four times a day. Doxycycline has the disadvantages of potential antibiotic side effects and possibly fostering the worldwide development of bacteria resistant to the antibiotic. Pepto-Bismol is virtually without side effects, but the large amount needed daily is inconvenient for most travelers.

The diarrhea is generally self-limiting, lasting about three to five days, and needs no specific therapy. However, symptoms can often be relieved with Pepto-Bismol. If the diarrheal flow contains blood or mucus, is more frequent than ten stools per day, or lasts longer than five or six days, a physician should be consulted.

Immunization

Although immunizations are usually associated with childhood, immunity to diseases such as tetanus and diphtheria can be lost with age and may need periodic boosters. Also, because several diseases, including influenza and pneumococcal pneumonia, tend to be more severe in the elderly, this age group may benefit from special protection. Furthermore, as international travel becomes increasingly popular for people of all ages, inoculation may sometimes be required for such diseases as yellow fever, typhoid fever, cholera, and polio.

There are a few precautions to consider before being immunized. Persons with egg allergies should avoid vaccines prepared in eggs. Taking several vaccines at the same time does not affect the efficacy of any one of them, but may combine their side effects. Minor illnesses do not necessarily preclude vaccination, but people who are sick should put it off until recovery is complete. This precaution will avoid the possibility of mistakenly identifying a complication of the preexisting illness as having been caused by the vaccine. Because gamma globulin may interfere with the response of certain vaccines, it is best to complete vaccinations several weeks before a gamma globulin shot, or wait several months following such a shot.

Tetanus and diphtheria continue to occur in the United States. They are very severe infections with high mortality rates. Everybody should have a primary series of three injections (usually administered in childhood) and a booster every ten years to combat these two diseases. Doses at other times are not usually necessary, but may sometimes be needed in cases of injury.

Influenza vaccine is recommended annually for persons with certain chronic illnesses, including valvular, hypertensive, and atherosclerotic heart disease, advanced tuberculosis, diabetes mellitus, and chronic kidney disease, and for those over 65 years old. The vaccine is made yearly and should be administered in the fall.

A vaccine has recently been approved for use in the United States for the prevention of infection with *pneumococcus*. This bacterium is a frequent cause of pneumonia and can sometimes be implicated in meningitis, sinusitis, arthritis, and endocarditis. While a pneumococcus infection can occur at any age, it tends to be more severe in older persons. The vaccine is especially recommended for all persons 50 years or older. Duration of protection is still unknown, but is anticipated to be many years, so that a single injection is considered adequate.

Since October 1977, there has not been a case of smallpox anywhere in the world outside of a laboratory. Because of this, most countries, including the United States, no longer require smallpox vaccination for travel (smallpox vaccination of infants has not been required in this country since 1971). As of June 7, 1979, approximately twenty countries have not yet changed their regulations (and still require) a smallpox vaccination certificate for travelers arriving directly from the United States:

Africa — Angola, Benin (for stay greater than two weeks), Botswana, Cameroon, Central African Republic, Chad, Comoros, Congo, Djibouti, Egypt, Equatorial Guinea, Ethiopia, Guinea, Ivory Coast, Lesotho, Libyan Arab Jamahariva, Madagascar, Mali, Mozambique, Namibia, Rhodesia, Sao Tome and Principe, Seychelles, Sierra Leone, South Africa, Sudan, Uganda, Upper Volta, Zaire.

Asia — Brunei, Democratic Kampuchea, East Timor, Iran, Lao People's Democratic Republic, Mongolia, Nepal, Philippines, Ryukyu Islands (unofficial), Saudia Arabia (during pilgrimage), Viet Nam.

Americas — Belize, Bolivia.

Since October 1977 there has not been a case of smallpox anywhere in the world outside of a laboratory accident. At the World Health assembly in May 1980, the World Health Organization declared the world completely free of smallpox. There are *no medical reasons* for smallpox vaccination for international travel (smallpox vaccination of infants has not been required in this country since 1971). Further, only two countries—Chad and Democratic Kampuchea—currently require a certificate of vaccination. For travel to all other countries a smallpox vaccination is not required or necessary. Because of the significant risk of complications from the vaccination to both vaccinees and their contacts, travelers to Chad and Democratic Kampuchea can avoid vaccination with a written statement from a physician indicating that vaccination is contraindicated for health reasons.

Typhoid and cholera vaccines do not fully protect against these diseases. They reduce the risk, but prudent travelers should still be careful about what they eat and drink. Travelers to certain areas of South America and Africa should be vaccinated against yellow fever. Polio vaccination is not routinely recommended for adults in the United States, but it is recommended for travelers to areas of the world where the disease still frequently appears. Although the injectable polio vaccine tends to have fewer serious side effects, the oral vaccine is generally preferable.

Additional immunizations may be desirable or required for travel in some countries. Consult your physicians and the authorities of the destination countries (embassies or consulates, for example) while making travel plans.

HEAD AND THROAT DISORDERS

Joseph P. Atkins, Jr., M.D.

Head Clinical Professor of Otorhinolaryngology
Pennsylvania Hospital

William M. Keane, M.D.

Clinical Assistant Professor of Otorhinolaryngology
Pennsylvania Hospital

Since head and throat problems tend to increase as we grow older, they are often needlessly accepted as inevitable or incurable. This attitude can delay the seeking of medical attention and only make matters worse.

For example, there is a natural tendency to assume that just "growing old" causes every difficulty with hearing or the sense of smell, and that a sore mouth is probably due to loose dentures or a sore throat to too many cigarettes. On the contrary, hearing loss often results from an easily corrected wax buildup, and inability to smell may be due to nasal breathing or sinus problems that are curable. Soreness may or may not be due to the assumed causes.

A great hindrance to the proper care of head and throat disorders in older people is the fear that the soreness they feel is really cancer and the belief that it can only lead to either death from the disease or disability from the treatment. This belief is simply not true. Cancers in this area are among the most curable of all types. When diagnosed and treated early, over 80 percent of all patients with such cancers are permanently cured.

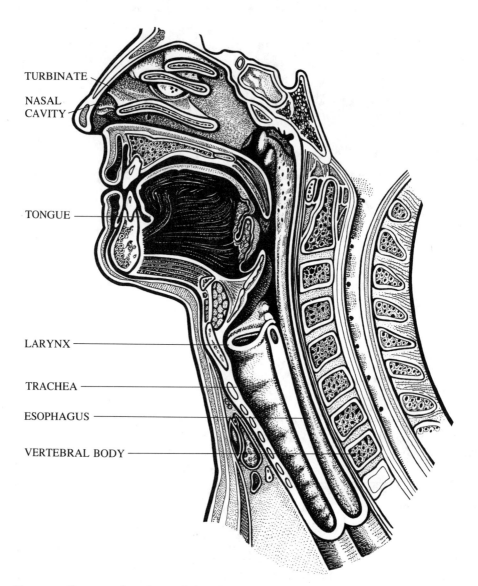

TURBINATE

NASAL
CAVITY

TONGUE

LARYNX

TRACHEA

ESOPHAGUS

VERTEBRAL BODY

Figure 1. Cross section through head and neck.

Other factors that delay treatment of older people are expense (''I just can't afford a specialist''); self-medication with over-the-counter drugs (''I'll see the doctor when it gets worse,'' or ''I don't want to bother the doctor''); and transportation problems, such as difficulty in walking, lack of a private car, and the inconvenience of traveling by public transport.

Proper care in the early stages of head and throat diseases not only insures treatment of the illness but also helps to prevent deterioration. It's true that the resiliency of youth fades with age, that we can't regrow lost teeth or damaged nerves, and that we can't restrengthen neglected muscles without difficulty. However, the real villain is a failure to seek help quickly when sickness strikes or to achieve rehabilitation after illness has been treated. This underscores the physician's aim to "treat early and treat conservatively."

Mouth and Throat

Teeth

The most common mouth problems of older people are those related to loss or deterioration of teeth (see chapter titled *Dental Care*). Poor or ill-fitting teeth can be responsible for soreness of the mouth, either excessive saliva or dryness, irritation of the tongue, pain felt in the ear, recurrent headaches, throat pain, and even mouth cancer (other cancer-causing agents include smoking and alcohol).

Some mouth disorders are due directly to gum infection and some to loss of proper occlusion. Occlusion refers to the way the upper and lower teeth come together when the jaws close. If the teeth fail to align properly, or molars are missing, the jaw joints near the ear become poorly positioned and a form of arthritis develops. This is particularly true when the bite is unbalanced because of lost molars, and the gums come closer together on one side of the mouth while most chewing is done on the other side. The jaw is then forced to rotate unnaturally. This, together with muscle imbalance, produces changes in the secretion of saliva. Discomfort may be felt in the affected area or referred to other places where the muscles are attached to the skull or to bones in the neck.

Dry Mouth and Tongue

Many factors can contribute to a tendency toward mouth dryness in later years. For example, plastic-and-steel dentures may cause too little or too much tongue abrasion. The lining of the natural palate is slightly rough and helps to scrape off tissue that tends to grow on the surface of the tongue. When covered by an upper denture plate, the palate becomes a smooth plastic surface which has no sensation. In the absence of natural

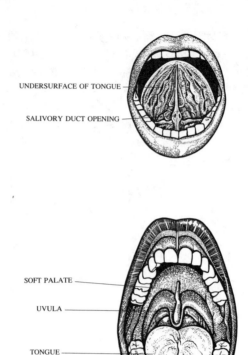

UNDERSURFACE OF TONGUE

SALIVORY DUCT OPENING

SOFT PALATE

UVULA

TONGUE

Figure 2. The oral cavity.

scraping action, the tongue may become coated with excess tissue, causing it to feel dry and—especially in smokers—to darken, a condition known as "black hairy tongue."

People with some mouth dryness will move their tongues constantly in an effort to produce more saliva. This leads to irritation and paradoxically increases dryness because it induces spitting or swallowing of saliva at a rate faster than the moisture can be replaced. This condition also occurs in people with neurologic problems such as Parkinson's Disease.

Vitamin deficiency can cause a dry, sore mouth, for example, following a respiratory illness such as influenza or after a prolonged hospital stay when nutrition has not kept up with the body's increased demands. Most commonly, the depleted vitamin is A, C, or D, but may also be B_{12} and folic acid. Diabetes and thyroid deficiency can also produce this condition. The symptoms therefore usually require both evaluation by a dentist, to rule out local causes and to correct teeth and denture problems, and a thorough medical checkup by a physician to rule out associated illness.

Local hygiene helps to relieve the condition. Brushing teeth, wiping or brushing the "hairy" tongue, and eliminating irritants are useful. However, strong salt or alkaline mouth washes should be avoided, as they tend to aggravate the condition. Multivitamin preparations that contain at least 5000 U of vitamin A and substantial quantities of B_{12} and folic acid must be taken twice a day for several months to be effective. A mouth wash composed of a half teaspoon of baking soda (sodium bicarbonate) in 8 ounces of water has been found to be soothing.

Sore Throat

Sore throats are common at every age. One of the most frequent causes of sore throat in the older person is a low-grade allergy that produces an irritating postnasal drip. However, many other disorders can cause throat soreness so that self-diagnosis is often difficult.

If a sore throat persists to the point of interfering with swallowing, examination by a physician is essential. If the soreness is associated with a respiratory infection (cold, or fever), the physician must determine if the infection is bacterial and can be expected to respond to antibiotics. If the symptoms do not subside, further examination is necessary.

Although chronic sore throat is most often due to postnasal drip, it can also be caused by excessive smoking, a vitamin or other nutritional deficiency, a systemic illness such as a blood disorder, thyroid abnormalities, and cancer.

The sore mouth or throat caused by throat cancer is often associated with ear discomfort. The pain is not severe, but rather a dull feeling of obstruction. A persistent throat pain accompanied by ear discomfort, especially in people who smoke, should be quickly brought to the attention of a physician.

Most types of throat cancer appear along the side gutters of the mouth and throat, the borders of the tongue, in the tonsils, and in the lower throat. They are most curable if detected early. Unlike victims of lung cancer and many other tumors, eight out of ten patients with small tumors of the floor of the mouth and the front part of the tongue are cured permanently. Surgery or radiation is used for small tumors in the mouth and throat, and a combination of both is used for larger tumors. The success rate is lower for large tumors, especially those that have spread to the lymph glands in the neck. Early diagnosis and aggressive treatment clearly make a difference in the outcome.

Although preliminary examination of the mouth and throat can be done by the dentist or general physician, a throat specialist may be needed to perform an adequate examination by mirror of the back of the tongue and lower part of the throat down to the larynx (voice box). If a suspect area is found that requires closer inspection, or if the examination is frustrated because the patient has an overactive gag reflex, a laryngo-scope (a hollow-tubed instrument) may be inserted under anesthesia. A special X ray, called a barium swallow, may also be taken of the parts and pathway used in swallowing, from the mouth to the stomach.

Hoarseness

Hoarseness, or change in the voice, occurs when the voice is strained by misuse or overuse. It is common in persons who inhale when smoking cigarettes and draw tobacco smoke over the vocal cords. Smokers may also have voice problems from viral infections which produce laryngitis, an inflammation and swelling of the vocal cords. Vocal-cord cancer almost exclusively afflicts those who smoke—or who formerly smoked—cigarettes.

The voice is generated by muscular contraction of the vocal folds to form two bands of tissue which vibrate when air is expelled past them from the lungs. When the tension is proper and the surfaces are clean and smooth, the vibrations are clear and resonant. If there is swelling of the tissue or excessive tension in the muscle due to loud or prolonged talking, irritation will develop, leading to generalized swelling. Continued use of the vocal cord during this phase may result in vocal-cord polyp or nodule,

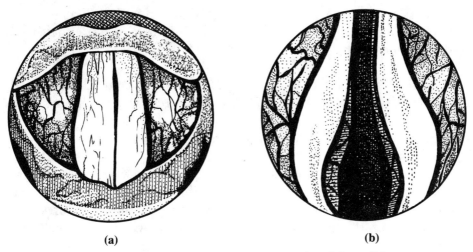

(a)   **(b)**

Figure 3. Vocal cords: **(a)** Open for breathing. **(b)** Closed for talking.

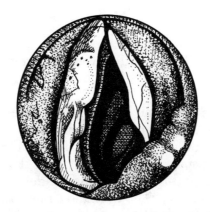

Figure 4. Polyp (arrow) on vocal cord, often caused by prolonged irritation.

the typical reaction of the body to any type of irritation. For example, irritation of the skin by the rubbing of a shoe on the heel will cause a blister, and continued irritation will cause the surface tissue to build up a callus. Similarly, vocal-cord polyps or nodules are the voice box's mechanism for creating callus. This abnormal surface prevents the vocal folds from fitting together and vibrating smoothly to generate a clear voice tone (Figures 3 and 4).

A hoarseness or voice change which lasts longer than three weeks is not typical of laryngitis; it is a sign that something basic is the matter with the vocal-fold vibration. Examination with a mirror will reveal abnormalities in the vocal folds due to any one of a number of causes, including a low-grade laryngitis or a thyroid deficiency. In the elderly, the vocal cords may atrophy (become thinner) due to muscle weakness or loss of muscle substance. This is commonly seen in those who use their vocal cords improperly.

A vocal-cord polyp or nodule may also appear as a raised white swelling, called *leukoplakia* ("white patches"), in response to chronic irritation, and may indicate a premalignant state. Malignancy will often develop if the irritation and white plaque persist.

Vocal-cord cancers are usually white swellings with irregular margins, resembling a wart or a miniature cauliflower. Occasionally, they are red and flat with a pearl-like surface. Accurate diagnosis requires close examination of the lesions on the vocal cords, which may include a biopsy.

Nose

Our noses clean, warm, and humidify the air we breathe, and allow us to smell and taste. They are thus very important to health and well-being.

The nose is made of bone and cartilage, covered on the outside by skin and on the inside by a lining of moist mucous membrane. It is divided into two cavities—*nares*, or nostrils—by the nasal septum. The *paranasal sinuses* (air spaces in the bones of the skull) communicate with and drain into the nose through openings under bony projections in the side walls of the nasal cavity. The nose and sinuses thus function together as a unit. The *eustachian* tube, which connects the middle ear with the nose, enters the rear lower part of the nasal cavity.

Postnasal Drip

The nose and sinuses normally produce two quarts of mucus each day, but infection and allergies change the amount and quality of the secretion. Extra mucus is formed in an attempt to wash out the offending substance. Often the mucus will flow down the throat instead of through the nostrils, producing a postnasal drip. This is especially common with low-grade infections, changes in weather, and irritation by allergies or smoking. Treatment aims to relieve the irritation with decongestant and antihistamine medication, and to destroy offending bacteria with antibiotics.

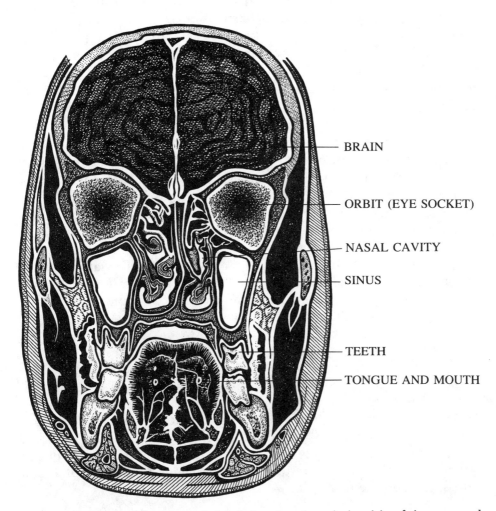

Figure 5. Vertical section through head showing the relationship of the nose and sinuses to the eyes and teeth.

Stuffy Nose

The nose may become stuffy and obstruct nasal breathing as a consequence of irritation. (Mechanical obstruction from a deviated septum may also produce a stuffy nose.) The mucus membrane lining, inflamed by irritants, becomes swollen with blood and tissue fluid. This is most commonly seen with a cold, a viral infection which produces a runny nose, postnasal drip, stuffiness, and often fever and chills. Rest, fluids, and decongestants usually bring relief within a few days.

A cold may become complicated with obstruction of the sinus openings and stagnation of secretions within the sinuses, possibly leading to bacterial infection and sinus inflammation. Pressure and pain develop around the eyes or over the forehead. Antibiotics are then required in addition to decongestants. Recurrent sinus infection suggests chronic obstruction within the nasal and sinus passages.

The nasal septum is almost never quite straight. Deviation may be present at birth or result from fracture. Usually, this is of no importance, but when the deviated septum causes obstruction, a simple corrective surgical procedure can relieve the condition.

Nasal polyps—soft jelly-like growths from the sinuses which extend into the nasal cavity—may also produce obstruction and stuffiness. They result from chronic, repeated inflammation of the nasal passages, and may lead to frequent infection and a decrease in the ability to smell. Medical management includes anti-allergy medication, such as decongestants, antihistamines, and steroids, and desensitization measures. Surgical correction of an obstructing septum and removal of polyps may be required. The polyps tend to recur if the underlying cause of the inflammation is not controlled.

People who have frequent stuffy noses tend to use nasal sprays. These provide temporary relief, but the swelling of the mucus membrane lining returns and is often more severe. This is termed a rebound effect. Sprays can also damage the lining of the nose.

Loss of Smell

Loss of smell, *anosmia*, may result from any of the conditions which produce a stuffy nose, but may also be due to brain injury from tumors, vascular disease, infection, or trauma. Loss of smell will typically interfere with taste as well. Medical attention should be sought to find and treat the underlying cause.

Nosebleeds

The nasal lining has many superficial blood vessels. Trauma to these vessels, as from nose picking, sneezing, direct punches, and inflammation, can cause nosebleeds (*epistaxis*). Most nosebleeds originate in vessels in the front of the nose and are readily controlled, but bleeding from the back of the nose is both less common and more troublesome. Lying down with the head elevated helps to control most nosebleeds, and squeezing the front of the nose will often stop the bleeding. Occasionally, cotton packing may be needed (Figure 6).

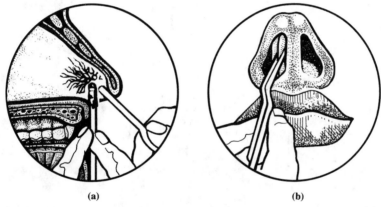

(a)   (b)

Figure 6. Nosebleeds may be stopped by (a) absorbent cotton packing or (b) cauterization of the broken blood vessels with a hot rod, electricity, or other means.

If bleeding persists, a physician should be consulted. Cauterization or special packing may be needed. In those unusual cases where bleeding is from the back of the nose, ligation (closing off) of the feeding blood vessels may be required. The physician should be informed of any other bleeding problems, or if anticoagulants or aspirin have been used by the patient.

Plastic Surgery

Changes in the outward appearance of the nose are occasionally sought by patients, especially when the shape has been altered by injury

or disease. Unusual development before birth and heredity are other
common causes of nasal disfigurement. A change in the shape of the nose
should be considered carefully by the patient and discussed frankly with
the surgeon to assure the right decision and satisfactory results.

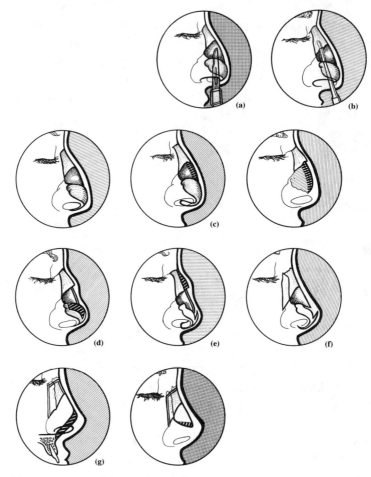

Figure 7. Nose reconstruction *(rhinoplasty)*: (a,b) Separating skin from bone
and cartilage. (c,d) Parts (striped areas) of cartilage being removed. (e) Bone
(striped area) under hump being removed. (f) Nasal bones are narrowed. (g)
Final result.

The surgical procedure involves the removal of excess tissue, bone,
and cartilage, and subtle remolding of the nasal framework. Results are
predictable when the work is done by a skilled plastic surgeon, and most
patients are pleased with the outcome (Figure 7).

The Ear

The ear is divided into three parts: the outer, the middle, and the inner. Each part is related to the others in the important function of hearing.

The outer ear consists of the *pinna* (the visible fleshy part) and the external ear canal, which gather and direct sound toward the eardrum. The ear-canal skin contains modified sweat glands which secrete ear wax (*cerumen*) that helps to trap dirt and protect the middle ear.

The middle ear is the space between the external and inner ears and contains the eardrum and three ear bones (*ossicles*): hammer (*malleus*), anvil (*incus*), and stirrup (*stapes*). The eardrum is a tightly stretched membrane separating the middle from the outer ear, which vibrates with the arrival of sound waves. Middle-ear structures receive sound vibrations from the external ear, amplify them, and transmit them to the inner ear.

The inner ear is the most complicated and important part of the hearing mechanism. It consists of two main parts: the shell-shaped *cochlea* and the semicircular canals. The cochlea contains the delicate organ of *Corti* from which project the hair cells which are the sensitive endings of the acoustic nerve. These nerve endings are bathed in a fluid which is stirred by arriving sound waves and, in turn, stimulates the nerve endings to generate impulses. The acoustic nerve relays these impulses to the brain for interpretation.

Hearing Loss

Since the outer and middle ear regions conduct sound to the inner ear, outer or middle ear defects can cause a conductive hearing loss. When the problem lies in the inner ear, sensorineural (nerve) deafness occurs. Occasionally, problems may arise in both areas, producing a mixed type of hearing loss.

A conductive hearing loss may be due to obstruction of the external ear canal by wax or foreign material. Infection or injury can open a hole in the eardrum or damage the delicate ear bones. The bones can also be immobilized by a bone growth (*otosclerosis*). When the hearing loss is conductive, the ears may feel full or plugged, and the voice will seem to echo in the blocked passage.

A variety of disorders can produce sensorineural hearing loss, including inadequate blood circulation to the inner ear or brain stem. Diseases, such as diabetes, which affect other nerve endings can also affect the ear nerve. Occasionally, medications may irritate the acoustic nerve and cause temporary or permanent hearing loss. For example, large dosages of aspirin can cause ringing in the ears and even temporary hearing loss. Sensorineural hearing loss can also be congenital (present from birth), or provoked by exposure to very loud sounds especially if prolonged or repeated. However, the most common cause is aging of the nerve endings, which can significantly impair hearing but rarely causes total deafness.

Someone with a sensorineural hearing loss may hear sound, for example, people talking, but be unable to comprehend what they are saying. Such an individual will have greatest difficulty in crowded rooms or in group discussion. Because the higher tones are most frequently affected, a man's voice will be better understood than a woman's.

A hearing loss should be properly evaluated by an ear specialist. The examination, including a hearing test, helps to determine the type of loss and to indicate appropriate corrective measures. If the loss is conductive, it may be remedied by simple removal of wax from the ear canal. A surgical procedure can free the small bones if they are immobilized.

If the hearing loss is nerve-related, correction may not be possible. Encouraging others to speak more clearly and loudly than usual will help the hard-of-hearing individual to both hear and understand. Relatives and friends may need reminding that they should make sure they have the attention of the affected person so that he or she can watch their lips and concentrate on listening. Lip reading is very helpful, but requires the speaker to make a special effort to communicate.

Helpful Devices

Special devices are available to help the hard of hearing. Adjustable telephone amplifiers make the incoming message louder, and the phone bell can also be made louder or tuned to an optimum frequency. Special vibration or lighted-alarm systems may also be used. Similar devices are available to make radio and television sound easier to hear and understand.

Hearing Aids

Hearing aids can greatly benefit many but not all of the hard-of-hearing. If the hearing is only slightly impaired, the hearing aid may be of little use. It may also be ineffective if the acoustic nerve is severely damaged. No device should be purchased before an ear specialist has determined the degree of need.

Every hearing aid requires special fitting and should be tailor-made for the individual. A variety is available, including some small enough to fit totally within the ear itself. Others can be mounted on eyeglasses, worn behind the ear, or, in cases where the hearing loss is more severe, hung around the neck. No matter which aid is selected, instruction in its proper use is advisable. Too often, the expectations of the patient exceed the capability of the instrument. A 30-day trial period is recommended before purchase.

Tinnitus

Head noise, or *tinnitus*, is very common. It may be constant or intermittent, its intensity may range from barely noticeable to very loud, and its pitch may vary. It may also be subjective, heard only by the patient, or objective and heard by others, and may or may not be associated with hearing loss. Most commonly, it results from an injury to the hearing nerve, and, just as pain is experienced when a pain nerve is injured, injury to a hearing nerve produces the sensation of sound.

Tinnitus can be related to problems in various parts of the ear. Wax, foreign bodies, or infection in the external ear canal can irritate the eardrum and produce a pulsating head noise. Middle-ear infection, or the collection of fluid in the middle ear due to infection or allergy, can both reduce hearing acuity and produce the sensation of noise.

Colds or allergies can block the eustachian tube. Since this tube serves to equalize the pressure between the middle-ear chamber and the outside air, a sudden pressure equalization, for example, in an airplane or a rapidly rising or falling elevator, can cause a popping sound in the ear. Objective (externally audible) tinnitus can be due to muscle spasms in the middle ear or eustachian tube, or to abnormalities in the blood vessels surrounding the ear.

Infection or varying blood flow in the inner ear can cause tinnitus. Any disturbance of the inner-ear fluid may stimulate the nerve endings which are delicate and vulnerable to damage. Other inner-ear events that can damage nerve endings and cause tinnitus include a systemic disease such as diabetes, sudden exposure to a loud noise, the use of an ototoxic (ear-disturbing) drug or one to which the user is especially sensitive, injury to the head as from a blow or an automobile accident, and tumors of the hearing nerve. Rupture of a small blood vessel that produces bleeding in the inner ear can cause both hearing loss and head noise.

The brain itself may be the source of tinnitus. Changes in circulation or nutrition may so damage brain structures that permanent tinnitus results. Tinnitus calls for examination by an ear specialist, though in most cases no medical or surgical treatment will eliminate it. Most of the time the patient will adjust to the noise so that it becomes less bothersome. Symptoms are usually more pronounced at night when surroundings are most quiet. A variety of medications have been tried to help control tinnitus, but these are usually ineffective. Sedatives may occasionally give some relief, and biofeedback and hypnosis have been used with some success. Small electronic devices, known as tinnitus maskers, generate a noise pattern which reduces the wearer's awareness of head noise, in effect substituting an external for an internal noise. This can be effective for some patients, but the masker should not be purchased until a trial period has shown it to bring relief. Surgical treatment of tinnitus can be frustrating, because cutting into the nerve endings produces nerve deafness but may not eliminate the tinnitus.

Dizziness

Dizziness may be defined as the subjective sensation of unsteadiness or imbalance, a disorientation in relation to one's surroundings. Balance is maintained by the interaction and coordination in the brain of nerve impulses from the inner ear, the eyes, the neck muscles, and the muscles and joints in the limbs. A disturbance in any of these areas can make one feel dizzy or unsteady.

Ear-caused dizziness results from disturbances in the circulation or fluid pressure in the inner ear chambers, or from indirect pressure on the balance nerve. The inner ear has two chambers: one for hearing (the *cochlea*) and one for balance (semicircular canals). These chambers contain fluid which circulates to stimulate nerve endings. Disturbances in the pressure of this circulation, or changes in local blood flow, may produce dizziness, hearing loss, or tinnitus. When the semicircular canals are thus affected, the reflexes that maintain balance are thrown out of gear, as also occurs with motion or seasickness. Meniere's disease, vestibular neuronitis, and ototoxic medication are some of the more common ear-related causes of dizziness.

Meniere's disease results from increased pressure of the inner-ear fluids. Any process which disturbs the delicate balance of the inner-ear fluid chambers may generate the disorder, which involves a variety of factors, including circulation, metabolism, allergy, and emotions. A typical symptom is a sudden onset of dizziness lasting several minutes to several hours, usually accompanied by hearing loss and head noise. Occasionally, hearing alone or only the balance system is involved. Treatment aims to control fluid pressure changes and underlying causes. Medical management, which may sometimes include surgery, is usually successful.

In vestibular or viral neuronitis, the onset is usually sudden and violent and lasts several days or weeks. It does not typically recur, and treatment with medication to quiet the vestibular canals is effective.

A number of drugs and medications, including certain antibiotics and diuretics, are toxic to the balance and hearing systems. Any disturbance in the ears should be reported to your physician, especially when it seems to follow the taking of newly-prescribed medication.

Dizziness associated with the brain may be produced by circulatory insufficiency, metabolic allergic dysfunction, tumors, or injuries. Neck-related dizziness results from abnormal or uncoordinated nerve impulses sent to the brain from the neck muscles. This may be due to arthritis of the spine, injury, or pressure on nerves in the neck.

Visual disturbances may also cause dizziness. Focusing difficulty, for example, as experienced by people with cataracts, may upset the perception of spatial relationships and compromise balance. Persistent dizziness requires an evaluation of all systems that contribute to balance. A variety of medical and surgical treatments are available depending on the underlying cause of the dizziness.

Earache

Earache may be caused by infection, foreign bodies, or wax in the ear canal. The ear pain may also be related to pain in the teeth, tonsils, or jaw bone. Treatment depends on the cause of the pain. In cases of swimmer's ear or external ear infection, cleansing of the ear canal and application of antibiotic eardrops are effective. If the infection is in the middle ear, pain may be accompanied by a decrease in hearing and occasionally drainage. Treatment then includes antibiotics administered by mouth.

While diseases of the head and neck have varied signs and symptoms, most are readily diagnosed and treated. With proper care, the important functions of the head and neck can be preserved.

EYE PROBLEMS

Harold Cameron, M.D.

Formerly Post-Graduate Fellow of Ophthalmology

Thomas R. Hedges, M.D.

Head, Ophthalmology Section, Pennsylvania Hospital
Professor of Ophthalmology, University of Pennsylvania

The eye is no more immune to aging than other parts of the body. As we grow older, fewer and fewer of us can do without some aid to vision. Those who have worn glasses before find it necessary to progress to bifocals and even trifocals. Also, although vision is the primary concern about the aging eye, some disorders can cause discomfort without necessarily affecting sight.

We will deal with six of the most common and bothersome eye problems associated with aging, what they are, why they occur, and what can be done about them. These are the dry or watery eye, cataracts, macular degeneration, glaucoma, vitreous floaters, and retinal detachment. It will be helpful first to know something about the anatomy of the eye and how it works.

The eye has often been compared with a camera (Figure 1). Light rays enter through the clear cornea (analogous to a camera filter or first lens), pass through the pupil (the adjustable aperture), and are focused on the retina (the film) by the crystalline lens (similar to the camera's

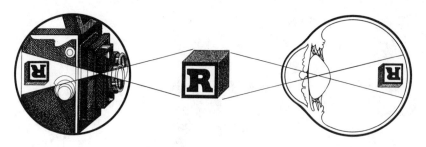

Figure 1. The camera and the eye form images in much the same way.

glass lens). In some ways, the eye is more like a television than a photographic camera because the received image is transmitted as electric impulses to the brain by the optic nerve, which is like a cable in a TV camera circuit. There is one cable for each eye and it connects to about a million separate cells (called rods and cones) in the retina. As with a camera, the image on the retina is upside down, but our TV brain interprets what we see as right side up.

The eyes are moved by six muscles attached to the eyeball's thick white outer coat (*sclera*). Both eyes normally move together and the slight difference between the two perceived images gives us stereo vision when they are processed by the brain. Some diseases associated primarily with older age groups can affect eye movement.

The eye has three chambers (Figure 2): the *anterior*, between the cornea and the iris; the *posterior*, between the iris and the lens; and the *vitreous*, between the lens and the retina. The anterior and posterior chambers are filled with a watery liquid (*aqueous humor*) which circulates through the posterior chamber and out through a filter-like meshwork in the cornea into a canal near the point where the cornea meets the iris. The canal makes direct contact with the veins of the eye so that the aqueous humor drains off along with the blood.

The vitreous chamber is filled with a gel (*vitreous humor* or gel) which is supported by a network of fine strands (*collagen fibrils*) that crisscross the chamber. A ring of fibers (*zonules*) encircles the disc-shaped lens and suspends it in the middle of the light path. The zonules are very strong in the young, but weaken with age.

A delicate membrane called the *conjunctiva* lines the inner surface of the eyelids and covers the front, exposed part of the eyeball. It contains

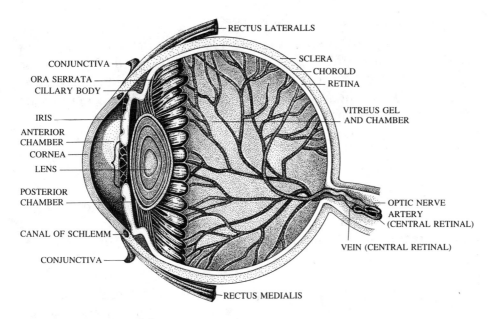

RECTUS LATERALLS

CONJUNCTIVA

ORA SERRATA
CILLARY BODY

SCLERA
CHOROLD
RETINA

IRIS

ANTERIOR
CHAMBER
CORNEA
LENS

VITREUS GEL
AND CHAMBER

POSTERIOR
CHAMBER

OPTIC NERVE
ARTERY
(CENTRAL RETINAL)

CANAL OF SCHLEMM

VEIN (CENTRAL RETINAL)

CONJUNCTIVA

RECTUS MEDIALIS

Figure 2. Structure of the eye.

mucus-secreting cells that play an important role in spreading tears into a protective film.

Dry or Watery Eyes

Eyelids not only protect the eye but their blinking produces a thin film of tears that nourishes the surface of the cornea and keeps it smooth. If there is an abnormality of the lids, the tears may not be evenly distributed and areas of the cornea may dry out. This causes irritation followed by a reflex action that produces more tears. One such common problem of aging, called an *ectropion*, is a laxness of the skin around the eyes. The lower lid droops and does not completely cover the eye. Simple surgical procedures can usually restore a more normal lid action.

If the eyelid muscles become tight or spastic at the same time that the skin becomes loose, they can actually curl the edge of the lid inward so that the lower lashes rub and irritate the cornea. This is called an *entropion*. It also causes reflex eye watering and can lead to infection and ulceration of the cornea. Simple surgery, usually with local anesthesia, can also correct this problem.

The tear film is made up of three layers (Figure 3): the inner (*mucin*), the middle (*aqueous*), and the outer (*oily*), produced by different gland cells in the eyelids. The watery middle layer is produced by a large tear gland located beneath the outer part of the upper lid and by accessory tear glands in the inner surface of the lids. The accessory glands are believed to supply most of the ordinary (basal) tears that are always present, and the large tear gland primarily produces tears in a reflex response to eye or nose irritation and emotional reactions, but these functions probably overlap.

"Goblet" cells of the conjunctiva produce the inner mucin layer which acts as a wetting agent that enables watery tears to spread evenly over the cornea. The outer oily layer normally coats over the water layer and prevents rapid evaporation.

Gland deficiencies can develop with aging and affect the associated layers in the tear film. The consequence can be chronic irritation, watering, or dryness.   Deficiencies in the inner layer can cause incomplete wetting so that the middle watery layer does not adequately cover the cornea. Deficiencies in the outer layer can allow the middle layer to evaporate faster than it can be replenished with tears. Both deficiencies can thus result in drying of portions of the cornea, irritation, and reflex tearing.

As we age, the basal rate of tear production decreases, often to the degree that some drying takes place and the cornea is irritated. If the tearing reflex is still intact, the result may be continuously watery eyes, even though the primary problem is a lack of enough tears.

If the basal tearing rate is severely deficient, as often happens with rheumatoid arthritis and some other disorders, reflex tearing may also be insufficient to keep the eyes wet. The result is then chronic dryness and irritation. Although more commonly associated with arthritis, this can also happen with non-arthritics.

The rate of tear production, both basal and reflex, can be measured by placing the end of a small strip of filter paper (Figure 4) behind the lower lid, with or without anesthetic drops, and observing how far down the strip the tears move in 5 minutes. More fundamentally, an ophthalmologist can examine the tear film under a slit-lamp microscope to detect abnormalities, sometimes first coloring the film with a dye and examining the cornea under blue light to bring out details. Staining also reveals damaged corneal cells. If the cornea is found to be inadequately coated by the tear film, or the tears evaporate too quickly, the eyes are treated with "artificial tears" of appropriate composition and at varying intervals as required to protect the cornea against drying and irritation.

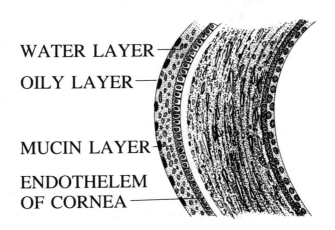

Figure 3. Cornea coated by three-layer tear film.

Another problem that can cause chronic irritation and tearing is *marginal blepharitis*, or inflammation of the rims of the eyelids. This is usually a chronic infection of the eyelash follicles and the glands in the border of the lid. It is characterized by granulation (somewhat like dandruff) on the lashes and itching and burning of the eyes. It is usually worst in the morning, clearing somewhat as the day goes on. This is in contrast to dry eyes, which are usually best in the morning and then get worse. Some blepharitis cases, if severe, may require periodic application of antibiotic drops, but many can be controlled by good hygiene such as cleansing the lids and lashes each night before retiring.

Another cause of watery eyes concerns tear drainage. Tears are not a stagnant pool but are constantly being produced, swept across the eyes, and drained into the nose through a system of tubes. Canals (Figure 5) carry tears from openings in the upper and lower lids near the nose to *nasolacrimal sacs* on either side, and the sacs are drained by nasolacrimal canals into the nose. Here, they run down to the throat where they are swallowed.

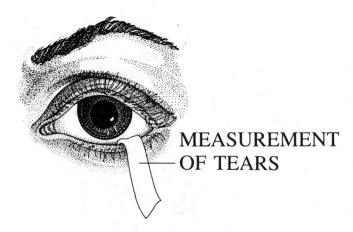

MEASUREMENT
OF TEARS

Figure 4. Rate of tear production is measured by timed absorption in filter paper.

A block at any point in the drainage system can back tears up into the eyes and make the eyes watery. Most often, the block forms at the canal openings in the lids due to shrinking of tissues. Many cases are cleared up by simple dilation and flushing in the ophthalmologist's office. However, sometimes the block is caused by formation of a stone at a further point of the drainage system. X rays may then be required to locate the cause and indicate appropriate treatment. The obstruction can be removed in some cases, but in others a new opening must be made through the bone to connect the nasolacrimal sac directly to the nose. This is a surgical procedure usually performed under general anesthesia.

Although surgery may be necessary if the eyes tear continuously, the risks of surgery and general anesthesia should be avoided when tearing is only occasional due to minor irritation such as the wind blowing against the eyes. The relative risks and benefits of surgery and the possibility of other alternatives should be discussed with the ophthalmologist.

Cataracts

A cataract is any opacity in the crystalline lens of the eye sufficient to impair vision. It is the leading cause of blindness in the world. In the United States, cataracts are the underlying cause in 15 percent of all individuals considered legally blind.

There are many types of cataract and they vary in their cause, the rapidity with which they develop, and their ultimate effect on vision. They may be congenital, a part of the aging process, or caused by toxic substances or injury. Although they may occur at any age, the great majority are associated with aging and are known collectively as senile cataracts.

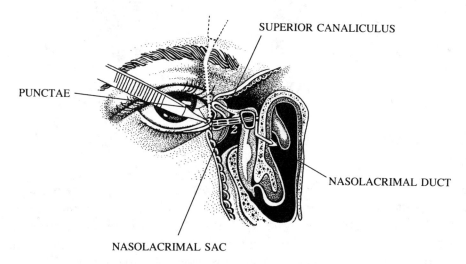

SUPERIOR CANALICULUS

PUNCTAE

NASOLACRIMAL DUCT

NASOLACRIMAL SAC

Figure 5. Small canals *(canaliculi)* drain tears form the eyes into the nose.

The most common type of senile cataracts is called *nuclear sclerosis* (hardening of the center of the lens). It arises from the natural growth of the lens which proceeds from the outside toward the center. The center, or nucleus, of the lens is therefore always older than the periphery (Figure 6). As the nucleus ages, it begins to harden and turn yellow (Figure 7). This happens earlier in some individuals than in others, but all of us, if we live long enough, will develop this type of cataract.

With further hardening, the nucleus becomes a darker yellow, then greenish, and finally brownish in color. At first, the eye becomes more nearsighted (or less farsighted) since the harder lens bends light rays more sharply than the younger, softer lens. This is the basis for "second sight" which enables some far-sighted people to stop wearing glasses for distance vision in their sixties, and others to read with bifocals or reading glasses for the first time since their mid-forties.

Mild nuclear sclerosis may not interfere significantly with vision, so that many people may go for years with no therapy other than a slight

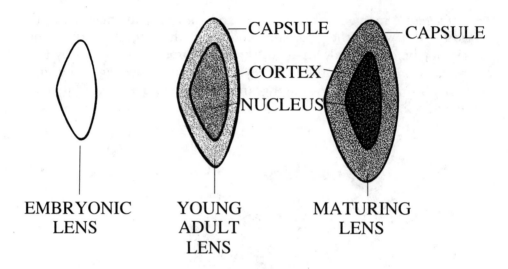

Figure 6. The nucleus is the oldest part of the eye's lens.

change in the strength of their glasses. As the condition worsens, however, distance vision diminishes, and many people see halos around lights
and significant glare if the lights are bright. Near vision is not affected as
much as distance vision in this type of cataract, and, depending on the
needs of the patient, surgery may be unnecessary for many years.

Cortical cataracts are very common in aging lenses and take many
forms, such as vacuoles (cavities), plaques (flat patches), and water clefts
(narrow splits) due to degeneration of the cortex (outer layer) of the lens
(Figure 8). Cortical cataracts, unlike nuclear sclerosis, do not cause near-
sightedness since they may not change the lens's refraction, and may actually make the eye farsighted. However, they tend to distort vision and
cause more glare than nuclear sclerosis does. Both types of cataract often
occur together.

The type of cataract that most rapidly decreases vision is the posteri-
or subcapsular cataract, an opacity of the lens which usually starts at the
center just beneath the membrane covering the back of the lens and
spreads to form a thin sheet resembling frosted glass. Because of its
nature and location, it causes early distortion of vision out of proportion
to its size, and often affects near vision as much as, or more than, distant
vision. Glare appears early with this type of cataract, and a change of
glasses will not improve vision as it often does with nuclear cataracts.

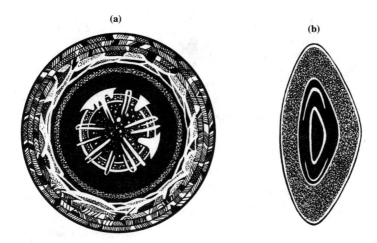

Figure 7. The tendency of the aging lens nucleus to harden and yellow *(nuclear sclerosis)* can cause a common type of cataract.

If one develops a cataract, at what point should it be removed? No blanket answer can be given, since each individual has different visual requirements. For some, their occupation (for example, truck driver or architect) makes it imperative to maintain the best possible vision in both eyes. In such cases, surgery may be indicated when visual acuity is reduced only two or three lines on the near or distant examination chart, even if only one eye is affected. Other individuals may function perfectly well with visual acuity down to 20/40 or 20/50 levels in their better eye, despite very poor vision in the more affected eye. This is especially true in the case of nuclear cataracts which do not affect near vision as significantly as they do distant vision. Surgery is normally recommended when a cataract has developed to the extent that it interferes with the patient's life style.

Do cataracts have to be removed? In other words, is it dangerous to leave a cataract in the eye? In most cases the answer is **NO**, it is not dangerous to the eye to leave a cataract in it. However, there are some exceptions. Although most individuals will develop cataracts in both eyes at approximately the same rate, occasionally one eye will become afflicted much earlier than the other. If vision becomes severely limited in one eye so that it perceives only light and gross hand motion, that eye may begin to drift in sight direction since it can no longer see well enough to line up with the better eye. If this condition is allowed to go on long enough, it may worsen so that eventual removal of the cataract may require additional surgery on the muscles of the affected eye to line up the eyes again and prevent double vision. In this case, even though an individual may still be functioning well with the better eye, it might be advisable to proceed with cataract surgery.

The other exception is when a cataract begins to beome "over-ripe," that is, degenerate and swell. This can lead to inflammation and *glaucoma* (damage due to high pressure inside the eye). *This does not happen in early or even moderately advanced cataracts, and is a cause of concern only in advanced or "mature" cases*. Most ophthalmologists would then recommend cataract surgery regardless of the condition of the other eye.

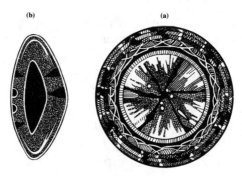

Figure 8. Cortical cataracts are caused by degeneration of the outer layer of the aging eye which produces holes, flat patches, and splits.

At present, there is no treatment for cataracts other than surgery. However, the many recent advances in cataract surgery have made it safer and more predictable than in past years. Probably the best form of cataract surgery for most patients is the classical approach in which an incision is made around the upper curve of the cornea into the anterior (front) chamber of the eye (Figure 9a). The cornea is pulled forward and the entire lens is removed from the eye (Figure 9b). The incision is then closed with very fine sutures made of nylon or absorbable synthetic material (Figure 9c). An enzyme, *alpha-chymotrypsin*, may be used to weaken the lens-supporting zonules so that the lens may be easily extracted. This procedure is almost always done with local anesthesia only and with minimal sedation. The surgery is greatly aided by the use of an operating microscope and newly developed micro-instruments and suture material, all of which make for tight and exact closure of the incision and comfort and safety for the patient.

Some new techniques have been developed recently which, although promising, may not be the ultimate or best for everyone, as some of their proponents would have us believe. One of these is *phacoemulsification*, removal of the cataract with the aid of a probe inserted through a small incision at the top of the cornea. The probe contains an ultrasonic vibrating tip which emulsifies (fragments and floats) the lens material. By means of irrigation and suction, the probe then removes the emulsified material from the eye. The advantages of this method claimed by its proponents are that the incision is smaller and thus safer, and the rear membrane covering the lens is left in place to hold the vitreous gel in its normal position. Results to date, however, do not prove that this procedure has fewer complications after surgery.

A disadvantage of the method is that the required instruments are very expensive and the techniques difficult to master. Thus, it may be less safely performed by some surgeons than by others. Another disadvantage is that in older patients with very hard lenses, especially in those over the age of 65 or 70, the long time required to fragment the lens with the ultrasonic vibrator may lead to damage to the cornea which may show up years later. Because this is a relatively new procedure, it has been recommended by some ophthalmologists that its use be limited in patients over 65. Also, in certain individuals the *endothelium*, the delicate inner lining of the cornea, may not be normal. In such cases, the ultrasonic vibrations or the impact of lens fragments against the inner surface of the cornea may cause damage which can limit vision. Such damage is very difficult to treat, and, if severe, may require a corneal transplant to restore vision.

In those individuals with no contraindication to the use of phacoemulsification, the technique's greatest single advantage is that the smaller incision permits shortening or eliminating the hospital stay. Also, there is little or no restriction on the patient's activity during the postoperative period. It should be noted, however, that use of the newer suture material and the operating microscope in the classical operation has already shortened the hospital stay to two or three days in most cases. Moreover, restrictions on activity are so minimal that the life style of very few patients over the age of 65 is affected in any significant way.

Two frequently reported claims for cataract removal techniques should be refuted. First, the laser beam which is useful in the treatment of certain diseases of the retina, especially complications of diabetes, has no place in the treatment of cataracts. Second, there is no way to "peel off" a cataract without entering the eye. Many patients have unfortunately misunderstood some of the talk about phacoemulsification and have the erroneous idea that it can remove cataracts without surgery.

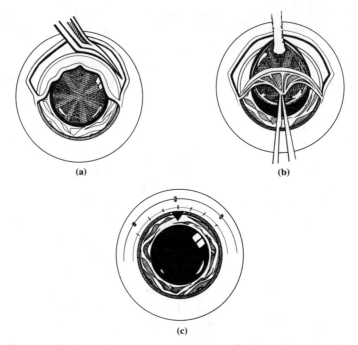

Figure 9. Surgery is the only present treatment for cataracts. (a) An incision is made along the upper curve of the cornea. (b) The cornea is pulled forward, and the lens is removed. (c) The incision is closed with very fine sutures.

Another recent development being used more each year is the artificial lens implant (Figure 10). These plastic lenses are inserted into the eye after removal of the cataract to replace the refractive power of the lost lens. If artificial lenses are properly implanted in carefully selected patients, good results can be expected, with the advantage that the patient does not have to wear contact lenses or thick bothersome cataract glasses. However, if a complication does arise, the results for the eye can be devastating. There are some contraindications to the implantation of these lenses, including some inflammatory and degenerative diseases of the eye, long-standing *diabetes mellitus*, and some retinal problems, especially previous retinal detachment in either eye. Because of the relatively short experience to date with implanted lenses, we do not yet know their long-term effects. For this reason, most surgeons have avoided lens implantation in patients under the age of 65, except in special circumstances.

Contact lenses for correcting *aphakia* (the condition existing after the lens is removed from the eye) have improved significantly over the last few years, but unfortunately a permanent-wear hard contact lens has not yet been developed. Because the cornea is less sensitive after cataract surgery, many people easily adapt to soft contact lenses and can wear them comfortably for weeks or months at a time with excellent correction of vision. Others, however, are unable to tolerate such long wear.

The other substitute for the removed lens is *aphakic* (cataract) glasses. Although some advances have been made in these relatively thick glasses, making them lighter and less distorting at the edge, all magnify the perceived image. Some wearers have difficulty adapting to the enlarged image. A special problem arises when only one cataract has been removed. The wearer of the cataract glasses cannot use both eyes at the same time because they present images of unequal size. This is not the case with the artificial lens implant or a contact lens—a great advantage in the use of either of these methods to correct aphakic vision. Most patients are able to adapt to aphakic glasses with little effort, thus avoiding the risks of artificial lens implants or contact lenses.

What about the complications of cataract surgery? Although up to five percent of cataract extractions have a complication of some kind during or after surgery, most can be managed successfully and good vision usually results. Poor vision following cataract surgery usually occurs as a secondary effect of unrelated problems such as glaucoma, corneal dystrophy, or retinal degeneration.

Swelling of the retinal area that provides central vision (*macular edema*) is a frequent occurrence after cataract surgery. This can delay visual recovery but usually clears up spontaneously. Even in severe cases, the edema is gone in half the patients within six months, and the recovery figure rises to 70 percent in one to three years. Retinal detachment, discussed later, is a possible late complication of cataract surgery.

Macular Degeneration

The *macula* is the specialized area of the retina associated with central, or reading, vision. It has a high metabolic rate which requires abundant blood circulation to the underlying area responsible for bringing in nutrients and carrying away waste products. In some patients with arteriosclerosis (hardening of the arteries), the blood supply becomes diminished and is no longer able to keep up with the demands of the macula. When this happens, the tissue begins to degenerate. This degeneration affects only the central area of the retina (Figure 11a). Although reading vision may significantly diminish, peripheral vision generally is not affected.

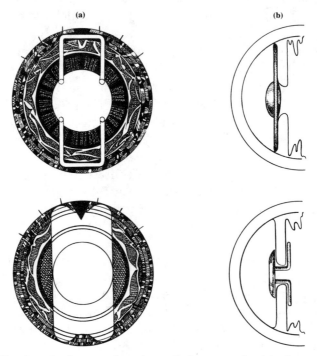

Figure 10. Plastic substitutes of various designs can be implanted to replace a lens removed during cataract surgery.

Unfortunately, there is no treatment for this condition once it has developed. One can only try to prevent the underlying vascular disease from developing at an early age. It must be emphasized, however, that only reading or central vision is affected; the individual will almost always maintain peripheral, or walking, vision. If the area involved is small, magnifying devices can be used to enlarge images so that they extend to and can be recognized by the unaffected area of the retina (Figure 11b). Low-vision clinics in many U.S. cities help a significant number of individuals with macular degeneration to see better with such optical devices.

Glaucoma

Glaucoma is defined as "increased pressure in the eye of sufficient force to cause damage to the visual function of the eye if left untreated." It is predominantly a disease of people over the age of 40, and accounts for 12 to 20 percent of all blindness in the United States. It has been estimated that the prevalence of glaucoma in people over 40 may be as high as two percent, and that glaucoma will eventually impair the vision of one out of every 200 people. There is also evidence that glaucoma runs in families. Studies show that the incidence of glaucoma over age 40 rises to 15–20 percent in the offspring of parents who had glaucoma.

Normal pressure is maintained in the eye by the constant production and reabsorption of the clear watery *aqueous humor*. The transparent aqueous plays a role in the eye similar to that of blood elsewhere in the body by circulating across the lens and back surface of the cornea, bringing nutrients to these bloodless structures and taking away waste products. If red blood were to do this, our vision would not be clear.

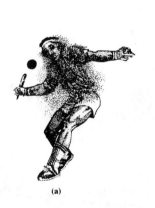
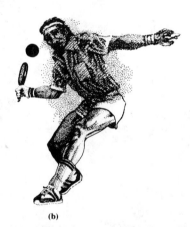

(a)   (b)

Figure 11. (a) Reduction of the retina's blood supply by arteriosclerosis can cause macular degeneration, affecting images formed on the central, or reading, area of the retina. (b) Magnifying the image so much of it falls on intact peripheral portions of the retina can improve vision.

The aqueous humor is produced by the ciliary body and is drained off through the veins of the eye by way of a fine net of fibers called the trabecular meshwork and a passage called Schlemm's canal (Figure 12). Normally, the rates of production and drainage are balanced, so the pressure inside the eyeball remains constant. In glaucoma, something goes wrong with this balance, and the pressure rises. For example, a partial block in the drainage path will increase the resistance to outflow and raise the balance to a new and higher pressure level. If the block is total, the pressure will rise to the point at which no more aqueous can be forced into the eye. Whatever the mechanism, the higher pressure is distributed throughout the eyeball. The tissue most vulnerable to pressure is the delicate nerve fibers that carry messages from the retina to the brain. If the pressure remains high for a long time, the nerve fibers can be permanently damaged and vision lost.

There are many different types of glaucoma, including congenital glaucoma and those secondary to eye inflammation or injury. The glaucomas which most commonly affect people over 40 can be separated into two groups: acute angle-closure glaucoma and chronic open-angle glaucoma.

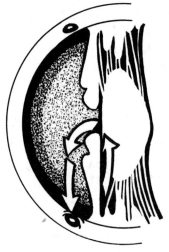

Figure 12. Clear, watery aqueous humor washes over the lens and back of the cornea (arrows) and drains off into the veins through Schlemm's canal. Blocked drainage increases eyeball pressure and can cause glaucoma.

Acute angle-closure glaucoma is a painful disorder of rather sudden onset which classically occurs in farsighted individuals over the age of 45. The sudden increase in pressure is due to a block in the normal flow of aqueous from the posterior chamber into the anterior chamber, caused by the edge of the pupil pressing against the front surface of the lens (Figure 13a). The iris is forced forward by the aqueous collecting in the posterior chamber, and the angle of the anterior chamber is closed off (Figure 13b), blocking the escape of aqueous from the eye. The pressure then rises precipitously, resulting in pain, clouding of vision, and a red, inflamed eye.

Although most cases of angle-closure glaucoma start suddenly, some may appear as recurring partial closures, usually in late afternoon or early evening, which cause some temporary blurring of vision with or without significant pain. The more common sudden attack leads to very high pressure in one or two hours. Classically, the eye in acute glaucoma has a red conjunctiva, a cloudy cornea, a shallow or absent anterior chamber, and an oval-shaped pupil which does not change size when light shines into the eye (a normal pupil would contract).

The first step in treatment of angle-closure glaucoma is to bring down the pressure by reducing the fluid in the eye with intravenous injections of mannitol or other drugs. Pilocarpine eyedrops are used to constrict the pupil, thus pulling the iris away from the angle and opening the drainage outflow. The definitive treatment is surgical, usually a *peripheral* iridectomy (removal of an outer part of the iris) to create a bypass from the posterior chamber into the anterior chamber and so prevent a pupillary block (Figure 14).

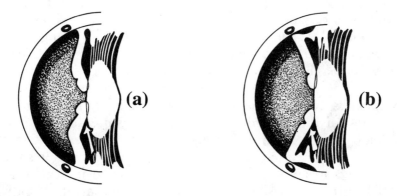

Figure 13. In acute angle-closure glaucoma, eye pressure first rises because the edge of the pupil presses against the lens and blocks normal liquid flow between the posterior and anterior chambers (a). The pressure on the lens side pushes the iris forward against the cornea, closing off the angle between the two (b). This prevents the escape of aqueous from the eye and causes a secondary sharp pressure rise accompanied by pain, clouded vision, and redness.

If the attack of acute glaucoma can be broken with medications, it is usually best to keep the eye quiet for two or three days before proceeding with surgery. However, if the pressure cannot be brought down to normal within a few hours by medical means, the peripheral iridectomy may have to be performed despite the high pressure and venous congestion. This involves the risk that sudden loss of pressure may cause retinal hemorrhage. Without treatment, however, loss of vision almost certainly will be permanent, and the eye itself might be lost.

When a patient manifests angle closure in one eye, the other eye must be examined for existing or potential glaucoma. It has been estimated that 50 percent of those with acute angle-closure glaucoma in one eye will have an attack in the other eye within one year. Therefore, most ophthalmologists will advise a prophylactic iridectomy in the second eye approximately one week after surgery in the first eye.

In contrast to angle-closure glaucoma, chronic open-angle glaucoma is a painless disorder in which vision is gradually lost over a period of months or years. The cause is a chronically elevated pressure, usually due to increased resistance to outflow of aqueous. The origin of the increased resistance is not clear.

Many people will have this disorder for years before they find themselves bumping into things they did not see or are involved in an accident while driving a car and then realize they have lost side vision. Unfortunately, if the disease goes unnoticed and untreated for a long time, many victims will not become aware that they have glaucoma until even central reading vision has been significantly diminished.

Vision loss from glaucoma is usually permanent. This is unfortunate because most of this loss could have been prevented or arrested if discovered and treated at an early stage. A routine eye examination every two years is recommended, including measurement of eye pressure, evaluation of the appearance of the optic nerve, and, if indicated, a test of visual field (width of vision). Although four percent of all individuals over 40 will have higher-than-normal pressure, fewer than two out of ten of this group will actually develop vision loss. On the other hand, those patients who manifest elevated pressure on periodic examination will include most who have or will develop glaucoma. A glaucoma suspect, that is, a patient with elevated pressure but no evidence of glaucoma, should be examined at more frequent intervals to detect symptoms early if they do appear. Such examination should be made three or four times during the first year, then every six months thereafter.

It must be emphasized that *one normal examination does not insure that glaucoma will not occur later in life*. Routine examinations every two years should not be neglected.

Treatment of chronic open-angle glaucoma controls the pressure with eyedrops, oral medications, or combinations of the two. Some of the most commonly used eyedrops are pilocarpine, epinephrine, and the relatively new drug, timilol. Stronger medications are used less often because of potential side effects such as an increased incidence of cataracts. However, if the glaucoma cannot be controlled in any other way, these medications may be employed.

(a)   (b)

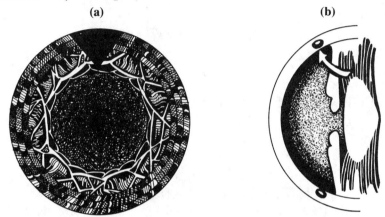

Figure 14. Peripheral iridectomy, the surgical removal of part of the iris (pie-wedge cut in a), bypasses (arrow in b) the pupillary block and relieves angle-closure glaucoma.

A test of the visual fields (Figure 15) complements the periodic checks of eye pressure and inspections of the optic nerve by detecting the extent and possible progression of vision loss. If, in spite of maximal medical therapy, eye pressure remains high and/or the visual fields progressively narrow, indicating a continuing loss of vision, surgery may be required to lower the pressure by establishing a new drainage route for the aqueous. Although surgery for glaucoma is successful 80 to 90 percent of the time, risk is involved, including possible infection and secondary cataract formation, so that ophthalmologists resort to surgery only when necessary because other means have failed. However, recent advances in surgical techniques and improvements in procedures allow much safer and predictable control of glaucoma than in the past. Consequently, earlier surgery is now more common when patients do not respond well to initial medical treatment so that vision loss is reduced.

A brief word on marijuana in glaucoma treatment may be in order. There is evidence that an ingredient in marijuana helps to lower pressure in the eye, but the mechanism of the effect is unknown. Also, there are side effects to the drug that make it undesirable for routine use. Much more research is needed before a final decision can be made regarding its usefulness in treatment of glaucoma.

The final word on glaucoma is PREVENTION. The visual loss for this disease is preventable with early diagnosis and treatment. HAVE ROUTINE MEDICAL EYE EXAMINATIONS!!!

Vitreous Floaters

The vitreous chamber of the eye contains a clear gel supported by a network of fine strands of *collagen* (a protein). Often, particles of collagen are visible as small floaters in the gel, especially against a light background. The great majority of floaters are harmless, but can be bothersome.

In the young eye, the gel completely fills the vitreous chamber. With increasing age, however, the gel shrinks and pulls forward to its region of strongest attachment. Occasionally, a sudden shower of floaters erupts, sometimes accompanied by flashes of light. This is caused by detachment of the shrinking gel (vitreous separation or detachment) from its relatively weak adhesion to the retina. Since a small percentage of vitreous detachments also tear the retina, people who experience these symptoms should be thoroughly examined by an ophthalmologist.

It should be emphasized that most floaters are harmless and merely annoying. They require no treatment since most will eventually settle to the lower part of the eye out of sight.

Retinal Detachment

The retina is not firmly attached to underlying tissue (*choroid*), but adheres to it much the way a vinyl plastic lining adheres to the cement bottom and walls of a swimming pool. Just as water seeping through a tear in the vinyl can gradually separate the lining from the cement, so liquid in the eye can seep through a tear in the retina and, in a few days or weeks, gradually float it off the underlying tissue (Figure 16). The detached retina loses its ability to see because it received much of its nourishment from the rich blood supply in the choroid with which it is no longer in contact.

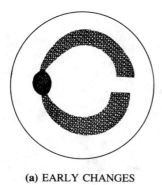 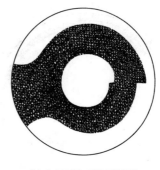

(a) EARLY CHANGES   **(b)** LATER CHANGES

Figure 15. Visual field tests complement eye pressure measurements in glaucoma management. If early losses (narrow dark band in **a**) worsen and progressively narrow the field (**b**), surgery may be indicated.

As described above in *Vitreous Floaters*, a retina sometimes becomes torn when the vitreous gel separates from the eye wall, in which case the retinal tear is heralded by a shower of floaters and flashes of light. After the retina tears and begins to detach, the patient may notice formation of a dark cloud, wall, or curtain, depending on which area of the retina is affected. The earlier treatment is started, the more normal the vision that is retained. Left untreated, the eye will become blind.

Because forward movement of the vitreous can tear the retina, two conditions increase the risk of detachment by this cause. First, the extremely nearsighted eyeball is longer than normal, so its ends are more curved, exerting a stronger pull on a thinner retina. Second, the removal of the lens in cataract surgery takes away a front restraint on the vitreous, allowing it to bulge forward and pull on the retina at the rear.

A third predisposition to retinal tear and detachment is *lattice degeneration* of the retina. A condition which may be hereditary, it is characterized by fine grey or white lines that intersect at the periphery of the retina. Although lattice degeneration does not inevitably lead to retinal detachment, it does increase the risk that the retina will detach after vitreous detachment, cataract extraction, or minor head injury.

Early treatment of retinal tears before detachment includes sealing off the tear with a laser beam, or freezing the external surface of the eye over the tear (*cryopexy*). Treatment after retinal detachment has occurred is surgical and is called *scleral buckling* (Figure 17). In this surgery, freezing is also used to seal the tear in the retina. However, because the retina

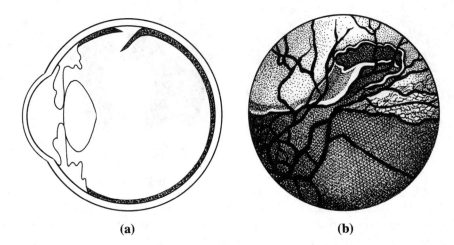

(a)   (b)

Figure 16. (a) Liquid in the eye can seep through a tear in the retina and (b) lift part of the membrane off underlying tissue.

is loose, a buckle or fold, must be made in the overlying *sclera* (tough white outer coat of the eye) to press the area of the tear against the underlying tissue until the seal becomes permanent. A permanent seal takes about two weeks and consists of scar tissue formed by damage due to the freezing or to the laser beam.

Once the hole has been sealed off, fluid can no longer seep under the retina. Any fluid that remains will be absorbed by the eye so that the retina will remain flat after surgery. Because the silicone sponge and sutures used to buckle the sclera usually have no long-term effect on the eye, they are left in place unless inflammation or infection demands their removal. Patients undergoing surgery of this type usually require general anesthesia. The risks any general anesthesia involves are a significant reason for not removing the materials used for the buckle unless some complication occurs.

In retinal detachment, earlier treatment gives greater assurance that the final result will be satisfactory. A sudden shower of floaters and flashes of light, or the appearance of a curtain, cloud, or wall in one eye is a warning that should not be ignored. It is much better to have an ophthalmic examination and find nothing wrong than to delay and risk the impairment or loss of vision.

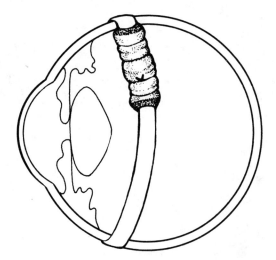

Figure 17. After a detached retina is repaired with a laser beam or by freezing, scleral buckling with a belt of sutures and silicone sponge dimples the tough white outer layer of the eye inward to press the mended area against underlying tissue until the seal becomes permanent.

SKIN DISORDERS

Paul Gross, M.D.

Assistant Professor of Dermatology, Pennsylvania Hospital

The skin is the body's largest and most visible organ. For years physicians regarded the skin merely as a protective covering of the more important vital organs within the body, but we now know that the skin is a vital organ in its own right. It helps regulate the body's temperature by sweating and by changing the degree of constriction of the blood vessels; it is an important medium for absorption of medications and toxins into the whole body; and it protects the body from infection, dehydration, and heat damage. The skin is also an important route for excretion of chemical waste products.

Aging is usually first detectable in the skin. Most of the aging changes are preventable, and many are treatable. Some are determined by the genetic makeup of the individual (inherited characteristics) together with environmental factors. In addition to significant cosmetic and medical aspects of the aging skin, there are obvious psychological considerations. People feel better when they look attractive. Anyone who feels ugly or abnormal in appearance to the world is likely to be depressed.

Some skin diseases are due specifically to aging, while others are merely more common in the elderly but not necessarily related to the number of years one has lived. Some common skin conditions actually become less severe as one ages, for example, contact dermatitis from irritants such as poison ivy or poison oak.

Wrinkles and Other Cosmetic Changes

The most common skin problems associated with aging include the familiar wrinkles, loss of tone, brown and red discolorations, and crusted growths. These are due largely to the effects of years of exposure to ultraviolet light from the sun. Extremes of heat and cold can also contribute to these changes. The harmful effects can be clearly seen by comparing the exposed skin of the face and back of the hands with the normally covered skin of the trunk or under the chin. It will be readily apparent that protected sites have aged much less than exposed areas. The skin of individuals with light complexions tends to age more from sun damage than does the skin of people with darker complexions because skin pigment absorbs a large proportion of the harmful ultraviolet rays. Because severe sun damage requires 20 to 30 years to show itself in the skin, it is important to protect oneself as much as possible from excessive exposure while young.

At one time it was felt that suntan was "healthy." Now we know that this is largely a culturally conditioned judgment. In fact, in past centuries, the upper classes were proud of their clear skin because it contrasted with the freckled skin of those who had to labor in the fields. Now, a "glorious tan" is seen by many as evidence that its bearer can afford a costly vacation in a sunny climate or weeks at the beach, while the less fortunate must languish in an enclosed office or factory.

Years ago, sunlight was necessary for the production of vitamin D in the skin. Today, this vitamin is prepared synthetically and is available in enriched foods such as milk or in multivitamin preparations. There is no longer a medical benefit to be derived from exposing the skin to sunlight.

Ultraviolet light alters deep layers of the skin, thickening and clumping its elastic fibers, and causing it to lose its normal resiliency or tone. The result is sagging, wrinkles, and loss of normal support for the skin's blood vessels, causing them to become fragile. This leads to a condition known as *senile purpura*, unsightly black and blue marks that appear after minor injuries due to breaking of weakened blood vessels in the skin.

Scaly brown flat or slightly raised spots result from the overgrowth of several different types of skin cells. Most of these are benign, but can sometimes develop into skin cancers. Other red spots may be due to the growth of superficial vessels in the skin, and, in most instances, are merely a cosmetic problem.

Treatment for these cosmetic conditions normally consists of a combination of surface coverings and certain surgical procedures. While face lifting is an increasingly popular way of eliminating wrinkles, it is not a permanent solution. The basic damage to elastic tissue remains, and wrinkles reappear after several years. Chemical peeling and dermabrasion can also remove superficial wrinkles and pigment changes but their effect also lasts only for several years.

Protection from avoidable harm to the skin is best achieved by not risking excessive sun exposure. Solar rays are most damaging when the sun is overhead, between the hours of 10 a.m. and 3 p.m. Protective clothing and hats can be worn, and effective chemical sun screens can be purchased without prescription. When applied once or twice a day, these skin coatings will screen out most of the damaging ultraviolet rays. Some permit a significant amount of tanning. However, it is wrong to suppose that burning rays are different from tanning rays in damaging the skin. The degree of exposure is the critical factor. Sun screens containing *para-aminobenzoic acid* (PABA) in alcohol bases are usually considered to be the most effective. *Benzophenones* are available in creamier preparations which may be less irritating to the skin than alcohol-containing solutions. However, they are slightly less effective screens, and also must be reapplied more frequently.

Dry Skin and Itching

Another problem of aged skin is dryness, accompanied by scaling and itching. Water is normally held in the outermost skin layers, and a thin natural oil film tends to trap this water and keep the skin moist. As the years go by, the oil glands of the skin become less active, reducing the natural lubrication. Then, when the humidity is low, for example, in the winter when indoor heat is on, our skin surfaces tend to lose moisture to the surrounding air. Bathing in very hot water and the use of strong soap aggravate the drying by removing protective oil. The resulting dry skin can be extremely itchy, even to the point of interfering with sleep. Scratching and secondary skin infections or rashes can develop. When our bodies fail to produce enough oil to slow down moisture evaporation and drying, it is often necessary to use a moisturizing cream or lotion.

Simple treatments for dry, itchy skin include less frequent bathing, use of gentle or super-fatted soaps, and short tepid baths or showers, rather than long hot ones, as well as creams or lotions if dryness persists. While there are many types of moisturizing preparations, all work the same way by depositing a layer of grease on the surface of the skin to prevent water from evaporating. Since such preparations do not add moisture to the skin, less expensive preparations are just as effective as the more expensive brands. Moisturizing creams will not prevent wrinkles, except for the superficial cracking that occurs when the skin is extremely dry.

Ordinary petroleum jelly, although too greasy for many, is one of the most effective agents for the prevention or treatment of dry, itchy skin. Lanolin and plain cold creams are also good. In general, bath oils are not as effective as lotions or creams. Results are best when the lotion or cream is used immediately after the bath while the skin is still moist. They may have to be applied several times a day, and some portions of the body may need more frequent lubrication than others. Areas most damaged by years of sun exposure may require more extensive treatment than protected parts of the body. It should be noted that the drying-out process tends to be more severe in the lower legs. Anesthetic creams and lotions for relief of itching should be avoided because they are effective for only a short time and frequently provoke allergic reactions.

Generalized itchiness in normal skin, not associated with a rash, may have any one of a number of causes. It is easy to blame ''nerves,'' especially since the anxieties experienced in daily life often generate psychosomatic symptoms. However, if persistent, unexplained itchiness is attributed to psychic stress before a careful search is made to exclude possible underlying medical problems, a serious disease may be overlooked. Systemic diseases which may produce severe itching include diabetes, kidney failure, liver obstruction, over or underactivity of the thyroid gland, reactions to medications, and various malignancies, especially Hodgkin's disease (a cancer of the lymph glands). A physician should be consulted in cases of severe and prolonged itching which is not relieved by simple precautions and lubrication.

Hair

Hair problems are usually not serious matters of general health, but can be distressing all the same. Some are remediable, others must simply be lived with.

Baldness

Aging causes some thinning of scalp hair for almost everyone. Typical male baldness, a familiar sight, starts with thinning at the temples followed by a gradually enlarging circle of bare scalp on top. This tendency is inherited. Early signs appear when a man is twenty or thirty years old and progress through his later years.

In women, the thinning of scalp hair may be general and relatively uniformly distributed, or the male balding pattern may sometimes occur. Male-type baldness in women is more evident after menopause because such hair loss depends on both heredity and on the local effect of male hormones on hair roots. These hormones are produced by the adrenal glands, and their influence usually becomes apparent only after the ovaries stop functioning.

The female pattern of hair loss rarely causes complete baldness and can usually be made less noticeable by such means as modification of hair styling to cover thinned areas. Permanent waving embrittles hair and may cause it to break, but does not cause permanent hair loss.

Men often resort to the use of hair pieces. Hair transplantation—-actually skin grafting—can transfer hair from the back to the front of the head for cosmetic improvement.

Greying

Greying of the hair is accepted as a common consequence of aging. It is caused by the diminished activity of pigment cells in the hair root. Dyeing the hair to hide the greyness will not cause the hair to fall out unless there is a severe allergic reaction to chemicals in the dye, and then the result is usually a rash and possibly temporary loss of hair. Whatever affects the outside of the hair shaft, whether it is dyeing, straightening, or curling, does not disturb the hair root, which lies about one-half inch below the skin surface. The root is more susceptible to internal changes such as shifts in hormone levels, high fevers, and the effects of drugs.

Natural Loss and New Growth

Combing or brushing does not permanently change the hair. The hairs that come away are some of the 50 to 100 strands lost naturally each day. These hairs are distinguished by a white bulb on their tips, and are replaced by new growing hairs. Shampoos and conditioners may affect the texture of the hair, but do not generate new growth. Only in cases of scalp disease, such as psoriasis or severe dandruff with infection, can scalp applications or medicated shampoos promote regrowth. Vitamin supplements or therapy will not prevent or recover genetically determined hair loss.

Facial Hair in Women

Male hormones produced by women are responsible for the development of coarse dark facial hair, especially during or following menopause, and usually with a genetic predisposition. Darkly complected women of Mediterranean origin may have significant facial hair from early adolescence. Such hair is often cosmetically undesirable and can usually be removed without harm unless it grows out of a mole. Mole hairs should be trimmed with scissors. Unwanted hair may be bleached, plucked, or trimmed as desired. Shaving or snipping does not cause hair to grow back faster or darker, but does produce sharp, stubbly ends. Depilatory creams should be tried with caution, as they often irritate the skin. Removal with wax is also effective. However, electrolysis is the only safe way of permanently eliminating unwanted facial hair. Because this must be done by a trained technician, it can be costly, but it need not leave scars and the hair will not usually regrow.

Nails

Fingernails and toenails thicken and become more brittle with age, especially if nearby joints are arthritic. Toenails may also become thick, brittle, and yellow due to common fungous infections which can often be successfully treated with prescribed medications.

Ridging of the nails is also common and usually not treatable. Peeling of the nails is often due to nail polish remover or strong detergents, and is unlikely to be remedied by diet, including vitamins or increased eating of gelatin. Commercial nail hardeners may be effective but tend to induce allergic reactions which can range from irritation to complete loss of the nail. In most cases, simply hiding unsightly nails under several coats of polish is harmless.

Skin Tumors

While many growths, or tumors, may appear on the skin as one ages, most are benign and of only cosmetic significance. However, some display a low degree of malignancy and others are highly dangerous.

The more common benign tumors are freckle-like lesions that normally appear on the back of the hands or on other exposed areas. They may be tan or brown and are usually flat, occasionally scaly, and sometimes slightly thickened. *Seborrheic keratoses,* another type of benign skin tumor, often referred to as "liver spots," are unrelated to the liver. They may occur anywhere on the body, but are more common in areas which have been exposed to sunlight. They are usually greasy and wartlike. Occasionally, they may be irritated by clothing or by being picked at, and may itch at times. However, despite their unpleasant appearance, they are harmless and never become malignant. They can be removed by freezing with liquid nitrogen, local surgery in the doctor's office, or cauterization with acid applications. Bleaching with commercial bleaching creams is rarely successful.

Premalignant growths known as *actinic* or *solar keratoses* also usually appear on exposed portions of the body such as the face or the back of the hands. Although they are usually redder and more irritated than seborrheic keratoses, expert examination is required to distinguish reliably between the two. The premalignant growths may sometimes bleed or build up a crust (*cutaneous horn*). If left untreated, they may become squamous-cell skin cancers. These rarely spread (metastasize) to other parts of the body, but invade nearby tissues.

The same is true of the most common skin cancer, *basal cell carcinoma.* These are slightly raised skin nodules with a central depression and a tendency to bleed or form a scab. They also appear on skin habitually exposed to the sun. Untreated, they grow slowly for years. They are especially troublesome around structures such as the eyes or the nose. Although they do not spread through the body and almost never kill, they should be removed while they are small and before they have invaded deeply into the skin. These carcinomas can often be treated in the doctor's office, but may sometimes require hospitalization for skin grafting.

They may also be treated by freezing with liquid nitrogen or by X-ray therapy.

While most skin cancers result from years of sun exposure, some may appear after X-ray treatments or ingestion of arsenic compounds. More rarely, they may arise in old scars, for example, from burns, or in vaccination marks. Carcinomas are more likely to appear on light skins than on dark ones and occur more often and at an earlier age in those who spend much of their lives outdoors. They are also more common in such parts of the country as the southwest where sunshine is more abundant and exposure greater than in other areas.

The most dangerous skin cancer is the malignant *melanoma* which develops in moles or appears like a mole in normal skin. It is characterized by a brown or blue-black color and is suspected in lesions or spots which begin to grow, bleed, itch, or hurt. Any mole changing in this manner should be evaluated by a physician, who will usually recommend a biopsy. If diagnosed and treated in an early stage, a melanoma is normally curable, but if it has grown deeply into the skin or ulcerated, cure is more difficult.

Lentigo maligna melanoma is a rare skin cancer which occurs mostly in elderly individuals. It is characterized by a flat, slightly scaly, brown growth, several inches in diameter, on the upper back, chest, or face. After several years, parts of the growth rise, darken, and may ulcerate or bleed. Although it is less dangerous than other types of malignant melanoma, it should be promptly removed.

Dermatitis (Skin Inflammation)

Contact Dermatitis

Contact dermatitis is the result of irritation by or allergy to substances that touch the skin. The most common example is poison ivy which causes an itchy rash. Frequently, a rash may be a reaction to medication prescribed by a physician or purchased over the counter for treatment of other types of skin irritation such as leg ulcers. Topical anesthetics, benzocaine, for example, are notorious offenders, but other agents such as merthiolate, neomycin (an antibiotic), and iodine, may also cause a rash. The rash usually subsides promptly when the irritating substance is no longer used. However, a physician may prescribe medication to relieve unbearable itching, or a cortisone-type cream to hasten the elimination of a lingering rash.

Seborrheic Dermatitis

In its simplest form, *seborrheic dermatitis* is dandruff of the scalp. This usually responds promptly to treatment with medicated shampoos containing coal tar, zinc, or salicylic acid. Some people seem predisposed to having dandruff, especially when emotionally stressed or physically run down. In such cases, it may spread to the face (forehead, eyebrows, chin, and sides of the nose), and may also affect the ears and the chest. However, this condition is not serious and can usually be controlled with a cortisone cream.

Chronic Neurodermatitis

Although "nerves" may be blamed for almost any condition, some types of rash are universally recognized as being of psychic origin. *Chronic neurodermatitis* is one of them. It is a red, thickened, scaly, itchy patch, which becomes more itchy when scratched, and usually appears on the back of the neck, the wrist, or the ankle. It is neither malignant nor contagious and responds quickly to treatment, but is likely to recur at times of stress.

Leg Ulcers

Stasis dermatitis, or eczema, is an itchy, scaly, red-brown rash on the lower legs. Often the feet and ankles swell, especially late in the day. This rash results from varicose veins and slow leakage of venous blood into the skin. Treatment includes support stockings, staying off the feet as much as possible, and application of appropriate prescription creams. The treatment described above for dry skin may be tried for a week or two. However, if the rash is not treated, or if scratching causes infection, the skin over the ankles may become severely ulcerated.

The rash and possible ulcerations that can develop from varicose veins are less serious than the problems stemming from an insufficient supply of arterial blood to the legs and feet. This blood supply decreases when arteriosclerosis narrows the blood vessels. The feet then become cold, cramps may develop in the calf muscles during exercise, the toes lose hair, and the skin on the legs appears thin and shiny. Since injured skin requires an increase in blood flow to facilitate healing, and the narrowed arteries prevent such an increase, minor irritations, such as fungal infections between the toes and blisters from rubbing of shoes and socks against the feet, may cause ulcers which do not heal. Damage which would normally be trivial may worsen. If not promptly treated, it may lead to severe infections that penetrate to the bone, ultimately resulting in gangrene and loss of a foot or even a leg.

Infection must be controlled under the care of a physician. Surgical reconstruction of the arteries may be required to increase the blood supply, although, unfortunately, surgery is not always possible. Nevertheless, most leg ulcers will heal eventually with proper treatment.

Psoriasis

Psoriasis, a common skin condition, affects two to three million people in the United States. It tends to run in families, although it does not exactly follow the genetic laws of inheritance. The usual age of onset is in the twenties and thirties, but may also range from infancy to over seventy.

The condition typically appears as thickened red patches of skin on the elbows and knees, usually with a silvery scale. On the scalp, it may appear to be severe dandruff with heavy scaling. The nails may become thickened, discolored, pitted, and separated from the underlying nail-bed. Periods of emotional stress tend to aggravate the symptoms, while vacations or hospitalization tend to relieve them. Contrary to TV advertisements, most psoriasis victims do not have severe itching. The disease is not life-threatening, but can be greatly distressing and even disabling if it spreads over a wide area of skin. It may also be associated with a painful, deforming type of arthritis.

Treatment is sometimes simply an application of bland petroleum jelly to lessen excessive scaling and shedding of skin. Other old but reliable aids include coal-tar ointments and lotions and medicated shampoos. Steroid (cortisone) creams can help, but they are expensive and their effects may be short-lived. Non-prescription salves should be used with care because they may cause local allergic reactions and make the rash temporarily worse. Physicians sometimes prescribe systemic steroids (related to cortisone) or even anti-cancer drugs such as Methotrexate® for severe psoriasis.

The disease is not curable, but periods of remission may occur either naturally or as a result of treatment. Because natural sunlight has a beneficial effect, treatment can sometimes be suspended during the summer.

Fungal Infections

Fungal infections are common in the general population, but also appear to increase in frequency with advancing age, probably because of circulatory changes that reduce the skin's ability to protect itself. These infections typically produce a dry, itchy, scaly rash on the soles of the feet or fissures between the toes (athlete's foot). Especially in warm weather, tiny blisters or pustules tend to appear on the soles of the feet, on the hands, and, in time, on any part of the body. These infections are often treatable with prescription creams, and in severe cases, with an antibiotic, *griseofulvin*, taken by mouth. A non-prescription medication, *tolnaftate* cream, may also be helpful. Keeping the skin area clean and dry is an important part of treatment. Socks need not be white but should be changed during the day as required to avoid the damp conditions in which the fungus thrives. The infection is usually chronic and is not contagious in ordinary circumstances.

Fungal infections of the toenails are difficult to treat because no medication applied to the surface of the nail is effective. The oral medication, griseofulvin, will clear up a fingernail infection in about three months, but may take 12 to 24 months for infected toenails, and the infection may reappear after treatment has ceased. Unless a toenail infection is unusually painful, no special treatment is necessary. In most instances, the result is thickening and a white or yellow discoloration, or crumbling away of the nail with only cosmetic significance. If a chronic toenail infection is left untreated, it is advisable to use a medicated foot powder to keep the toes dry and to prevent spread of the infection to surrounding skin.

Drug Allergies

Almost any drug taken internally can produce an allergic rash in some people. Often, the rash may be merely annoying and slightly itchy, but the reaction can sometimes be severe and even life-threatening.

While drugs can produce almost any kind of rash, the most common are hives and red, measle-like eruptions. The rash does not appear when a drug is first taken, because it takes one to two weeks of exposure to develop a sensitivity to the substance.

Allergic reactions are almost always very itchy and usually affect wide areas of the body. However, in a rare type known as *fixed-drug-reaction* (most often caused by the laxative agent, *phenolphthalein*), the effect is localized and recurs at the same skin site each time the offending drug is taken.

Fortunately, *digitalis,* a widely prescribed heart medication, rarely produces drug reactions. However, antihypertensive drugs, diuretics, and even aspirin frequently cause skin problems. For this reason, unless there is an obvious other cause for a rash, allergic drug reaction should be considered.

People who suspect they are having an allergic reaction to medication should not stop taking it without first consulting their physicians because abrupt withdrawal is dangerous under some circumstances. The physician may be able to determine that the offending drug is not really needed or may find an appropriate substitute.

Allergy rashes are treated symptomatically with cool baths, bland applications, and antihistamines to relieve itching. Steroid drugs may be needed in severe cases, especially if blisters develop or the lining of the mouth or eyes is affected.

Since there are no standard tests for drug allergies, a suspected drug may have to be given cautiously to determine if it does produce a rash. This practice is restricted to cases where the drug is essential and no substitute is available. Surface skin tests for allergy are sometimes performed with penicillin and some other antibiotics, but the results are not conclusive. A negative outcome does not assure that the drug will not produce a rash when injected or swallowed. Also, medication taken regularly for a long period can produce a belated allergic reaction, misleading the taker into believing that the rash must be due to another, more recently introduced drug. Clearly, drug reactions are variable. The best course is to take only drugs that are absolutely necessary and only for the shortest possible time.

Shingles

Shingles, known medically as *herpes zoster,* is a reactivation of the same viral infection that causes chickenpox and occurs more frequently in the elderly than in the young. It is dreaded because it tends to produce severe pain which may be disabling for long periods, even after the rash has disappeared.

Typically, it begins with pain near one of the nerves in the skin, often affecting a narrow band on one side of the back and chest, down an arm or leg, or over the scalp and front of the face. The pain is often described as sharp and electric, rather than a dull ache. Usually the cause is not apparent at first, but in a day or two, groups of blisters appear which, in severe cases, may be blood-filled or rapidly ulcerate. Typically, the rash lasts about three weeks without treatment, but frequently leaves deep ulcers which heal with scars. Although the pain may sometimes be mild and respond to simple aspirin or non-narcotic pain relievers, it can also become severe enough to demand stronger medication. It is not true that simultaneous shingles on both sides of the body is fatal, nor is it true that a recurrence, which is rare, is more severe or dangerous than the initial attack.

Shingles is not contagious except to children who have not had chickenpox. In them the disease may appear after an incubation period of two or three weeks following exposure. The usual treatment of shingles is pain killers, as needed, cool compresses, and bland lotions to speed drying up of the rash.

Shingles rarely spreads from the original site. (When it does affect the entire surface of the body, it is actually chickenpox.) The appearance of three or four blisters outside the primary pattern of skin nerves is not a cause for concern. They will simply progress through the usual stages of crusting and peeling and then be gone. However, if dozens develop, they may indicate poor natural immunity, possibly associated with certain systemic diseases, particularly malignancies of the blood, bone marrow, or lymph nodes. The most serious complication of shingles is scarring of the cornea of the eye or even blindness, which can result if the disease affects the forehead or the tip of the nose and is not promptly treated by a skilled ophthalmologist.

Unfortunately, many elderly victims have severe persistent pain long after shingles has healed. Their skin may remain chronically hypersensitive, so that the weight of normal clothing is unbearable and they lose sleep and become depressed. The physician can prescribe drugs that help ease the pain, but they are potent and prolonged use can cause addiction. Because the pain can develop along nerve paths after the shingles is gone, many physicians elect to treat the early stage with cortisone or related synthetic drugs in an attempt to forestall the later problems. If there is no medical contraindication, early administration of high doses of these drugs can provide relatively rapid pain relief, speed the healing process, and prevent the later development of prolonged and painful nerve inflammation. Therefore, patients should seek prompt attention for shingles even when they feel certain they have correctly diagnosed the condition themselves.

Blistering Diseases

Pemphigus vulgaris and *bullous pemphigoid* are two blistering diseases, probably of auto-immune cause, also seen more often in the elderly than in the young. Auto-immune means that patients become immune or ''allergic'' to their own skins. Their immune systems try to reject their skins as alien, much as a heart transplant might be rejected by its recipient.

Pemphigus was formerly almost invariably fatal, but is now controlled by appropriate medication. It typically begins in the mouth with painful erosions and ulcers, then spreads elsewhere on the skin in the form of thin-walled, short-lived blisters and crusts which rapidly become infected.

Pemphigoid usually produces fewer blisters than pemphigus, but they have thicker walls and so last longer. Also, there may be considerable itching, but less tendency for involvement of the mouth and other mucous membranes, and patients do not become as sick as with pemphigus.

Cortisone-type drugs are routinely used to treat both these conditions. Although these medications are strong and tend to produce side effcts, they permit most patients to live relatively normal lives. In some cases, immunosuppressant drugs, like those used for arthritis patients, may be administered to minimize the side effects.

DENTAL CARE FOR THE OLDER PATIENT

Jonathan Nash, D.D.S.

Assistant Professor, University of Pennsylvania
School of Dental Medicine

Joseph T. Thompson, D.M.D.
Joanne Warnalis, R.D.H.

Meadowbrook, Pennsylvania

Oral health contributes significantly to a sense of well-being. Loose, missing, or unsightly teeth, oral infections, and similar discomforting conditions can be sources of much personal distress. In contrast, a healthy mouth encourages social ease and confidence. The myth that tooth loss is inevitable is unfortunate, for we are not fated to lose our teeth as we grow older. Cavities and gum disease are preventable, and it is possible for most individuals to keep all their teeth for their entire lives. However, since most of us need dental care, it is well to be an informed user of dental services, with a basic understanding that will permit intelligent selection and evaluation of such services.

As we age, the normal changes that the body undergoes, such as dry and occasionally discolored skin and graying and thinning hair, include changes that make teeth, bones, and mouth surfaces more vulnerable. The slightest pressure may cause ulceration, and tissues supporting the teeth become less resistant to disease. Many older patients lack the motivation or even the physical ability to keep their mouths clean. Poor oral hygiene increases susceptibility to dental disease. Nutrition may be inadequate, commonly as a result of a high carbohydrate diet which fosters gum disease and tooth decay. Lack of regular professional care may also be a contributing factor.

Many adults lose most or all of their teeth by their 65th year. In the United States, 23 percent of adults between 45 and 64 are toothless. Nationwide, 50 percent of those over 65 are completely toothless, with some surveys indicating 70 percent. It has also been estimated that over 90 percent of all adults have periodontal disease in some form.

As we grow older, many of our tissues atrophy. Tissues and organs may shrink or waste away, reflecting a failure of nutrition. Resilience is lost as the body grows less able to replace cells and repair tissues. The supporting structures of the mouth, including the jawbones, are subject to constant wear and tear, and aging reduces their ability to withstand these stresses. Thus, gum disease and loss of bone support are common in the older person. Chronic low-grade infections of the gums, easily tolerated by younger persons, begin to take their toll, resulting in a shrinking of the bone supporting the teeth.

As the kidneys age and become less efficient, the oral tissues become dehydrated. Aging also causes a progressive thinning of the mucous lining of the mouth. These conditions combine to make oral tissues more susceptible to injury, and mouth sores develop easily.

The diets of many older people are deficient in essential nutrients, which adversely affects tissues already compromised by aging. Vitamin B deficiencies are commonly associated with cracks in the corners of the mouth (*angular cheilosis*), abnormal taste, and a burning tongue. Vitamin A deficiencies cause the mucous lining to tear and abrade easily. Inadequate levels of vitamin C result in poor wound healing, especially after a tooth extraction. Calcium deficiencies may contribute to loss of bone support.

An additional factor is the effect of the extensive hormonal changes that accompany the ''change of life.'' Although not fully understood, these changes appear to affect mouth tissues directly, occasionally causing significant problems. Many individuals experiencing the emotional stresses of the change of life find it difficult to tolerate dental procedures and appliances.

Obviously, the older patient is confronted with a number of potentially debilitating factors: an aging body and less resilient tissues; nutritional deficiencies associated with improper diet; decreased cellular
metabolism; hormonal changes; and psychological problems. Awareness
of these factors is essential to maintain a healthy mouth and to minimize
potential problems.

Dental Diseases

Two forms of dental disease are most commonly found in the older
individual: *periodontal* (gum) disease, and dental *caries* (cavities). The
major contributing cause of both diseases is the same—a substance
known as *plaque* (pronounced "plack").

Dental plaque is a mass of bacteria in a sticky coating on the teeth
and in the space between teeth and gums. Mouth bacteria alone are not
dangerous, and in fact are needed in the mouth. But when different
types accumulate to form plaque, they become disease producers. As the
bacteria grow and multiply, they break down sugary foods into acid,
which concentrates and combines with bacterial poisons to cause periodontal disease and caries.

Periodontal (Gum) Disease

In periodontal disease(Figure 1), the first effect of plaque is inflammation and bleeding of the gums. This occurs as a result of microscopic
ulcerations and breakdown of gum tissue by the products of bacterial activity. This weakens the tissue and reduces the ability of the gums to support the teeth.

Plaque that is not removed by daily brushing and use of dental floss
forms a thick, crusty deposit on the teeth and under the gums. The deposit, called *calculus,* hardens—or calcifies—to the point where brushing
or flossing cannot remove it. Scaling, a procedure performed by a dentist
or dental hygienist, is necessary to remove the calculus and relieve the irritation caused by the deposits. If the calculus is allowed to remain under
the gums, the inflammation not only causes bleeding, but also leads to a
weakening of the area where the gums attach to the teeth. Pockets of diseased gum tissue then form around the teeth, which can cause recession
of the gums and exposure of root surfaces.

As periodontal disease progresses, it becomes more difficult to reverse. When the disease affects only soft tissue, it can be controlled and to some extent reversed or cured by professional dental and home care. However, when the disease has involved the bone support of the teeth, causing teeth to loosen, the loss of support may be permanent. Such bone loss occurs gradually and may go unnoticed unless detected by X ray. When aging individuals notice that their teeth have rotated or drifted over a period of years, it is usually a sign of advanced, chronic periodontal disease. This condition accounts for a majority of tooth loss in older people, much more so than cavities.

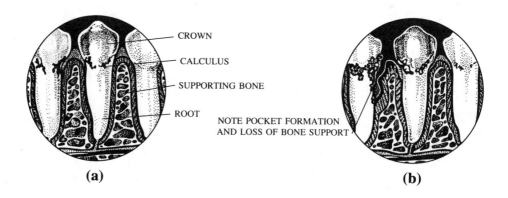

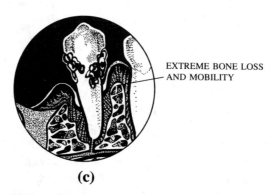

Figure 1. The progression of periodontal (gum) disease (a) beginning stage; (b) moderate; (c) extreme bone loss and mobility (from *The Chairside Instructor*, American Dental Association, 1975).

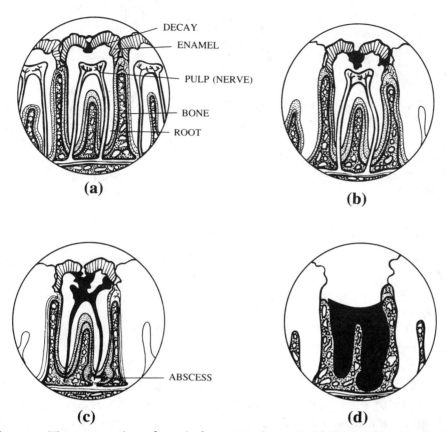

Figure 2. The progression of tooth decay **(a)** plaque holds bacterial acids on the tooth, dissolving enamel; **(b)** dentin decays rapidly and the cavity enlargens; **(c)** decay reaches the pulp and causes an infection; an abscess is formed at the tip of the root; **(d)** post-extraction — this tooth was lost due to extensive decay (from *The Chairside Instructor*, American Dental Association, 1975).

Dental Caries (Cavities)

The prevention of dental caries also depends to a great extent on the control of plaque. Acid produced by the bacterial breakdown of sugar in foods and liquids dissolves the tooth surface. Persistent exposure to sugar leads to a breakdown of tooth structure and formation of a cavity. Thus, the three factors involved in the development of a cavity are sugar, plaque bacteria, and a susceptible tooth. Since resistance to dental caries is strengthened by fluoride in the tooth surface, a susceptible tooth is one lacking a proper amount of fluoride (Figure 2).

The Dentist

Choosing a Dentist

The special dental and medical problems of the older patient make selection of a qualified dentist especially important. It is often a good idea to solicit advice from sources such as local dental schools or dental societies, nearby dentists, a knowledgeable friend or relative, or your personal physician. Certain names are likely to be repeated, and from this group you can then choose the dentist best suited to your special needs.

What to Expect of Your Dentist

The first visit to the dentist's office should include a thorough health history; a complete set of X rays to detect or rule out problems that are not visible on normal examination of the mouth; palpation of the soft tissues of the mouth, head, and neck to screen for cancer and other abnormalities; palpation of the joint connecting the jaw to the skull, and associated muscles; examination of gum tissues for periodontal disease; and inspection of the teeth for cavities, defective restoration, or poor position. The examination may also include a check of blood pressure and pulse for signs of medical problems that might impede dental work or require referral to a physician. A comfortable and convenient environment is also important for dental treatment.

The dentist should be committed to prevention as well as elimination of disease and should encourage the patient to cooperate in a preventive program. Periodic examinations should be scheduled for at least once each year.

To insure up-to-date care, the practitioner should routinely attend continuing education courses. While these tend to be costly, attendance indicates interest in professional improvement and concern for the patient.

Because dental fees vary, and the fee may have little connection with the quality of the service, the dentist should frankly and agreeably discuss treatment and fees from the very beginning. The patient has a right to be fully informed about the proposed treatment and possible alternatives.

The dentist should be willing to treat emergencies promptly and thoroughly, even if this requires seeing the patient outside of normal office hours. If the regular dentist is not available, a pre-arranged alternate should be accessible without delay.

Most dentists employ auxiliary personnel to improve the efficiency and economy of dental services much as a physician works with a nursing staff. Like the physician, the dentist performs the complex tasks that require a high degree of professional skill, while simpler procedures are handled by dental hygienists and dental assistants. The dental hygienist has had at least two years of college-level training, is licensed by the state, and is normally responsible for cleaning teeth, treating gums, and educating patients in self-care. The training of the dental assistant may vary from formal schooling at the college level to on-the-job training by the dentist. The assistant usually performs routine office chores, assists the dentist at chairside, and, depending on state laws, may also take X rays and work directly in the mouth.

A modern dental facility is usually a sign—but not a guarantee—of an up-to-date practitioner. A well organized and efficient office will provide for patient comfort and effective treatment, and will convey an impression of cleanliness and sterility. Most dentists today work while sitting, with the patient in a relaxed position in a reclining chair.

Because it is more difficult to chew well with fewer teeth, a good dentist avoids extraction and saves teeth whenever possible. It is especially important to save strategic teeth to serve as anchors for removable and fixed prosthetic replacements for missing teeth. Treatment complications may require the attention of a dental specialist.

Dental Specialties

The *periodontist* specializes in treating the tissues that support the teeth, that is, the surrounding bone and gums, and is trained in oral medicine, the study of oral diseases, and their treatment. Periodontal disease can be likened to a smoldering fire that insidiously consumes bone and healthy gum tissue. Symptoms are usually absent until the disease is in an advanced stage which may be painful. Fastidious oral hygiene and both preventive and corrective treatment are essential to prevent periodontal disease from becoming a recurring problem.

Periodontal treatment involves scraping away plaque and calculus from the teeth, adjusting the teeth to give an even bite, and surgical removal of diseased tissue. The surgical procedure causes only moderate discomfort, and should not make the patient unduly apprehensive.

The *orthodontist* (literally "teeth corrector") usually is associated with teenagers, braces, and poor bites. However, there is no age limit for orthodontic treatment, and in recent years more and more adults have come to accept braces to improve their appearance, or to reposition strategic teeth to give better support to replacements.

Endodontics—root canal treatment—makes it possible to save teeth that would otherwise be extracted because cavities had penetrated the nerve. The endodontist removes the infection and diseased tissue by cleaning out the nerve from the crown and root with fine instruments through a hole drilled in the back or top of the tooth. Once cleansed, the tooth begins to heal itself. The procedure usually requires more than one office visit and can be completed with little discomfort.

Occasionally a patient has a condition that defies restoration and is made worse by medical complications. Removal of teeth in such cases may require the special skills of an *oral surgeon*. An oral surgeon is trained to operate in all areas involving the mouth, jaws, and related structures, including biopsies, removal of cysts and mouth cancers, reduction of fractures, and other complex procedures.

In difficult cases requiring rebuilding the mouth, a *prosthodontist* may be consulted. A prosthodontist is a specialist skilled in complex rehabilitation of teeth which requires the design and replacement of appliances to replace missing teeth. Such services are normally both lengthy and costly.

The older patient who suffers from chronic dental disease and neglect will often require advanced dental treatment. The most common need is the repair, relining, or total replacement of full or partial dentures. Although the older patient may need such extensive dental treatment, it is important not to exceed an individual's tolerance level. Research has shown that "only those who are well oriented to their general needs, who are flexible in daily living, and who are essentially self-motivated and have adjusted well to the changes of old age should receive comprehensive dental care.'' Many patients, especially those who are institutionalized and advanced in years, are poor candidates for new dentures or major dental rehabilitation.

Common Medical Problems

Diabetes

The aging individual should be aware that medical disorders originating elsewhere can affect the mouth, and that oral disease can have a debilitating effect on general health. Diabetes is an example of a disease that can complicate mouth care.

A common disease in the elderly, diabetes is a metabolic disorder which prevents the body from using sugar properly. Classic symptoms include general malaise, weakness, weight loss, poor appetite, frequent urination, excessive thirst, and delayed or poor healing of injuries. Because diabetics have lowered resistance to infection, and their mouth tissues tend to deteriorate and peel away when irritated or injured, they do not respond well to dental treatment. Periodontal disease progresses much faster in diabetics than in other patients, and is usually more severe. If a diabetic needs gum surgery or tooth extraction, the dentist must take special precautions. Surgery must be coordinated with sugar balance in the controlled diabetic patient, and doses of antibiotic before and after surgery may be necessary to prevent infection. High doses of vitamins B and C help to promote healing.

Hypertension (High Blood Pressure)

Some dental procedures require the use of drugs or other medications that may adversely affect the hypertensive patient. It is important to inform the dentist if blood pressure is abnormally high so that necessary precautions can be taken. A hypertensive's blood pressure should be routinely monitored during dental treatment.

Rheumatic Fever, Heart Murmurs, Prosthetic Valves

If a dental patient has had rheumatic fever, has undergone heart surgery to install an artificial valve, or has an organic heart murmur, the dentist must exercise special care. Routine dental procedures can allow bacteria to enter the bloodstream, lodge in the heart valves, and cause endocarditis, a serious heart infection. This is prevented by administering a specific antibiotic before and after the dental procedure.

Debilitating Diseases

Arthritis, stroke, and Parkinson's disease complicate dental treatment and diminish patients' ability to care for themselves. Patients with these conditions often need help in keeping their mouths clean, and the use of an electric toothbrush or Water-Pic will usually be beneficial.

Constipation

One of the most common maladies in the elderly, constipation may be related to teeth problems. It has been found that patients with faulty dentures or chewing difficulty tend to avoid roughage and eat only soft foods. Properly constructed dentures improve the ability to chew and to eat necessary roughage, thus reducing or eliminating constipation.

Preventive Dentistry and Home Care

The maintenance or restoration of oral health is achieved in large part through preventive dentistry. However, dental professionals cannot do the job alone. In the prevention of disease, the patient plays a vital role by practicing good dental hygiene. Conscientious brushing and use of dental floss to remove the plaque are the primary elements in maintaining the health of the mouth.

Toothbrushing

Because the toothbrush is the principal instrument for regular removal of plaque, it is essential to choose the right type from the many different kinds that are marketed. A soft nylon brush with rounded ends is recommended. The soft bristles bend easily and get into the space between the teeth and gums so that they are effective in cleaning the area near the gumline. Also, a soft brush is less damaging to gum tissue than a medium or hard brush, so that vigorous brushers won't harm their teeth and gums. Instruction in the best brushing technique for each individual can be given by the dentist or dental hygienist.

Because bacteria tend to accumulate in the ridges and grooves of the tongue, mouth hygiene should include tongue brushing. This is done with the tongue extended. The sides of the bristles are placed on the back of the tongue and the brush is drawn forward with light pressure. The motion should be repeated three or four times.

Dental Floss

Research has established that toothbrushing alone fails to remove all plaque and that the use of dental floss immediately after brushing removes most remaining plaque. For this reason, floss is strongly recommended as part of the daily routine for plaque control.

Two kinds of floss—waxed and unwaxed—are available. Unwaxed floss is often recommended because its thinner thread permits it to slip between close teeth with little or no pressure. However, waxed floss is best when teeth or dental work shred or tear unwaxed floss.

Use of dental floss before brushing is best for most people because previous removal of plaque from surfaces between teeth permits the fluoride in toothpaste to reach these surfaces for cavity prevention. Flossing is simpler and easier when done before a mirror.

Other aids for removing plaque include white knitting yarn used like floss for wide spaces between teeth, cotton strips to clean the sides of teeth, and plastic floss holders for those who have limited finger dexterity. Still other aids may be recommended by the dentist or dental hygienist for use in especially difficult situations.

Care of Dentures and Bridgework

The success of a dental appliance depends heavily on the patient's daily cleaning and plaque control of remaining natural teeth. Cleaning needs and techniques vary with different types of appliances.

A fixed partial denture, or bridge, requires angular brushing and flossing of the bridge area to remove the plaque and debris that tend to collect under the bridge. Specially designed threaders made of nylon or plastic help to place floss under the bridge so that it can be used in the same manner as with natural teeth.

Full dentures need daily cleaning to remove plaque, stains, and debris. Three methods commonly used are rinsing under water after meals, brushing with water and a mild cleansing agent, and soaking the denture in a chemical detergent. Most denture wearers use immersion (soaking), brushing, or a combination of these methods. When full cleansing is impossible, rinsing after eating is suggested. Immersion cleaning has the advantage of reaching all surfaces of the denture and also reduces the danger of dropping it. It is especially helpful to handicapped individuals with limited ability to manage a brush.

Brushes designed for denture care are widely available. When brushing is the method selected, special care must be taken to avoid dropping the denture. Damage can be reduced by holding the denture over a sink lined with a wash cloth or towel to act as a cushion. All surfaces of the denture should be brushed with warm water and a mild soap, avoiding strenuous brushing that may scratch or alter the fit of the denture.

When the denture is removed for cleaning, attention must be given to the underlying tissue by rinsing the mouth and massaging the gum with fingertips or a soft brush. Massage helps to stimulate circulation and increases resistance to injury.

A loose or defective denture should always be brought to the attention of a professional; no attempt should be made to make repairs at home. A denture that has been properly fitted should not need pastes or adhesive powders to keep it in place. An ill-fitting denture can sometimes be relined by the dentist in a short office visit.

Immersion and brushing are also appropriate for cleaning partial dentures, with special attention to brushing. Since brushing clasps and other metal parts of dentures can damage fine toothbrushes, a brush designed to clean these parts is available.

Nutrition

Nutrition is a critical factor in the prevention of dental disease and in maintaining dental health. Restricting intake of sugar reduces acid production by bacteria, which in turn helps to minimize cavities and gum disease. Protein, vitamins, and other nutrients are vital to the health of gum tissue and bones, as well as to other tissues throughout the body. The gum tissue's resistance to disease can be reduced by deficiencies of vitamin B complex, vitamin C, and protein.

The consistency of foods is also a factor in prevention. Soft foods tend to cling to the teeth and gums, encouraging the buildup of debris, while fibrous foods help to clean away loose debris. Chewing stimulates circulation in mouth tissues.

Elderly individuals are often inclined to be careless with diet, consuming too much carbohydrates and not enough other essential nutrients. A balanced diet is important to all aspects of good health.

Fluorides

Fluoride is a mineral that is extremely effective in promoting resistance to dental decay. It is available from a variety of sources, including professional gels, mouth washes, tablets, toothpastes, and community water supplies.

Gum recession which exposes the root surfaces of the teeth is common in aging individuals and often leads to sensitivity of these surfaces. It has been found that fluoride reduces such sensitivity by mineralizing and hardening the affected parts of the teeth. The obvious benefits of fluoride make brushing with fluoridated toothpaste advisable for individuals of any age, but especially for those of advanced years.

General Considerations

Although older people tend to be more susceptible to dental diseases, many of these maladies can be prevented. It is also important to be well informed about the various available treatments. An informed consumer has a definite advantage in any marketplace, and dental care is no exception. Proper home care, good nutrition, and periodic dental visits can help to assure good oral health.

FOOT HEALTH

Neil J. Kanner, D.P.M., F.A.C.F.O.

*Associate Professor of Community Health, Pennsylvania College of Podiatric Medicine,
Consultant, Diabetes Treatment and Education Center, Pennsylvania Hospital, and
Philadelphia Veterans Administration Hospital*

The foot is probably the most neglected part of the human body. This can be verified by a stroll through the home remedy section of any pharmacy. The range and variety of such preparations reflect the neglect and mistreatment that are the common lot of the foot.

As a result of aging, common foot problems often tend to worsen, making good foot hygiene essential to the well-being of the elderly. Proper foot care can keep the aging individual moving about with ease. Inability to get around, to perform personal errands, and to visit friends or family are likely to cause depression and to impair the ability to cope successfully with normal daily stress. Such immobility may make the aging individual a burden to the family, and to society as well. While the ambulatory patient often remains self-sufficient, the non-ambulatory patient may require institutionalization. Also, inability to walk freely often brings a decline in well-being that may be irreversible.

Because many of the chronic diseases of the elderly appear first in the lower extremities, the podiatrist may be the first health professional to detect major medical problems. Chronic diseases such as arthritis, stroke, diabetes, peripheral vascular and cardiovascular conditions, kidney and liver disease—all can have ramifications in the lower extremities. It is therefore important both for detection of disease and for therapy that older people receive proper foot care.

Foot problems are common among the elderly for a number of reasons. As a weight-bearing organ, the foot is constantly subjected to injury. When the deleterious effects of aging are added, the foot is especially vulnerable to troublesome problems. Such effects may include a decrease in circulation, peripheral vascular changes which tend to weaken the bones, and atrophy of the skin and muscles. Also, the fat pad beneath the ball of the foot commonly shifts or deteriorates, making walking more difficult and often painful. Degenerative joint diseases can cause toe and other foot bone deformities. Pre-existing biomechanical imbalances tend to increase with aging.

The podiatrist often plays an important role in the health care of the aging individual. Because the foot is affected by so many diseases, the initial visit to the podiatrist will include a thorough physical examination and a medical and podiatric history. In some cases, both the podiatrist and the physician work together to treat medical foot problems. These problems may affect the skin, toenails, muscles, or bones and sometimes several areas at the same time.

Skin

Dryness and Itching

The sweat glands of the feet produce moisture, fats, and oils which moisten and lubricate the skin, making it soft and supple. With age, and especially with the onset of vascular and neurologic problems such as those that accompany diabetes mellitus, the number of sweat glands and the amount of secretions decline. The skin tends to become dryer and thinner, lose some of its hair and elasticity, and itch.

Itching induces scratching, and scratching the feet may break the skin, permitting bacteria commonly found on the feet to cause infection. Also, dry skin is brittle and cracks easily. The cracking of chapped skin also opens a path for bacterial infection. Heel fissures are a common problem among the elderly, especially when the blood supply is inadequate. Deepening of the normal skin creases can lead to cracking and the likelihood of both pain and infection.

Treatment of dry skin aims to replace lost moisture, fats, and oils by application of an emollient skin cream. The cream should be rubbed in well over all parts of the feet *except between the toes*. In severe cases, the feet should be soaked for five or ten minutes in lukewarm water, then patted almost dry before cream is applied. The remaining dampness will help to moisten the skin and allow the cream to penetrate faster.

Although many good creams are available, it should be kept in mind that price is not a reliable index of quality. Also, because of the variability of the human skin, a product that works well for one person may not be satisfactory for another. Thus, several trials with different brands of cream may be necessary before one is found that is adequate. Use of petrolatum (petroleum jelly) and lanolin should be avoided as these are basically greases. When applied, they coat the skin but do not replenish moisture or oil. While greasy skin appears to be soft and supple, removal of the coating will reveal skin as dry as it was before the grease was applied.

The heels should be generously covered with skin cream because of their tendency to crack easily as a result of persistent dryness. Occasionally, heel fissures may require additional therapy, including bath oil soaks, protective petrolatum gauze dressings, and heel cups.

If, after several weeks of regular applications of cream, the foot has failed to respond satisfactorily, a professional examination is in order. Many skin conditions such as dryness, scaling, and peeling may be more than just dry skin. A break in the skin in particular is a sign to consult a podiatrist or physician without delay, because it may be associated with circulation changes which reduce the amount of blood reaching the foot and render it more vulnerable to infection. Such infection is much more easily prevented than treated.

The skin between the toes—toe webs—is usually moist, no matter how dry the rest of the foot may appear. It is important to keep the toe webs as dry as possible at all times, and this is most easily done by daily use of foot powder. Ordinary cornstarch is best because it absorbs more moisture than the talcum powder used in commercial preparations. It is also much less expensive.

Fungal Infections

The fungal infection *tinea pedis,* commonly known as athlete's foot, is a frequent complaint of the elderly. It is caused by a parasitic fungus closely related to bread mold, and is found everywhere. Contrary to popular belief, athlete's foot is not a sign of poor foot hygiene, and should not be a cause for embarrassment. However, while the fungus is widespread, some people are immune because of an unknown factor in the skin which prevents the fungus from growing.

The fungus feeds on a protein, *keratin,* supplied by dead cells on the top layer of skin. For this reason, athlete's foot is invariably confined to the outer skin. Our concern arises from its tendency to increase the risk of infection by breaking the skin, either directly through the effect of the fungus on the skin, or indirectly by causing itching which provokes scratching.

The first, or acute, stage of athlete's foot is characterized by cracks and wet, softened skin between the toes. Small, clear blisters may appear which leave a pattern of rings when they break and give off a strong yeasty or musty odor. In the chronic stage, circular scaly patches develop on the skin.

Treatment of athlete's foot is based on depriving the fungus of the warm, dark, damp environment (like that inside shoes and socks) it needs to grow. Moisture is kept to a minimum by the regular use of foot powder, wearing natural materials (cotton socks) on the feet, and exposing the feet to the air whenever possible. After competent diagnosis, which may be confirmed by culturing and microscopic examination of skin scrapings, medication may also be applied.

While the most effective medications for treating athete's foot require prescriptions, over-the-counter commercial preparations such as Desenex and Tinactin are also useful. Both come in liquid, cream, and powder forms. However, it should be emphasized that any persisting foot problem should be brought to the attention of a podiatrist or physician to insure proper diagnosis and treatment.

Corns and Calluses

The formation of a corn or a callus is simply the skin's reaction to friction and pressure. When such friction or pressure persists over a period of time, the outer layer of the skin thickens as a protective measure to prevent irritation of the tissues underneath the affected area. The same thickening (*hyperkeratosis*) takes place in the formation of both corns and calluses, but the locations differ. Calluses usually appear on the bottom of the feet, and corns, which are much thicker than calluses, cover smaller areas on the tops of the toes.

Treatment of corns and calluses is normally confined to determining and removing the cause of friction or pressure. Pain (''My corn is killing me.'') does not result from the thickening of the skin's outer layer, but rather from an inflammatory reaction beneath the corn or callus. Some inflammations (*capsulitis* or *bursitis*) may have to be treated with injection of an anesthetic and a corticosteroid solution. Regular surgical trimming of the corn or callus and the use of cushioning pads will also relieve pain and discomfort. Pads made to be worn in the shoe also help to make walking pain-free for elderly people with such foot problems.

Self-treatment with commercial corn or callus removers is hazardous. These are acids which digest the thickened skin. Since their action is not restricted to corns and calluses, they can also burn healthy skin. Picking at corns and calluses or cutting them with a razor or scissors should also be avoided because they can break the skin and result in infection.

The source of friction or pressure that generates corns and calluses may be external, for example, a tight or otherwise improperly fitted shoe. It may also be internal, an abnormality in the foot itself such as hammertoes, rotated toes, bunion deformities, and bending of the big toe over the others (*hallux valgus*), or a deforming disease such as rheumatoid or degenerative arthritis.

Soft Corns

Soft corns are found between rather than on top of the toes. They are identical to other corns and calluses except that they absorb the moisture always present between the toes and swell and soften. Treatment is the same as for other corns and calluses.

Plantar Warts

The plantar wart (*verruca plantaris*) is a virus-induced benign tumor that grows on the bottom of the foot. Physicians sometimes confuse it with a deep-seated corn or other persistent growth on the sole, but when they remove it, it returns again and again. Although the plantar wart usually goes away by itself without treatment in two to five years, especially in the young, larger warts can be painful and interfere with walking. They must then be chemically or surgically removed.

The plantar wart is most often found in the young, but also afflicts the elderly for whom it can represent a more serious problem, particularly if it grows large enough to require surgical removal. Since older people tend to have poorer circulation to the foot, the surgical wound may heal very slowly because of an inadequate blood supply to the injured tissue.

Ulceration

Foot ulcers can have serious consequences for older people, making it difficult to walk and possibly requiring hospitalization, surgery, and, in the most severe cases, amputation. Ulcers may develop under a corn or callus if the affected tissues are not receiving a sufficient supply of blood. The elderly are especially susceptible because a reduced blood supply to the feet is a common effect of aging. The susceptibility may be increased by neurological and pathological factors, which also often accompany aging, that dull the sensation of temperature change and pain. Thus, the aging individual may not feel the rubbing and pressure that precede the ulceration and consequently fail to take corrective action that might prevent it. Systemic conditions such as diabetes and arteriosclerosis, which can seriously reduce the blood supply to the feet, tend to promote the development of ulcers and rapidly spreading infection.

It is essential that treatment of foot ulcers by the podiatrist or physician be aggressive. The ulceration is thoroughly cleaned, infected tissue cut away, and cultures taken to identify the infecting bacteria so that an effective antibiotic can be prescribed. When the ulcer has been caused by excessive pressure on a bony area of the foot, all pressure must be removed. No therapy and no amount of antibiotic will effect a cure where pressure is sustained.

Sweating and Odor

Although older people are more likely to have dry than sweaty feet, some do have the problem of excessive perspiration. Bacterial breakdown of the abundant fats and oils produced by the overactive sweat glands produces a characteristic odor. Treatment consists of keeping the foot as dry as possible through the use of foot powder (cornstarch works well) and cotton socks or stockings. Application of a solution of 10 to 15 percent formalin in rose water will also help. If excessive perspiration is caused by nervousness, a mild sedative or tranquilizer may be beneficial. The odor will diminish with reduced sweating.

Toenails

While the tips of fingernails may be cut in a rounded arc because the fingers do not carry weight, toenails should always be cut straight across. This keeps the nail from growing into the skin of the toe and causing inflammation and swelling. If the toenail is cut round, the pointed corners between the front and the sides grows against the skin, eventually punctures it, and creates the characteristic ingrown toenail. Ingrown toenails can also develop from abnormally shaped nails or from any other deformity that causes the nail to rub, irritate, and inflame the skin. An ingrown toenail should be treated by a podiatrist. Neglect or improper self-treatment can lead to serious infection and needless pain and discomfort.

The healthy toenail is thin and flexible, with a slight curvature at the edges where it meets the nail grooves. With age, toenails tend to harden and, in some cases, to thicken, and so become more difficult to cut. Soaking the feet in lukewarm water will usually help soften the nail and make cutting easier.

Thickened toenails can also result from injury, as when the toe is stubbed or a heavy weight dropped on it. Such thickening is a cause for concern because the increased pressure on the nail bed may lead to ulceration.

Various fungal infections thicken, whiten, and embrittle the nail and loosen it from the nail bed. The infection can serve as a reservoir to contaminate the skin, and the thickened nail can contribute to ulceration of the nail bed. The nail may also catch on a sock, stocking, or bed sheet and be pulled away from the skin.

Treatment consists of trimming away the deformed toenail and applying therapy to the nail bed as needed. A culture will determine the organism causing the infection and indicate specific medication to combat it.

Muscle and Bone Abnormalities

Foot discomfort in the elderly individual is often due to abnormally high weight-bearing stresses and deviations from the foot's normal anatomy. Most of such complaints fall into one of three categories: structural, functional, and a combination of both.

Structural abnormalities can generate excessive friction and pressure, as when a hammertoe rubs the inside of a shoe. Twisted toes, enlarged bunions, or a big toe bent to the side can cause pain in weight-bearing areas. Destructive diseases such as rheumatoid and osteoarthritis can deform bones and joints. Also, structural losses such as atrophy of the fat pad at the ball of the foot can lead to local pain.

When functional problems are the source of pain, the foot structure may be normal, but excessive movement and associated stress and strain can cause inflammations such as *tendinitis* (tendons), *myositis* (muscles), *fascitis* (tissue covering the muscles), *bursitis* (lubricating sac), and *capsulitis* (ligament sacs around the joints). Painful heels—whether related to bursitis under the bone or to heel-bone spurs—are ultimately due to muscle movement pulling too much at the heel bone. Pain in the bones over the ball of the foot is usually due to inflammation in the surrounding area or to bursitis in the joints that connect the toes to the main part of the foot.

In many cases, problems are both structural and functional, and it is difficult to determine which came first. It is generally believed today that abnormal function is the primary cause, especially in the feet of older people.

For many years, various structural deformities were thought to be caused by improperly fitting shoes. For example, when the big toe is bent over the others toward the little toe (*hallux valgus* deformity), it looks as if a tight shoe has squeezed the toe into its abnormal position. However, careful study has indicated that abnormal function over a period of years gradually shifts the foot's bones and leads to pain in later life. Some podiatrists now believe that persistent muscle pull is the major cause of hammertoes and other deformities.

Although shoes may not cause many structural deformities, they can aggravate them. For example, a hammertoe that rests at a 45-degree angle on top of its neighbor is no problem to a bare foot but will rub against the inside of a shoe and raise a corn. Similarly, a bunion deformity will cause a callus or bursitis only if the bulge is irritated by friction with a shoe.

Before treatment of a foot problem, X rays should be taken with the person standing so the feet are bearing weight. This helps to determine the extent of bone deformity and joint involvement. Podiatric examination of the foot in action helps to reveal how much functional abnormality contributes to the symptoms.

Initial therapy should be conservative, including removal of hard corns or calluses, the use of cushioning pads or special shoe inserts (orthoses) to relieve or redistribute pressures. If a deformity is too gross for ordinary shoes, shoes can be specially molded to fit the contours of the foot. Injection of a corticosteroid is beneficial for severe inflammations such as bursitis, capsulitis, and tendinitis. Surgical intervention is considered only if more conservative measures fail to give satisfactory foot comfort.

Footwear

Because shoes are made on a last, and last sizes vary with different manufacturers, shoes should be bought by fit not by size. A shoe that does not fit comfortably when tried on for the first time should not be purchased, nor should the shoe be stretched or pads added in attempts to make a proper fit. It is best to purchase shoes at the end of the day to allow for normal swelling that occurs with the day's activities. Shoes made of natural material, such as leather, are preferable to synthetics or plastics. Natural material permits the free passage of air and moisture, while synthetics tend to keep the foot hot and damp. Shoe soles should be at least quarter-inch thick leather, and older women should select broad heels to provide stability. Wedges and padding can be added to increase stability and to help the gait. The wearing of flimsy slippers at home is to be avoided because a good supportive shoe is needed throughout the day.

"Orthopedic shoe" is a much misused term. Shoes alone cannot correct a deformity, but can only attempt to accommodate it. Individuals should have a thorough podiatric examination by a trained professional before purchasing any "corrective" shoe or device to be added to the shoe. The shoe salesman is *not* competent to diagnose a foot problem or to advise about proper treatment.

RADIOLOGY

William J. Tuddenham, M.D.

Professor of Radiology, Pennsylvania Hospital

Radiology is the medical specialty that deals with the use of X rays and gamma rays in the diagnosis and treatment of disease. It plays an important role in virtually every branch of medical practice. About seven of every ten Americans will have some sort of radiologic examination during the coming year, and about one of every four medical decisions is said to be based on radiologic diagnosis. Nevertheless, radiologic practice is not well understood by the general public, perhaps because it is so different from the popular idea of "bedside medicine." Some explanation of the nature and effects of X rays (and other radiation) and of common radiologic procedures may be useful.

Nature and Effects of X Rays

What Are X Rays?

X rays are part of a broad spectrum of electromagnetic energy that also includes light, radio waves, gamma rays, and other forms. The forms differ only in frequency. However, frequency is related to energy and determines the penetrating power and effect on biological tissues and other matter. X rays and gamma rays are more energetic (higher in frequency) and more penetrating than visible light.

Effect on Matter in General

When X rays pass through a substance, parts of the beam collide with electrons surrounding the nuclei of the atoms in the beam's path. A collision knocks an electron out of position, electrically unbalancing (ionizing) the atom, and also weakens the X ray and deflects it out of the forward beam. More collisions occur when X rays pass through solid muscle or bone, in which atoms and their electrons are more closely packed, than through a gas, in which atoms are more widely scattered. More collisions occur in thicker than in thinner layers of the same material, regardless of composition. Also, atoms of metallic elements like calcium contain more electrons, and therefore absorb more X rays by collision, than do atoms of elements like hydrogen, carbon, nitrogen, and oxygen (human tissues are largely made of these elements).

Since electrons play a major role in the attachments between atoms that determine the structure and properties of all substances, displacement of electrons disturbs the structure. Sometimes this is useful, for example, in photographic film. The disturbance of the substances in the film by collisions with X rays remains as a darkening after the film is developed. This indicates the relative intensity of the beam and creates the conventional X-ray picture (radiograph). In complex biologic tissues, however, the effect is likely to be harmful, but the harm depends very much on the amount of exposure among other things.

Effect on Human Tissue

Since radiation hazards are very much in the news, let us consider the effects on human tissues of the small doses of ionizing radiation used in diagnostic radiology. Some understanding of cell processes is necessary.

Virtually all cells of the human body periodically reproduce themselves by cell division. Normally, the process is self-controlled, new cells merely replacing dead cells to maintain a biologic status quo. The structure and function of the newly created (daughter) cells are determined by the sequence of chemical structural units in the long string (the famous double helix) that makes up the molecule DNA. The sequence is a code transmitted from the dividing parent cell to each of the daughter cells that enables them to exactly duplicate the parent.

Radiation collisions can interfere with the mechanics of cell division so that the transmission of DNA is defective. They can break DNA chains so that the pieces become scrambled when the breaks are healed, alter chemical linkages so that the sequence of units is changed, and otherwise vary the genetic code so that the daughter cells develop different characteristics (mutations) from those of the parent cells. Virtually all mutations are undesirable, and geneticists believe that the survival of the human species may be threatened if the frequency of mutations is markedly increased. Since radiation can cause mutations, excessive exposure of people who may later have children is regarded as potentially hazardous to mankind as a whole.

The problem must be seen in perspective. We are all constantly exposed to a low level of ionizing radiation from naturally radioactive materials in our environment (soil, bricks) and cosmic rays from outer space. Also, mutations can occur spontaneously and can be induced by certain drugs and chemicals. Thus, medical radiography is only one of several sources of possible mutations. However, it is the only radiation we can readily control, and the medical profession and the government are working together to minimize exposure in medical practice.

Until very recently, it was assumed that genetic changes in the cells of an adult (other than germ cells from which children may be born) probably did no harm if the exposure level was low. Some scientists now argue that any amount of radiation, however small, may cause changes in body cells that develop into certain diseases and shorten lives after many subsequent generations of cell division. One of the suspected diseases is cancer, which is ironic, since radiation is one of the most effective cancer treatments now available.

Thus, even small doses of radiation may have undesirable effects on human tissues, especially in young adults and children. The risks are very small, but probably not zero, for older adults. For these reasons, the radiologist follows two important rules in planning and performing radiologic studies:

1. Make sure the potential benefit exceeds the hazard. The decision is usually easy with older patients because the hazards are almost negligible and the importance of prompt diagnosis and treatment is indisputable.

2. Expose the patient to as little radiation as possible consistent with the diagnostic objectives.

X-Ray Equipment

How Are X Rays Made?

An X-ray tube is a glass-and-metal vacuum bulb, similar to an over-size old-fashioned radio tube. Near one end, a hot tungsten filament emits negatively charged electric particles (electrons) which are attracted to a positively charged metal target near the other end by a very high voltage difference (40,000 to 150,000 volts). When the speeding electrons are halted by the target, their energy is converted into heat (the target temperature rises) and X rays. Since the X rays radiate in all directions from the target, the tube is encased in a heavy metal housing which allows rays to emerge only through a small window. The rays are further confined by a metal cone (collimator) so that a useful beam is obtained with a well-defined width and direction.

The high voltages require relatively massive auxiliary equipment, mainly a heavy voltage-raising transformer. An X-ray machine also includes control circuits, meters, protective devices, and means for forming and sometimes displaying the X-ray image.

How X-ray Images are Formed

When X rays pass through the human body, the beam that emerges varies in intensity from point to point depending on the nature and thickness of the tissues through which each part of the beam has passed. Historically, the first method used to convert this variation into a viewable image was fluoroscopy. When the beam was allowed to strike a screen coated with fluorescent crystals, the crystals glowed with a brightness that varied with the beam intensity. Where the beam had lost little energy because it had passed through only open space or soft tissue, the screen was bright; where the beam had lost more energy in bone and denser tissue, the screen was dimmer or dark. Since the display was continuous, it permitted not only a view of internal organs but also a study of their motion (heartbeat, stomach contraction, joint movement).

One drawback to fluoroscopy was that the screen gave off little light and had to be viewed in a darkened room. Today, the screen can be replaced by the photoelectrically sensitive surface of an image amplifier tube. The brightness is then electronically magnified thousands of times and displayed like a television picture in normal room light. Although fluoroscopy is still used in radiology, it is further limited because it creates no permanent record and does not allow comparison of images from different times to follow the progress of disease. The image amplifier system permits recording on movie film or video tape (with instant replay like a sports broadcast), a process called cinefluorography which is important for diagnosing some forms of heart disease.

The more traditional and most common method of obtaining a permanent X-ray record is to allow the emerging beam to strike a sheet of photographic film encased in a box called a cassette that seals out light but not X rays. Although the film must be processed in a darkroom, automated processing now takes only 90 seconds, including drying, and the method produces the best diagnostic images. Like the negative in ordinary photography, the X-ray film is darkest where the beam was brightest. In a chest X ray, for example, the air-filled soft lung tissue appears relatively black (the beam passes through almost intact), denser heart and mid-chest structures are gray, and bones and other calcifications are nearly white. This is the reverse of the fluoroscope, which is more like a photographic positive, or print. X-ray film is used in the vast majority of all radiologic examinations.

Contrast Media

Although lungs, bones, and muscles (including the heart) absorb X rays differently enough to be distinguishable in a chest radiograph, this is not true of the soft tissues of the digestive organs, urinary tract, and blood vessels in the abdomen. To make such organs more distinct, substances are introduced that are relatively opaque to X rays.

Powdered barium sulfate suspended in water and swallowed or given as an enema makes the esophagus, stomach, small intestine, and large bowel visible on an X ray. Since there is no direct access to the gallbladder, a compound containing radiopaque atoms is swallowed or injected, and the body's own metabolism is allowed to concentrate the X-ray absorbing material in the gallbladder. Similarly, a substance known to be excreted through the kidneys is combined with an iodine compound and administered intravenously to reveal the details of the urinary tract. Iodinated substances can also be introduced into the blood stream through needles and catheters to make arteries and veins of particular organs stand out. By a similar principle, the internal structure of the brain was once (and occasionally still is) imaged by injections of air into the ventricles (the air inflates spaces so they appear less opaque than before). The air, barium sulfate, and iodinated compounds are called contrast media (or agents), and their use with X rays is called contrast radiography.

Equipment Variations

While all X-ray units have the same basic elements, they are arranged differently to facilitate different types of examination.

General Radiography. In the most common applications, the X-ray tube is suspended from the ceiling over a fixed table. The film cassette is slipped into a tray under the table.

Fluoroscopy. For digestive tract studies, the table can be tilted to permit examination with the patient either horizontal or erect. The X-ray tube is placed under the table, and a fluoroscopic screen or image amplifier system is mounted above the table. The image may be viewed directly on the amplifier display or scanned by a television camera for display on a remote monitor. The room may also have a ceiling-mounted X-ray tube.

Chest Radiography. Most radiology departments have special equipment for chest X rays with a tube that emits a horizontal beam, a vertical cassette holder, and no table.

Skull Radiography. Head bones are exceptionally complex, and precise positioning is essential for accurate diagnosis. A special head stand has been developed in which the cassette tray is mounted on a vertical column, an extension arm pivots the X-ray tube about the cassette tray, and both tube and tray can be independently tilted precisely to any angle.

Dental Radiography. Compact, movable X-ray units that operate at relatively low voltages have been designed specially for examination of jaws and teeth.

Mammography. Compact, low voltage, vertical X-ray units are designed specially to permit positioning and compression of the female breast and accentuation of important shadows in the radiograph. The tube head can be rotated through an arc around the subject to vary the viewpoint of the radiograph, and the tube may contain a molybdenum instead of a tungsten target.

Sectional Radiography. Since X rays cannot be focused as light can, it is difficult to distinguish between structures or abnormalities that lie above or below each other in the X-ray path. Special equipment called a tomograph helps to overcome this problem. It consists of a lever arm attached to a fixed table, with an X-ray tube at one end of the arm and a film cassette at the other. The lever arm pivots about a point that can be adjusted to lie in the same plane as the area of interest in the patient's body. As the arm revolves during an exposure, the tube and cassette move in an arc, always facing each other at opposite ends of a diameter with the patient in between. The radiograph shows only the desired plane in sharp detail, isolating the imaginary slice of tissue from the blurred areas above and below it. A machine based on a similar principle takes panoramic views of the jaws and teeth.

Vascular Radiography. A radiographic study of the arteries and veins of a particular organ, accentuated by injection of a contrast medium, must be taken in short exposures because the blood flow soon sweeps the medium out of the target area. This is done with rapid serial film changers instead of standard cassette trays. The changer either advances the film between exposures (as in a movie camera) or shifts the cassette position to permit exposures at intervals of a fraction of a second. Special tables are usually employed so that fluoroscopic observation can be used to guide placement of the catheter through which the contrast medium is introduced into the blood vessel under examination. X-ray tubes must also be specially constructed to withstand the great heat generated by a rapid series of X-ray pulses.

Computerized Imaging. The most recent technical advance in radiology is the computerized (sometimes called computer-assisted) tomographic (CT or CAT) scanner (Figure 1). In this device, the subject lies on a table which passes through the hole in a large ring. The X-ray tube moves around the ring, always pointing toward the center through the subject at an X-ray detector at the opposite end of the ring diameter. The tube position is changed in small steps and many successive exposures are made with a thin pencil of X-rays, each at a different angle but in the same plane of the subject's body. The X-ray ring can be moved in small steps along the table to examine different body sections and can also be tilted to change the angle of the plane. A computer processes the large

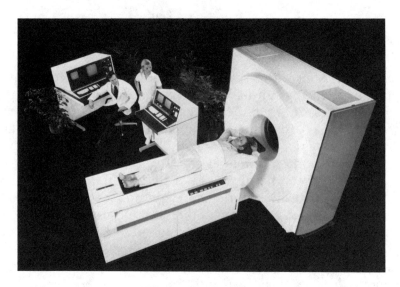

Figure 1. CT or CAT Scan. Sliding table top is used to position patient within "doughnut" housing where a rotating pencil-like beam of X rays passes through a thin "slice" of the patient's body at all angles. A computer transforms the multiple exposure into a detailed cross section displayed on the TV-like screens and permanently recorded on film.

amount of information and converts it into a screen display and film record of a thin cross section of the subject's body. The system reveals details previously inaccessible without surgery.

Other Imaging Systems

Since the X-ray beam passes through the body, the taking of X rays is also known as transmission radiography. Internal organs can also be studied by placing radioactive substances in them and detecting the emitted gamma rays. This is called emission or gamma-ray imaging.

Emission Imaging

The substances most commonly used for emission imaging are short-lived radioactive forms (isotopes) of iodine, technetium, and gallium. They are chosen for the convenience of the gamma rays they emit, the absence of toxicity and side effects in the concentrations used, and their short life which minimizes exposure to radiation. For example, the technetium isotope emits little radiation 24 hours after injection. The isotopes may be incorporated in drugs or in substances that normal body processes concentrate in the organs or tissues to be studied.

The images are formed and recorded by means of a gamma-ray, or Anger, camera or a rectilinear scanner. In both, fluorescent crystals emit light when struck by gamma rays. The sensitive surface of a gamma-ray camera is large enough to produce the image of an entire organ, and the patient and camera remain stationary while the image is being recorded. The sensitive surface of a scanner is small and must be moved back and forth over the stationary patient until the organ of interest has been "scanned" and the image recorded. Although the gamma-ray camera has become more popular because of its greater speed and resolution, rectilinear scanning has the advantage that its image has exactly the same size as the scanned organ. This is helpful, for example, in thyroid studies where the gland location and size of a contained nodule are important factors in determining treatment.

Emission images are usually displayed on a television-like screen. They are much less detailed than X-ray transmission images, but do show specific organs by themselves. Also, since the distribution of the radioactive isotopes in the body is related to the activity of the organs, emission images give functional information not available from conventional X rays. The lungs, liver, thyroid gland, bones, and brain are among the organs most commonly studied by emission imaging.

Ultrasonography

In recent years, an imaging technique called ultrasonography has been developed (Figure 2). It is based on a sound-echo system like that of sonar used to track enemy submarines and does not involve ionizing radiation. High-frequency, inaudible sound pulses, projected into the body through a probe (the transducer) pressed against the skin, reflect from boundaries between different tissues and are received by the same probe acting as a receiver. The location and timing of the echos are converted electronically into a visual display of internal organs. The technique can distinguish between a fluid-filled cyst, which does not cause pronounced echos, and a solid tumor, which does. Like fluoroscopy, it can also display movement. Since sound does not travel efficiently through air, the device is not useful for lung studies. The images are also not as detailed as a conventional X ray. However, they contribute other unique and useful information because they derive from a different principle. Because the relatively weak sound signals are considered harmless to the developing fetus, ultrasonography is widely used in obstetrics.

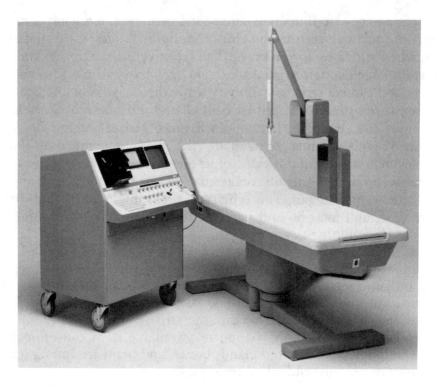

Figure 2. Ultrasonograph. Probe on end of traveling arm transmits high-frequency, inaudible sound pulses into the body and receives echoes reflected by changes in tissue such as the boundaries of organs. As probe is moved over the body surface, electronic circuits convert the echoes into an image of the internal anatomy displayed on the viewer screen. The image can also be recorded on film.

The Radiologic Patient: What to Expect

Now let's look at what happens when you, the patient, are to be examined by X-ray or other imaging procedure. Almost all X-ray departments (whether in a hospital or private office) schedule some examinations in advance, usually those requiring the participation of a physician or the availability of a special piece of equipment. Most often these are gastrointestinal studies (upper GI's), barium enemas, kidney studies (IVP's), gallbladder examinations, and tomograms.

Your personal physician may make the appointment or leave it up to you. Make sure you know who will do it. It can be frustrating to report for your examination and discover you are not expected and can't be taken. Also, many radiographic studies require advance preparation, particularly barium enemas and upper GI, kidney, and gallbladder studies. If scheduled for such studies, you should be instructed how to prepare yourself and which drugs, if any, to take.

X rays that can be completed quickly in a private office need much more time in a crowded hospital department. A simple chest X ray may take 30–45 minutes, a spine study will take an hour or more, and a half day must be allowed for GI (upper tract and barium enema), urinary tract (IVP), and gallbladder (cholecystogram) studies. Hasty rearrangement of an already tight schedule to accommodate a surprise patient may only result in patient anxiety and an inadequate study that will have to be repeated.

Because you will usually have to partially or completely disrobe, wear clothing you can slip out of easily. A tight girdle interferes with lung studies and must be removed even for a chest X ray. Rings, necklaces, bracelets, and other metal jewelry worn in the area being X-rayed must also be removed because they can obscure important clinical details. Since they are easily misplaced, it's better to leave them home. X rays will not damage a watch so you can wear one unless your wrist is to be examined.

Most likely you will want your insurance company or Medicare to pay the bill, so make sure you have your identifying numbers with you. Some radiologists may insist that you pay the bill and then have the insurance company repay you, but others will be happy to bill the third party, especially if it is Medicare.

The first one you see when you arrive for your appointment is the receptionist who not only greets you but also begins the record-keeping process that insures reports of X-ray results to your physician and accurate filing of information for future retrieval. Details will include your name, address, birth date, referring physician, and others such as your identifying insurance numbers. Some may seem irrelevant, but they are usually intended to add identifying features to your radiographs that will distinguish them from those of other people with the same or similar names. Give your full and correct names. Nicknames or the use of a first name on one visit and a middle name on another can play havoc with record-keeping systems. The receptionist will also answer questions about how much the X rays will cost.

An escort, who may also be a technologist, will show you to a dressing room, tell you which clothing to take off, and give you a gown to wear that will not interfere with the X rays. In some facilities, you lock the room and take the key with you. In others, you store your clothes in a locker and free the room for the next patient. In either case, take your purse or wallet with you!

You are then directed to a waiting area from which you go to the examining room when your name is called. Don't respond unless your name is called. Some patients who answered to the wrong name have been given the wrong examination.

After the X rays are taken, you will usually be asked to remain in the waiting area for any of several reasons: The technologist must check the films for technical quality, and may repeat some exposures if necessary. The radiologist may interpret the films immediately and request more to clarify a tentative diagnosis. The radiologist may wish to perform a limited physical examination while you are in the waiting area (you may also be examined before the X rays are taken). If your physician has requested an immediate interpretation (called a "stat"), the radiologist will discuss the results on the telephone and may order additional films after consultation. Do not leave until the technologist or radiologist tells you the studies are complete. More than one examination may have been ordered. If you are scheduled for another examination on a later day, confirm the schedule and preparatory instructions before you leave.

Unless your physician has requested an immediate interpretation, your X rays may not be studied for some hours after you leave, and the results may not reach your physician for several days. Allow at least a few days before calling your physician about the findings.

Specific Procedures

General Radiography

Skeletal (skull, spine, extremities, joints). These studies are usually not scheduled in advance since they do not require special preparation or equipment. However, if you were given barium sulfate for a gastrointestinal examination not too long ago, tell the technologist since it could prevent examination of your lower spine. You remove clothing over the area to be X-rayed. You don't disrobe for a skull examination, but must remove hair pins, jewelry such as earrings, and dentures.

For most of these examinations you will lie on a table under the X-ray tube and over the film, but for skull and cervical spine examinations, you may sit in front of a vertical film holder. A cast or splint on an injured arm or leg may have to be removed to obtain satisfactory radiographs. Two exposures usually suffice for long bones; joints may entail four to six exposures; and the skull and spine require up to six and sometimes more. Each exposure requires only a second or two, but careful positioning takes time. Thirty to forty-five minutes will be needed for arm or leg examination, and up to an hour for a skull or spine study. There are no aftereffects. X rays of the sinuses, mastoids, mandible, and facial bones require a procedure similar to skull examinations and are often combined with them.

Abdominal. Studies of soft abdominal tissues are conducted in much the same manner as a lumbar spine examination. They may sometimes consist of a single radiograph in a horizontal, face-up position, but often include both horizontal and vertical patient positions achieved with a tilting table. Additional views may include the patient lying on one side in front of a vertical film holder with a horizontally directed X-ray beam. Such studies help to detect gallstones, kidney stones, and sources of acute intestinal problems such as obstruction.

Chest. Chest examinations are usually not scheduled and require no preparation. You usually disrobe to the waist, but may sometimes have to undress completely, for example, if a tight girdle prevents full aeration of the lungs. You stand facing a wall-mounted vertical film holder, and the X-ray beam is directed horizontally from behind. Individual exposures require only fractions of a second and the entire study can usually be completed within 15 minutes. Because chest radiographs are the most sensitive and informative of all X-ray studies, they may be taken to detect early disease before symptoms have appeared. Survey studies in asymptomatic people up to age 50 usually consist of a single view; after 50, front and side views are usually exposed. In symptomatic patients or those with known disease, a chest examination may entail as many as four or five exposures. In some cases, the patient may swallow barium paste to outline the esophagus as an aid in studying heart problems. Chest X rays cause no aftereffects.

Mammography. Breast examinations are usually scheduled in advance because they are performed with a special machine designed for this single purpose. In most cases, the patient disrobes to the waist, sits in front of the machine, and the X-ray tube is moved to produce films at right angles. The breast is usually compressed during the exposure, causing some minor discomfort. Also, a small metallic marker may be fastened to each breast with transparent tape. Mammograms, like chest films, may be employed in asymptomatic patients in an attempt to detect disease at a very early stage. Mammography is one of the most effective weapons available against breast cancer and causes no aftereffects.

Contrast Radiography

Studies of abdominal organs differ in several respects from general radiographic procedures. They are most often conducted by the radiologist with the aid of a technician, and usually involve patient preparation such as the administration of a contrast agent. They also extend over a period of time and may have minor aftereffects.

Upper Gastrointestinal Series. This is probably the most common special X-ray study. It covers the esophagus (gullet), stomach, and duodenum, the first portion of the small intestine. It is performed to investigate a wide variety of indications and is particularly helpful for diagnosis of ulcer and hiatus hernia. Patient preparation is abstention from food or fluids after midnight before the day of the examination (food or fluid in the stomach can obscure evidence of disease). You disrobe completely for the examination and drink barium, a chalky fluid with a rather unpleasant consistency usually made more palatable with fruit flavoring. A tilting table is normally used to permit both horizontal and vertical patient positions. Ten to fifteen exposures may be made depending on the findings.

You normally wait following completion of the study until the films have been reviewed. The radiologist may request delayed films 30 minutes or more after a fluoroscopic examination. If an examination of the entire small bowel is needed, you drink another glass of barium, and radiographs are exposed and fluoroscopy performed at intervals until the barium has progressed through the entire length of the small bowel. This may require as little as 30 minutes or as much as four hours. Most people have no significant after effects, but barium tends to be constipating, and a mild cathartic such as milk of magnesia may be helpful for those who need relief.

Barium Enema. For examining the colon or large bowel, the barium suspension is introduced into the colon as an enema rather than administered orally. In this procedure, preparation of the patient is very important to the success of the study because all fecal residue must be eliminated from the colon to prevent defects in the barium shadow that simulate disease. If preparation is inadequate, definitive diagnosis is not possible. For this reason, radiologists apply vigorous catharsis. Some prefer castor oil while others use salt solutions as cathartics. Most suggest tap water enemas, and some insist on a low residue diet for a day or two before the study. Also, it is important not to eat anything or drink coffee prior to the examination since these stimulate peristalsis and may defeat the most careful preparation. To avoid the need to repeat the study, it is essential to follow the radiologist's directions meticulously. However, even the most careful preparation occasionally fails to cleanse the colon adequately, and a second examination is then necessary.

You disrobe completely for this study and lie face up on the X-ray table. An enema is administered, and the radiologist watches the flow of barium into the colon on the image amplifier. You are turned from side to side to open up bowel convolutions and several spot films are taken. At the conclusion of the study, the technologist usually takes additional radiographs (for better detail) with a ceiling-mounted tube. You may feel some cramping during the examination due to the distention of the colon. On request, the radiologist will stop the enema until the discomfort subsides. If you have trouble retaining an enema, the physician will order the use of a tip with a little balloon to help you. After the study, you are escorted to a private toilet to evacuate the enema fluid.

Occasionally, the radiologist will introduce air into the colon along with barium for double contrast. This is somewhat time consuming, requires rigorous preparation, and is likely to cause more discomfort than a conventional barium enema. For some problems, however, specifically the possible presence of polyps, it may be more revealing than a conventional barium enema. If preparation for a conventional enema has been adequate, an air study is seldom necessary.

In some facilities, the study may be performed by a technologist without the direction of a fluoroscopist. Since the technologist can only guess at the distribution of the barium within the patient's body, such studies are usually not of diagnostic quality. The technique is not considered adequate by most radiologists.

You may feel weak and tired at the completion of the study, as after any vigorous catharsis. However, there should be no other significant aftereffects. Any bleeding or persistent abdominal pain following the study should be promptly brought to the attention of your physician.

Cholecystography (Gallbladder Examination). This is useful in the detection of abnormal gallbladder function and gallstones. The study must be scheduled in advance and requires careful preparation, usually eating a lunch containing an abundance of fat to contract the gallbladder, and eating no fat thereafter until the study is completed. The night before the study, you take a number of pills or capsules containing a contrast agent to make the gallbladder visible on a radiograph.

You disrobe completely for the study, and radiographs are exposed while you lie on your stomach on an X-ray table and again while on your side in front of a vertically mounted film holder. Sometimes, the radiologist will expose additional spot films while you stand erect in front of a fluoroscope. After the initial radiographs have been reviewed, you may be asked to drink a preparation to make your gallbladder contract, and additional exposures will then be made.

The contrast material travels from the stomach to the gallbladder through a complex physiologic process, and many things can go wrong. If the gallbladder is not visible in radiographs after a single dose of contrast agent, a second dose is usually given and more radiographs exposed the following day. This study will probably require two to three hours.

A gallbladder examination is not uncomfortable for most patients, but a few may experience nausea after taking the pills and some will have burning urination for a few hours. The contrast agent contains iodine, and in rare cases patients have a delayed reaction to it. A rash or any other unexpected development should be reported to your doctor, even though it will almost certainly resolve itself without treatment.

Intravenous Urography (Kidney Examination). The intravenous urogram shows anatomic details and measures the functional integrity of the kidneys, ureters (the tubes that connect the kidneys to the bladder), and the bladder. It is almost always scheduled in advance. In the case of a conventional intravenous urogram (pyelogram or IVP), preparation usually requires only that no fluids be consumed for 12 hours prior to the examination. In some cases, you may be asked to take an enema, especially if barium has been ingested recently as part of a gastrointestinal study.

You completely disrobe for an intravenous urogram and lie on your back on an X-ray table. Usually, a survey radiograph is exposed and reviewed by the radiologist before the contrast agent is administered. You must lie still meanwhile since the survey radiograph is, in part, a guide to positioning. It also will reveal faint kidney stones that may be obscured in subsequent radiographs.

When the survey radiograph has been approved, a physician or, in some facilities, a nurse or technologist injects a contrast agent into a vein in your hand or elbow, and radiographs are taken at timed intervals. The table may be tilted for some of the films and a tight binder applied across the abdomen for others. There may also be a few slanting views before the table is finally raised to a semi-erect position. In all, five to eight exposures will be made over the course of 20 to 30 minutes. Then, while these are reviewed by the radiologist, you are asked to urinate before a final radiograph of your bladder is exposed. This usually completes the study, which normally takes an hour, but delay in the excretion of the contrast agent or an obstruction of the kidney may require the exposure of more films for several hours.

A variant of this procedure, used in emergencies or for patients with known kidney impairment, is the infusion of contrast agent as an intravenous drip over a brief period. More contrast agent is used, and the patient doesn't have to refrain from drinking water beforehand and is even encouraged to drink.

The contrast agent is an organic iodine compound that is selectively excreted from the body via the urine, just as gallbladder contrast material is excreted in the bile. A few individuals may be hypersensitive to such compounds, but, unfortunately, there is no reliable way to identify them in advance. Some adverse reactions are shoulder pain (due to spasm of the veins), nausea and vomiting, and hives, but, in rare instances, may include breathing difficulty, cardiovascular collapse, and even death.

Several precautions are taken to reduce the chance of a hypersensitivity reaction. First, you are asked if you have any known allergies (especially to seafood containing iodine) or a history of previous reactions to a contrast substance. If you have, you will probably be prepared for the intravenous urogram with small doses of oral steroids and antihistamines (drugs that diminish or prevent hypersensitivity reactions). Make sure you tell your doctor about your allergies when a contrast X-ray study is suggested. Second, the contrast agent will be injected in small amounts at short intervals to be sure that no symptoms appear before the remainder of the dose is administered. Third, in case symptoms develop, oxygen and a special kit of drugs to treat the reaction are kept at the ready, and most hospitals have special systems to mobilize experts to handle such problems within a minute or two. With prompt and vigorous management, the outcome is usually a happy one, though the reaction is uncomfortable and frightening. In many facilities, you are asked to sign a statement of informed consent that the risks and expected benefits of the study have been explained and that you are willing to undergo the procedure with full knowledge of the potential hazard. The risk is very much like that of individuals hypersensitive to bee venom. They may develop exactly the same symptoms, and death is possible but extremely rare.

Reactions to intravenous urography usually occur immediately upon injection of the contrast agent. Delayed reactions are rare and probably unrelated to the procedure. Except for minor burning urination for a few hours, there are no afteraffects.

Other commonly performed studies of the urinary tract include retrograde pyelography which, like intravenous urography or pyelography, gives information about the anatomy of the kidney. It is usually employed in cases of a nonfunctioning kidney that doesn't show up clearly enough with intravenous urography. In this instance, the contrast agent is injected into the kidney through a thin tube (catheter) inserted by a urologist during examination of the interior of the bladder. There is virtually no hazard from the contrast agent in this study, but there is some risk of infection, and the procedure is rarely performed today.

Cystourethrography is a study of the lower urinary tract in which dilute contrast material is injected through a catheter into the bladder. Such a study can detect back flow of urine from the bladder to the kidney (which may be a source of infection), and abnormalities of the urinary bladder such as small growths or diverticula (pouches or recesses). Radiographs made during urination give information about the urethra, the tube through which the bladder is emptied.

Tomography

Tomography, an X ray involving only a thin layer of tissue, is usually scheduled because it uses special equipment, but requires no special preparation (unless it is part of another study such as an intravenous urogram). It entails no risks and aftereffects. However, despite technologic progress, tomography remains a "cut-and-try" technique. For the patient, this means lying very still in one position for up to an hour while films are exposed, processed, and reviewed, and additional films of different slices or with different techniques are ordered. While the study is in no sense hazardous, it is tedious and can be very uncomfortable.

Special Radiography

Myelography. A myelogram is a study used to identify disease that may involve or compress the spinal cord, most notably a herniated disc. Contrast material is injected through a needle in the lower back into the space around the spinal cord. A tilting table is used to allow gravity to raise or lower the contrast agent as required. A water-soluble contrast agent does not have to be removed afterward, but an oily type is drawn out by suction after the study. The contrast agent poses some hazard, but less than for an intravenous urogram, and the injection (and removal, if any) may cause pain. The study is usually performed completely by the radiologist and is done with fluoroscopy and spot filming.

Angiography. Angiography is the study of the arteries and veins of various organs including the brain, heart, kidneys, adrenals, pancreas, intestines, liver, and extremities. It involves inserting a needle into an artery, usually in a groin, threading a fine guide wire with a flexible tip through the needle, and passing a catheter over the wire. The wire stiffens the flexible catheter so that it can be inserted, with fluoroscopic guidance, into the vessel being studied. The wire is then withdrawn, and contrast agent is injected through the catheter. A rapid (two or more per second) series of radiographs is exposed to record the flow of the contrast agent through the arteries and veins of the organ in question. This procedure can reveal tumors not demonstrable by other means, identify bleeding sites in the gastrointestinal tract, and has recently found dramatic application in studies of the coronary arteries of patients with angina pectoris. There is a hazard of hypersensitivity to an intravascular contrast agent, as in intravenous urograms, but the usefulness of the technique for guiding the planning of treatment most often outweighs the risks.

Venography entails the opacification specifically of veins, usually by injection of contrast agent through a needle into a superficial vein. Study of peripheral veins is useful as a guide to varicose vein surgery. The technique is occasionally applied to the inferior vena cava (a very large vein of the abdomen). Reaction to the contrast agent is again a possibility.

Bronchography. Bronchography is a technique for studying the trachea (windpipe) and bronchi (the airways within the lungs) which is useful in the evaluation of lung tumors and bronchiectasis (chronic widening of the bronchi). A contrast agent instilled into the trachea and allowed to flow into the major bronchi is observed fluoroscopically and then radiographs are exposed. The agent can induce violent coughing, making it necessary to suppress the cough reflex with drugs. The study is uncomfortable and is rarely performed today.

Pneumoencephalography. Since the advent of the CAT scanner, pneumoencephalography and ventriculography are very rarely performed. These studies employ air for contrast. In the case of pneumoencephalography, air is injected into the space around the spinal cord through a needle placed in the center of the lower back. The air rises into the ventricles of the brain as the patient is rotated full circle in a special tumbling chair. Ventriculography is similar, except that air is injected directly into the ventricles. The study is uncomfortable and usually brings on a severe headache that may persist for hours or several days.

Biopsy. The radiologist may also participate in biopsies, the removal of small amounts of tissue for microscopic study. In one technique, the radiologist passes a wire into a suspected tumor or infection in the lung through a catheter placed in the air passages under fluoroscopic guidance. The rough end of the wire picks up cells for examination. The procedure requires suppression of the cough reflex and the patient may spit some blood and be short of breath afterward. In another procedure, a needle is inserted directly into the diseased tissue under fluoroscopic guidance, and cells are drawn in by suction. This may also cause some bleeding and shortness of breath.

Angiograms, myelograms, bronchograms, pneumoencephalograms, and biopsies are essentially minor surgical procedures and require pre-medication. They are performed only on hospitalized patients.

Special Outpatient Studies

Arthrography. In this study, contrast material and air are injected through a needle into a joint space which is then X-rayed, usually in a search for torn cartilage in a knee but sometimes to examine a shoulder or ankle. Needle insertion and distention of the joint capsule are painful, but aftereffects are rare.

Sialography. Sialography is a radiographic procedure in which a contrast agent is first injected through a fine tube (*cannula*) into the duct draining one of the salivary glands in the mouth. If the opening of the duct is difficult to locate, it may be necessary to probe the soft tissues of the floor of the mouth, causing much discomfort for the patient.

Lymphangiography. In lymphangiography, a fine tube is inserted in a lymph channel in the foot. Contrast agent is then pumped into the tube very slowly, to avoid rupturing the fragile lymph vessel. It takes several hours to opacify the lymph channels and nodes of the leg and trunk, making the procedure lengthy and tedious for the patient.

Interventional Radiography

The radiologist may perform several so-called interventional proce-dures at the request of the attending physician. These studies are often substitutes for conventional surgical procedures and are frequently re-served for patients whose condition does not permit surgery. In one tech-nique, the radiologist inserts a catheter into a specific artery and fills the artery bed with a high concentration of the selected drug, while the rest of the body is exposed to a much lower concentration because of the drug's dilution by the circulation. The catheter may be left in place for an extended time to permit repeated infusions, as in the case of anticancer chemotherapeutic agents. The technique may also be used on an emergency basis to control gastrointestinal bleeding by injection of agents that constrict the arteries.

In similar fashion, a needle may be inserted into the liver and a catheter passed through it into the ducts draining the liver. Advancing the catheter beyond an obstructing stone or tumor opens a passage for the flow of bile and relieves jaundice.

Another technique involves the insertion of a catheter with a tiny balloon at its tip into a narrowed artery. The catheter tip is placed at the site of narrowing and the balloon is inflated to displace or flatten the plaque and so widen the vessel. This may restore normal blood flow without recourse to vascular surgery.

CT Scanning

CT scans distinguish between tissues of only slightly different densities much more readily than conventional radiographic techniques, and any part of the body may be scanned with only a slightly higher radiation dosage than usual. While such studies are scheduled ahead of time, advance preparation is not usually required.

For a CT examination, you lie on a table, usually face up. The table is then moved into a circular structure, which resembles a doughnut and contains the X-ray tube and detector, until the part of your body to be examined is in the path of the beam. You must remain still while the X-ray beam is scanning (rotating around the doughnut), and straps may be used to help prevent movement, the main cause of an unsatisfactory study. For scans of the chest and abdomen, you are usually asked to hold your breath, but soft breathing is permitted during a brain scan. Scan time varies with the machine, but the latest models take only a few seconds.

No pre-scan preparation is needed for examination of the head. For abdominal scans, you may sometimes receive an injection of a drug called glucagon immediately prior to the examination, to temporarily reduce bowel motion. You may also be asked to drink fluid containing a contrast agent which accentuates the image of the gastrointestinal tract.

For both head and body scans, you may be given an intravenous injection of contrast material to make abnormalities more detectable. This involves the usual small risk of hypersensitivity to the contrast agent. CT scans cause no significant aftereffects.

Ultrasonography

Ultrasonic studies are being ordered in increasing numbers. Although they do not involve X rays, they are usually performed by the radiologist. They are almost always scheduled in advance, but normally require no preparation. You may sometimes be asked to eat no fat for several hours before the study to distend the gallbladder, or to drink several glasses of water and postpone urination to fill the bladder, depending on the purpose of the examination.

You lie on an ordinary litter, usually face up, exposing only the area to be examined. The radiologist or a specially trained technologist presses a small probe about an inch in diameter against the skin and moves it back and forth with a rocking motion over the surface. An image of the underlying tissue structures appears on a television-like screen and is photographed for a permanent record. The skin is coated with mineral oil to improve sound transmission between the probe and the body. The examination causes little discomfort and no after effects.

Radionuclide (Emission) Imaging

Radionuclides are radioactive isotopes of chemical elements. For emission imaging, short-lived isotopes are specially man-made in nuclear reactors. Studies using these materials are neither complicated nor uncomfortable, but do require you to lie still for about two to ten minutes while an image is recorded. Most examinations are over in a half hour, but may last longer depending on the patient's ability to cooperate. They require no preparation, and you may eat and drink normally before and after the study. Activities are unrestricted. Most of these studies can be performed on outpatients.

Liver Scanning. For a liver scan, you receive an intravenous injection of a radionuclide that is selectively removed from the blood by certain cells of the liver. Eighty percent of the material normally goes to the liver and 20 percent is equally divided between the spleen and bone marrow. By showing the structure of the liver and spleen, the study can indicate whether the organs contain masses or are displaced from normal positions. The varying brightness of the image also shows the isotope distribution, an important factor in the evaluation of liver and spleen function. Front, back, and side images are obtained, augmented by slanting views as needed for clarification.

Lung Scanning (Perfusion). The object of this study is evaluation of the lung's blood supply. The radionuclide is attached to particles slightly larger than the smallest lung arteries which then trap them as the intravenously injected material flows through. Images of both lungs are obtained from the front, back, and sides. They indicate whether blood is adequately reaching all areas and outline abnormalities.

Lung Scanning (Ventilation). This study shows the distribution of air in the lung and is a useful adjunct to a perfusion scan. You sit with your back to the gamma-ray camera, wearing a face mask through which you breathe a mixture of oxygen and radioactive xenon gas, and then hold your breath while the image is formed. Most people tolerate the procedure without much breathlessness. Some institutions perform a practice run with the mask in place but without xenon.

Brain Scanning. Radionuclide brain scans screen for abnormalities such as tumors and the results of injury. If certain agents are used (pertechnetate), an oral dose of potassium perchlorate is given first to block the entry of the isotope into certain sites where it might be confused with disease. Otherwise, no preliminary medication is necessary.

Images may be obtained during the injection of isotope to permit a gross estimate of blood flow to and through the brain. About two to three hours after the injection, images of the head are taken from the front, back, and side. No food or activity restrictions are imposed during the waiting period.

Bone Scanning. An image of the skeletal system is obtained by intravenous or intramuscular injection of a radioactive technetium compound that accumulates in areas of active bone formation. Two to four hours are allowed for proper distribution of the radionuclide after the injection, and then the scanning instrument is passed over the patient lying flat on the table face either up or down. The bone scan alone cannot distinguish between benign and malignant causes of active bone formation, but a combination of radioactive scanning and conventional radiographs is suggestive.

Gallium Scanning. A gallium isotope tends to accumulate at sites of inflammation, abscess, and certain types of tumor, and is most effective 24 to 48 hours after intravenous or intramuscular injection. Because gallium also normally accumulates in the colon, an enema may be given before scanning.

Cardiac Scanning. Radionuclide studies of the heart take many forms, depending on the desired information and the suspected abnormality. Various radioactive agents are used for various purposes, such as to depict the damage to the heart wall after a heart attack, to determine if chest pain in certain patients is caused by diminished blood flow to the heart wall, and to study the activity of the heart muscle itself. Technical details vary widely.

Radiologic Personnel

It is useful to consider the background of the people who perform radiologic services.

The radiologist is a doctor of medicine or osteopathy who has completed four years of medical school beyond college, four years of postgraduate training largely in radiology, and perhaps one or more years of fellowship in a radiologic specialty. Most practicing radiologists are Diplomates of the American Board of Radiology, which requires passing a rigorous examination. Osteopathic radiologists are certified by the American Board of Osteopathic Radiology.

Most state laws permit not only radiologists, but any health professional, including medical and osteopathic doctors, dentists, podiatrists, and others such as chiropractors, to use X rays to diagnose and treat disease. The practice of radiology by nonradiologists is sometimes appropriate, for example, by a dentist, who is likely to be competent in the interpretation of dental radiographs, and sometimes unavoidable, for example, in remote areas where radiologic consultation is not readily available. Some medical specialists, such as orthopedists, also frequently perform their own radiologic studies. Generally, however, the radiologist can more dependably detect subtle abnormalities, recognize artifacts, and find evidence of disease without being limited by the boundaries of particular medical specialties. Evidence also indicates that physicians order twice as many X rays when they do their own interpretation than when they refer their patients to radiologists. This increases the cost of health care.

The radiologist is responsible for insuring that examinations are diagnostically useful, involve minimal risk, and are promptly and accurately interpreted, and that results are reported quickly to the referring physician, often with personal or telephone consultation. A radiologist's written report is the legally official interpretation of a diagnostic image. The radiologist also personally performs or monitors many studies, participates in teaching conferences and research, supervises the radiology department (which may have over 100 employees), and shares hospital staff duties with other physicians. Many, if not most, departments require more than one radiologist, and large teaching departments may have over thirty.

Among the others who contribute to the service are the radiographers (formerly called technologists or technicians) who actually conduct most radiographic examinations. A registered technologist (R.T.) must complete a 24-month course of instruction and supervised clinical experience and then pass an American Registry of Radiologic Technologists (ARRT) examination. Many now take a 3-year college program leading to an Associate degree, and often take additional training in special fields such as CT scans, ultrasonography, angiography, and radiation therapy. Ten states now require medical X-ray workers to be licensed. Proper supervision by a responsible professional minimizes the risks of service by unlicensed personnel. If you do have to use a radiology department, make sure that at least the supervisory radiographers have qualified as R.T.'s (look for registry pins).

Other personnel include two broad categories: those concerned with patient care, who, in large facilities, will be supervised by a Chief Technician, and clerical staff under an Office Manager. These supervisors can help you with any departmental problem you encounter.

The Radiologist's Bill

Questions often arise about the radiologist's bill and relationship to the hospital. A word of explanation may be helpful.

First, some radiologists practice in private offices as other consulting physicians do, maintaining no hospital connections. Most radiologists, however, practice in a hospital under various arrangements. The nature of the agreement between the radiologist and the hospital determines how you are billed. Regardless of the details, the charges reflect both technical costs (equipment, nonprofessional staff pay, and operating and maintenance expenses), and professional fees (to compensate the radiologist for professional time and expertise). In a sense, all practitioners charge for these items but usually combine them in a single bill. In a radiologic facility, the technical costs are proportionately far greater than in most other medical offices.

There are basically three ways in which you may be billed.

(1) If the radiologist operates a private office independent of a hospital, or pays the hospital for the use of space and equipment (a lease agreement), and also pays all department personnel, then both technical and professional operating costs are being carried by the radiologist. In this case, you will get a single bill in the radiologist's own name. Lease arrangements are relatively uncommon but have many desirable features, not the least of which is the straightforwardness of the relationship between the patient and physician.

(2) If the radiologist has a separate billing arrangement with the hospital, technical and professional cost components will be divided. The hospital pays for the space, equipment, and nonprofessional personnel, and bills for the technical (hospital) component of the charges. The radiologist bills separately and in his or her own name for professional services which may include those of associates. In this case, the relationship is analogous to that between the hospital and the surgeon who uses its operating room facilities–the hospital bills for the use of the operating room, and the surgeon bills for professional services. This system avoids many misunderstandings between hospital and radiologists and is favored by most radiologists today. However, it is sometimes confusing to the patient who receives two bills from different sources for the same radiologic study.

(3) If the radiologist is salaried, or receives some part of the income of the radiology department, the hospital will send a single bill for the examination. This may seem simpler to you, but

most radiologists object to this system, and federal health care planners share their feelings.

Whatever the arrangement or method of billing, the total fee is likely to be about the same—strongly influenced in most localities by the policies of third-party insurance carriers.

Commonly Asked Questions

1. *Why doesn't the radiologist tell me what the films show?*

The radiologic consultation is only one of many sources on which the physician bases an evaluation of the patient and a choice of treatment. The radiologic interpretation may be at variance with other data such as laboratory findings and the evidence of a physical examination. Taken alone, it may cause confusion. It is customary, therefore, for the radiologist to report to the patient's physician, who in turn weighs the various data and sorts out apparent inconsistencies.

2. *Why must the patient be referred for radiologic consultation by another physician—why can't the patient go directly to the radiologist?*

Radiologic examination is only one of many diagnostic tools available to the physician and involves some hazard associated with the use of ionizing radiation. X-ray examination should not, for this reason, be performed in the absence of specific indications. Your physician is best able to judge which diagnostic procedure is most likely to help in a given circumstance; many health problems can be resolved without recourse to X-ray examination. The requirement that a patient be referred for radiologic examination is a protection for the patient.

3. *Why doesn't the radiologist give the radiographs to the patient who paid for them?*

Technically, the radiographs belong to the radiologist not to the patient. The patient does not pay for the radiographs but for the radiologist's opinion based on the radiographs. In practice, it is to the patient's advantage to have the films retained for future reference in the event subsequent examination may be necessary. Radiologists are happy to forward radiographic studies to other physicians to help with the patient's health care, and some radiologists who have no facilities for film storage do give the radiographs to the patient as a matter of course.

4. Why must the patient wait after the radiographs have been exposed?

This is to be certain that the films are technically adequate, and that there are no ambiguous findings that might be resolved by additional radiographs. The exposure of radiographs remains something of an art. The technician does not have an accurate "finder" as you do in a camera to help direct the X-ray beam, and exposure factors are necessarily based on external measurements that may not take account of abnormalities within the patient's body. For these reasons, it is occasionally necessary to repeat an exposure. More often, a supplemental exposure is useful to establish the significance of a suspicious shadow.

5. My doctor read the films for me, so why should I pay the radiologist?

Radiographs are often released to the referring physician as a matter of convenience and to facilitate medical management of an acute problem. The supervision of the examination, however, and the ultimate interpretation are provided by the radiologist, not the referring physician. In hospital practice, the Joint Commission on Accreditation of Hospitals requires that radiographic studies be interpreted by a qualified radiologist as a protection to the patient.

6. Since I had the study two years ago, why must I have it again?

It is often important to study the course of a disease process over time. In fact, the interpretation of certain shadows may depend entirely on whether the shadow is static (has been present for some years) or changing (represents an active process). The human body is a dynamic system and subject to change. With the development of new symptoms, repetition of a previously performed study is often indicated.

7. How soon will my doctor have the report?

Your physician can obtain an immediate report by requesting a "stat interpretation." If this is not required, a written interpretation may not be received for three or four days after the completion of the examination. In most facilities, reports are distributed within a week.

HEMATOLOGY

John R. Durocher, M.D.

*Clinical Assistant Professor of Hematology
and Oncology, Pennsylvania Hospital*

Hematology is the study of the normal properties and disorders of blood and blood-forming tissues. A hematologist is a specialist in internal medicine who has had extensive training in blood disorders.

Blood is essential for life. A sudden excessive blood loss can cause shock and possibly death; a slow loss can cause anemia and poor health. On the other hand, too much blood in the body can lead to heart failure and consequent lung congestion. The average adult has about 12 pints of blood.

About half the blood volume is made up of three types of cells—red cells, white cells, and platelets—in varying proportions, which are suspended in a liquid called plasma. When the blood clots, the cells and certain other components settle out of the plasma, and the remaining cell-free liquid is then called serum.

Bone Marrow

Blood cells in an adult are made primarily by bone marrow in the pelvis, spine, ribs, breastbone, and skull. Blood abnormalities can result from suppression or other disturbances of bone-marrow activity by certain illnesses, drugs such as anti-cancer agents and alcohol, radiation (accidental or therapeutic), and invasion by cancer or other alien cells. *Aplastic anemia* is a general name for some conditions in which the bone marrow functions poorly or not at all.

Although blood tests are useful indicators of bone marrow activity, the hematologist may also test a sample of bone marrow itself, obtained by bone marrow aspiration. The suggestion that bone marrow be examined does not necessarily mean that leukemia is suspected. The test is often performed simply to determine general marrow activity and to check for deficiencies of vitamins and iron.

Aspiration consists of withdrawal of a small amount of marrow through a syringe needle, usually from the breastbone or rear pelvic bone, under local anesthesia. It is no more painful than other procedures involving local anesthesia of the skin and underlying tissue. The marrow, which resembles cranberry sauce, is smeared on a glass slide which is then stained to bring out details and studied under a microscope.

The hematologist may sometimes also perform a bone marrow biopsy, removing a sliver of bone about one inch long and as thick as pencil lead. The procedure is not painful and the bone rapidly grows back.

Any discomfort after bone marrow aspiration or biopsy is minor, local, and transient. Normal activities can be resumed immediately afterward.

Red Blood Cells

The main function of red blood cells (*erythrocytes*) is to carry oxygen from the lungs to body tissues. Oxygen combines temporarily with the red protein hemoglobin in the cells and is released where needed. Red blood cells survive about four months, after which they are destroyed and removed by the spleen and the liver.

The abundance of red blood cells can be determined by counting the number in a blood sample (red blood cell count), by measuring the hemoglobin content, or by gauging the volume occupied by closely-packed red blood cells in a given volume of whole blood (*hematocrit*). Normally, about 1 percent are newly formed red blood cells (*reticulocytes*) which can be counted after being made recognizable by staining. A low reticulocyte count indicates a sluggish marrow which may not be adequately replacing old red cells that have been removed. A high reticulocyte count indicates an active marrow compensating for blood loss or premature red blood cell destruction.

Elevated Red Blood Cell Count

If oxygen delivery by the blood decreases for any reason (most commonly due to a chronic lung disease such as emphysema which is usually caused by heavy cigarette smoking), the body compensates by increasing the quantity of red blood cells. If the increase, called *polycythemia*, is great enough, the blood becomes viscous, and the heart must pump harder and may fail. The slower blood flow also increases the risk of clotting (*thrombosis*) in the vessels which may lead to stroke.

Decreased Red Blood Cell Count

Anemia is an abnormally low red blood cell level. Symptoms depend on how rapidly the condition develops, but chronic anemia can cause fatigue on minor exertion, pallor, and shortness of breath. If the onset is slow, a marked degree of anemia can be tolerated without severe symptoms because body mechanisms compensate to support oxygen delivery to the tissues.

Since iron is an integral part of hemoglobin, anemia may sometimes be caused by an iron deficiency. Iron is present in meats and green leafy vegetables. However, adult iron deficiency is almost always secondary to blood loss, for example, menstruation and pregnancies in women, rather than diet. In men and older women, the cause is usually gastrointestinal bleeding, and the physician will look for abnormalities in the stomach and intestines.

Another common cause of anemia in adults is a chronic illness such as arthritis, infection, and kidney disease. Since the effect of the illness is suppression of bone marrow activity rather than loss of blood, iron or other supplements do not help.

Other dietary factors needed for the production of red blood cells include folic acid (meats and leafy vegetables) and vitamin B_{12} (meats and eggs). Malnourishment, especially due to debilitation or alcohol abuse, can cause a folic acid deficiency. Excessive drinking is even more likely to cause anemia by other routes, including gastrointestinal bleeding, than by folic acid deficiency. Despite popular opinion, vitamin B_{12} deficiency is rare, but may occur several years after total surgical removal of the stomach or in the uncommon illness called pernicious anemia.

Red Blood Cell Transfusions

Transfusions of red blood cells without plasma, rather than of whole blood, are used to quickly restore the red blood cell level of anemic patients. Physicians administer transfusions judiciously because they entail certain hazards such as a volume overload (too much blood) for elderly and frail patients, fever reactions, and, most importantly, hepatitis transmitted from infected donors. The hepatitis risk has been substantially reduced in the United States by the more selective use of voluntary donors and screening for the hepatitis virus, but has not been completely eliminated. If the anemia is caused by inadequate iron, and replenishment of red blood cells is not urgent, the physician may avoid transfusion and treat with iron alone.

Abnormal Red Blood Cells

The most common red blood cell abnormalities appear in the hemoglobin, and the major hemoglobin abnormality is sickle cell disease which affects approximately 1 out of 400 black Americans. Its consequences can be devastating, including chronic anemia, recurrent pain, leg ulcers, gallstones, jaundice, and a shortened life expectancy (sickle cell anemia is not usually a problem of the elderly). About 1 out of 10 black Americans are carriers of the sickle cell trait. Less than half of the hemoglobin in their red blood cells is abnormal, they exhibit no disease symptoms, and they live a normal life span.

Another hemoglobin abnormality is *thalassemia* (Cooley's anemia) which primarily affects people of Mediterranean ancestry. In this condition, the hemoglobin is not intrinsically abnormal, but its production is inadequate to fill the red blood cells. The disease can cause a significant anemia and is often fatal to children or teenagers. Carriers of the trait without the disease may have a mild anemia which resembles an iron deficiency. However, the blood iron level is normal, iron supplements are not beneficial, and the carriers otherwise live normal lives without unusual medical problems.

White Blood Cells

White blood cells (*leukocytes*) come in a variety of forms distinguishable under the microscope and generally help the body resist infection. A standard blood test will include a white blood cell count as well as one of red cells.

Elevated White Blood Cell Count

An abnormally high white blood cell level usually indicates infection, but for certain infections, the level may remain normal or even fall. Some drugs, such as steroids, used to counteract allergic disorders, can raise the white blood cell count. The most feared cause of an increase in white blood cells is leukemia.

Leukemia is a primary malignancy of the bone marrow in which the uncontrolled proliferation of malignant white blood cells crowds out the normal production of red and white blood cells and platelets. Not only does the blood become deficient in these other cells, but the proliferating abnormal white blood cells do not have the usual disease-fighting ability and therefore increase the risk of infection.

It is important to recognize that leukemia appears in many forms which vary in malignancy, required treatment, and prognosis. In fact, some forms of leukemia common in older people may have little effect on length of life. The hematologist must distinguish among the various forms to prescribe appropriate treatment and correctly inform the patient.

Decreased White Blood Cell Count

An abnormally low white blood cell level (*leukopenia*) may impair the body's resistance to disease and result in frequent infections and severe sore throats. Causes of a subnormal white blood cell count include severe bacterial or viral infections, adverse drug reactions, cancer chemotherapy, and radiation treatment. People with known leukopenia should contact their physicians immediately if they develop a high fever or shaking chill.

White Blood Cell Transfusions

It might be expected that white blood cell transfusions would help overcome leukopenia just as red blood cell transfusions alleviate anemia. Until recently, this supposition could not be tested because active white blood cells could not be practically extracted in sufficient quantities from stored blood. This is now practical, and large numbers of white blood cells can also be drawn from single donors by means of special machines. However, white blood cell transfusions are restricted to certain infections, and their efficacy has not been adequately proven.

Abnormal White Blood Cells

The most common white blood cell abnormality is leukemia, but other malignant processes such as *multiple myeloma* and *lymphoma* (including Hodgkin's disease) can also affect white blood or their precursor cells.

Platelets

Platelets (*thrombocytes*) are intimately involved in blood coagulation. Abnormal levels affect the ability to form clots and platelet counts are part of the battery of frequently performed blood tests.

Elevated Platelet Count

An elevated platelet count (*thrombocytosis*) may be a reaction to a chronic inflammatory disease or the result of a bone marrow malignancy. When the count exceeds 1,000,000, the risk of clotting in blood vessels rises significantly. Paradoxically, although the number of platelets may increase for certain bone marrow malignancies, bleeding may occur because the platelets are abnormal and do not provide the usual aid to clotting.

Decreased Platelet Count

A decrease of platelets (*thrombocytopenia*) is much more common than an increase. Symptoms are nosebleeds, spontaneous bleeding from the gums, bruising easily (purpura), and other abnormal bleeding. The condition may result from underproduction of platelets in the bone marrow due to drugs (for example, anti-cancer agents and alcohol), radiation, and marrow replacement by abnormal tissue in tuberculosis, cancer, or, more rarely, *myelofibrosis*. It may also be caused by increased destruction in the circulation by immunologic reactions and certain drugs, most commonly quinidine, a medication for heart patients. Often the cause is unknown, and the condition is called *idiopathic thrombocytopenia purpura* (ITP).

Aspirin is known to interfere with platelet activity, but the effect is normally not significant. However, if the platelet count is low, it is advisable to use non-aspirin analgesics such as Tylenol.

If the cause of a low platelet count is unknown, the condition may first be treated with *prednisone,* a synthetic cortisone-like drug. If no improvement occurs, removal of the spleen may be recommended.

Platelet Transfusions

Platelets may be transfused in an attempt to stop bleeding due to a low platelet count or to prevent complications before they start. However, recipients soon develop resistance to donation of alien platelets and may not respond with a rise in platelet count. Platelets from family members or other genetically similar donors may then be used with varying success.

Abnormal Platelets

In some instances, the platelet count is normal, but the platelets do not function normally (*thrombocytopathy*). The condition may be congenital, but is more often caused by aspirin, high doses of certain antibiotics, or kidney failure. It is tested by a measurement of bleeding time. A special instrument is used to scratch the forearm painlessly, and the interval between the start and cessation of bleeding is timed. Bleeding time is normally less than 8 minutes. Platelet counts below 75,000 may also prolong bleeding time, but longer times at normal platelet counts indicate abnormal platelet function.

Plasma

The liquid called *plasma* contains a variety of substances, including fats (lipids), sugar (glucose), and proteins, and makes up over half the blood's volume. The proteins can be broadly divided into albumin and gamma globulins. Albumin helps to keep the fluid from diffusing out of blood vessels (low albumin levels can result reflects the status of nutrition. A main concern of the hematologist is the gamma globulins which include, among others, two important classes of proteins: immunoglobulins and coagulation factors.

Immunoglobulins

The immunoglobulins work in conjunction with the white blood cells in complex ways to prevent or control infection. There are five main types, and some may appear in other body fluids as well as the blood.

Elevated Blood Levels of Immunoglobulins

The blood level of one of the various immunoglobulins may sometimes increase above its normal value. It is then called a *paraprotein*. The incidence of paraproteins increases with age. If their concentration becomes too great, the blood may become viscous and cause circulation problems. Paraproteins are occasionally associated with multiple myeloma, a malignant plasma cell disease. Although paraproteins are abundant, they are also abnormal and do not participate in immunologic reactions against infection. This is one reason that victims of multiple myeloma have frequent bacterials infection such as pneumonia.

Decreased Blood Levels of Immunoglobulins

Low immunoglobulin levels are usually unimportant in adults. However, in a disease such as multiple myeloma, the elevated levels of paraproteins may be accompanied by decreased levels of normal immunoglobulins, which significantly reduces resistance to infection.

Immunoglobulin Injections

Injections of immunoglobulins in the form of gamma globulin are used primarily to ward off hepatitis. Low immunoglobulin levels are not usually treated with gamma globulin injections, nor have these been shown to help multiple myeloma patients fight infection.

Coagulation Factors

Coagulation factors in the plasma work in conjunction with blood platelets to produce clots and keep blood from flowing out of injured vessels. The coagulation system can be activated by exposure to tissues surrounding the blood vessels, for example, by a local injury. A series of inactivators then prevents the coagulation from spreading beyond the site. The function of the coagulation system is assessed by such tests as prothrombin time (PT) and partial thromboplastin time (PTT). If results are abnormal, further tests may be performed by laboratories that specialize in blood coagulation studies.

Elevated Coagulation Factors

Elevated coagulation factors have been suspected of contributing to strokes by causing clotting in cerebral blood vessels. Although plausible, this has never been proven.

Decreased Coagulation Factors

Since many of the blood coagulation factors are made in the liver, severe liver disease may reduce their levels, result in bleeding, and require infusion of fresh plasma. Vitamin K is also required for the producton of some coagulation factors in the liver. A deficiency of these factors may therefore develop if less vitamin K is available due to inadequate diet, decreased absorption, or inhibition by anticoagulant medications such as warfarin or Coumadin. People with low levels of coagulation factors may find blood in the urine or at the rectum, and bruise easily.

Certain congenital diseases, most commonly hemophilia, are marked by deficiencies of certain blood coagulation factors. Hemophilia is rare and is usually identified before middle age.

Transfusion of Coagulation Factors

Transfusion of coagulation factors, most commonly in the form of fresh frozen plasma, can help to stop bleeding if reduced levels of the factors are a contributing cause. To preserve the properties of the coagulation factors, which tend to deteriorate under normal blood bank storage conditions, the plasma is separated from the red cells at the time of blood donation and quickly frozen. In some instances, such as the treatment of hemophilia, specially prepared fractions of plasma may be used.

PHYSICAL THERAPY
FOR THE OVER-55 PATIENT

Carolyn M. Scott, B.A.,M.S.,P.T.

Director, Department of Physical Therapy, Pennsylvania Hospital

The physical therapist is a health professional who specializes in the use of therapeutic exercise, heat, cold, electricity, and massage, to treat disorders and disabilities resulting from disease and injury. Physical therapy is especially helpful to individuals with orthopedic, neurologic, arthritic, vascular, coronary, and pulmonary conditions, and to those who have suffered amputations, strokes, or paraplegia. Millions of dollars are allocated yearly for rehabilitation of injured, diseased, and handicapped children, adults, and older people.

Elements of Physical Therapy

Heat

Heat increases blood circulation and facilitates the delivery of oxygen and removal of waste products in an injured area. Its beneficial effects include reduction of pain, relaxation of sore muscles, and enhancement of the healing process. However, heat should be used cautiously on patients who have blood circulation problems with the prior approval of the patient's physician.

Heat can be administered in several different ways, including moist hot (hydrocollator) packs, paraffin, ultrasound, and whirlpools.

Hydrocollator packs are fabric-covered pads filled with silica gel, which permits them to absorb and retain large amounts of water. The packs are kept in water-filled stainless steel tanks at a constant temperature of 77°C (170°F). When removed for use in treatment, they are wrapped in several layers of towel and applied to the affected body area for approximately 20 minutes. Hot packs are effective in relieving a wide variety of disorders, including muscle spasms associated with lumbosacral sprains, low back pain, acute tendinitis and bursitis of the shoulder, and arthritic aches of the shoulder, knees, and other joints.

The paraffin bath is similar to hydrocollator packs in that it provides moist heat and helps to relieve pain, especially the joint pain of arthritis. The patient dips the body part to be treated into a paraffin-mineral oil mixture heated to 52°C (126°F) and then withdraws it. An advantage of paraffin is that it forms a closefitting glove over body parts, such as hands and feet, with difficult-to-reach surfaces, and retains the heat for approximately 20 minutes.

Hot packs and paraffin baths are both available commercially for home use. Hot packs should be boiled in water for 30 minutes, wrapped in towels, and applied to affected body areas. Paraffin baths are purchased ready for use.

Ultrasound produces heat by transforming electrical energy into high frequency mechanical vibrations. It is frequently used in conjunction with hot packs and whirlpools because its heat penetrates into muscles and joints, and its effect can be restricted to a smaller surface area. Ultrasound provides effective therapy for lumbosacral sprains, low back pain, and tendinitis and bursitis of the shoulder.

Whirlpools are beneficial for their heating and cleansing action. They are available in various sizes to accommodate the different shapes of the body's parts. In the hubbard tank (a large whirlpool), the patient lies on a sloping canvas stretcher which permits immersion of the entire body. A motor agitates the water and produces a massaging effect.

A water bath heated to 37–39°C (98–102°F) produces an effect similar to moist heat, relaxing muscle spasms and relieving the pain of arthritic joints. Water is also effective in the treatment of burns and open wounds, where it aids the healing process by preventing infection.

Cold

Cold produces a physiologic response opposite to that of heat. It lowers joint temperature, inhibiting the transport of oxygen and removal of wastes by diminishing blood flow and partially anesthetizes painful areas. It is useful to reduce the pain, muscle spasm, spasticity, and swelling that follow injury.

Exercise

Therapeutic exercise is the most frequently used form of physical therapy. Its purpose is to increase strength and mobility with the ultimate objective of restoring normal muscle activity and maintaining a healthful state.

There are two basic muscle contractions: isometric and isotonic. In an isometric contraction, there is no movement and no change in the length of the muscle fibers. Such exercise is appropriate when preservation of muscle tone is desired but not movement—a common situation in arthritics and patients recovering from fractures. In contrast, isotonic exercise is characterized by a shortening of muscle fibers and movement of a limb, and is usually intended not only to preserve muscle tone but also to increase strength.

Exercise is classified into four types of movement: passive, assistive, active, and resistive. In passive exercise, the motion is induced by an external influence—the physical therapist—and there is no voluntary muscle contraction or energy expenditure by the patient. This type of exercise is helpful to prevent the loss of flexibility of joints and muscles and is often prescribed for the patient paralyzed by spinal cord injury or stroke.

Assistive, active, and resistive movements begin with the recovery of voluntary muscle function. Assistive exercises require the help of a therapist to complete movements that weak muscles can start but not finish. Active exercises are appropriate when muscles are strong enough to complete a motion without assistance. In resistive exercise, work against external forces such as weights and sandbags further strengthens the muscles.

The choice of the most suitable exercise is made by the therapist after careful consideration of the patient's diagnosis and physical condition. There are many kinds of therapeutic exercise of which the following are among the most commonly used:

> *Range of motion (ROM)* Passage of a joint through all its normal motions. This may be passive, assistive, active, or resistive.

> *Muscle re-education* Exercises which help a muscle to "relearn" its normal function. Loss of function commonly occurs in muscles weakened by paralysis, disease, or surgery.

> *Progressive resistive exercises (PRE)* Exercises to strengthen muscles. These are performed against measured increases in resistance in the form of weights or other apparatus.

> *Endurance* These are exercises in which repetition and low resistance are key factors. They serve to increase muscle endurance.

> *Coordination* Exercises which improve precision of movement. The objective is to enhance the ability to use the right muscle with the proper intensity to achieve the most efficient movement.

> *Breathing* Exercises prescribed in the treatment of chronic respiratory disease and following chest surgery. They help to restore maximum possible lung function, maintain the patient's normal posture, and shorten the period of convalescence.

Conditions Commonly Treated by Physical Therapy

Osteoarthritis

Degenerative joint disease (*osteoarthritis*) is often described as a "wear-and-tear" consequence of aging. Arthritis may also be associated with minor injury and obesity. Symptoms of the disease include pain and stiffness of varying severity, commonly in the large weight-bearing joints such as the hips, knees, lumbosacral spine, lower back, and cervical spine (neck).

The objectives of physical therapy for arthritis include maintenance of joint mobility, preservation of strength in muscle groups surrounding painful joints, relief of pain, and protection of joints against worsening of the disease. However, arthritic joint defects are inescapably permanent and progressive, so the therapist directs efforts toward educating the patient in a program which can be carried out daily at home. Heat in the form of hot packs, paraffin baths, or whirlpools is usually included in the program for its relaxing and pain-killing effect. This is followed by isometric and isotonic exercises to preserve joint mobility and muscle strength.

Rheumatoid Arthritis

Rheumatoid arthritis is characterized by joint swelling, pain, and deformity. It most commonly involves arm and leg joints in both right and left limbs simultaneously. Physical therapy for rheumatoid arthritis aims to preserve normal joint range of motion and relieve pain. During the acute phase of the disease, the patient is often hospitalized and given daily physical therapy. Sources of moist heat to relax muscle spasms and reduce pain include hot packs, paraffin, whirlpools, and hubbard tanks. Active and resistive exercises are prescribed, and the patient is taught to use energy economically in daily activities to minimize stress on the joint. After leaving the hospital, the patient continues the program at home to prevent further loss of strength and range of motion.

Amputations

Physical therapy plays a major role in rehabilitating the amputee has lost a lower limb. Treatment begins when surgery is complete and continues until the patient achieves the greatest possible independence. The level of independence varies with the patient's age, physical condition, and the site of the amputation. It is unrealistic to assume that all patients will become proficient in the use of an artificial leg.

In its initial stage, the physical therapy program includes positioning, stump wrapping, and gait training. Positioning is important to maintain normal range of motion, as there is a tendency for the joints of the amputated extremity to assume a bent position. The patient is therefore instructed not to place a pillow under the hip or knee when lying on his or her back, and to ensure preservation of hip extension by lying on his or her stomach at least one hour every day.

An exercise program must involve all limbs. The amputated lower extremity must have normal strength to be eligible for a prosthesis. The remaining lower extremity must also have normal strength and endurance because it must assume a heavier work load during walking. The arms must be sufficiently strong to manipulate crutches or a walker.

Gait training begins in the parallel bars within three to five days following surgery. Advancement to a walker or crutches, is possible once the patient feels comfortable and stable. Training is not complete until the patient is able to transfer independently to the bed, toilet, bathtub, and car and is proficient in climbing stairs, ramps, and curbs.

Proper stump wrapping following amputation gives support which minimizes swelling during the early phase of healing, when fluids tend to accumulate because of blood vessel damage. Stump wrapping is essential prior to fabrication of a prosthesis because it helps to shrink and shape the stump, reduces excess fat, and prevents formation of a roll of tissue along the inner side of the stump. The amputee is released from the hospital within two weeks after surgery, but prosthetic evaluation and training must wait until healing is complete, usually about two months.

Cerebral Vascular Accident (CVA), or Stroke

An individual who suffers a stroke that paralyzes one side of the body requires extensive physical therapy. Treatment begins during the acute phase. Passive exercise to maintain normal range of motion and proper positioning of the paralyzed arm and leg helps to prevent joint stiffness, muscle tightening, and deformity. The patient is usually permitted out of bed as soon as his or her medical condition stabilizes. However, if complications require continued bedrest, the non-paralyzed arm and leg are given active and resistive exercises to prevent weakness and muscle atrophy. The patient is also encouraged to use non-paralyzed limbs for activities such as feeding, grooming, and turning in bed.

Gait training, moving from place to place, and balance activities are begun about two weeks after the onset of the stroke. Balance exercises and placement and movement of the weak leg are practiced between parallel bars. As strength and endurance improve, the patient begins walking with a cane—usually a quad cane with four short legs. The quad cane is exchanged for a normal straight cane as performance improves and confidence grows. Training is complete when the patient becomes proficient in climbing stairs and is able to get about without difficulty.

Recovery of strength, coordination, balance, and endurance depends heavily on the success of an aggressive exercise program. Voluntary motion often appears first in the leg, then strength returns rapidly, and the patient starts resistive exercises with pulleys and weights. Return of function to the arm is often slow and incomplete. Voluntary motion appears in the shoulder before progressing to the elbow, wrist, and fingers, but use often remains limited because of diminished sensation and coordination.

Fractures

Physical therapy management of fractures depends on the limb, the surgical procedure, and the type and location of the fracture.

The arm is a non-weight-bearing limb which requires dexterity and mobility to function normally. Therefore, treatment by immobilization is minimized because soft tissue in the shoulder and elbow can change rapidly and result in permanent loss of movement and function. Early active movement to preserve normal shoulder motion takes precedence over complete bone healing. The patient begins active pendulum exercises under the supervision of a therapist, and strengthening exercises with pulleys and weighted sandbags are added when X rays confirm that the fracture is stable.

The leg, a weight-bearing limb, must retain adequate stability, length, and alignment, even at the cost of some loss of motion. For this reason, appropriate treatment often requires immobilization in a cast for a prolonged period.

The physical therapy program is designed to ensure that all joints not encased in plaster maintain their normal motion and strength, and includes isometric exercises to preserve tone in those muscles that are within the cast. Physical therapy is continued following cast removal to promote recovery of normal motion and strength.

Fractures of some bones such as the pelvis and compression fractures of the spine frequently do not require prolonged support. In these cases, the patient soon leaves bed with the help of a walker, crutches, or cane, and begins exercises under the supervision of the therapist to prevent joint stiffness and loss of strength. Care must be taken to avoid overly strenuous exercise. Any increase in pain or discomfort may be a sign that the pace should be slower.

Fractures that severely displace the bone ends will often require internal devices to hold the ends together during healing. The surgeon attaches a metal support to both sides of the fracture to permit early use of the limb and to prevent the complications of prolonged bed rest.

Gait training and strengthening exercises begin several days after surgery. Usually, the patient is able to bear some weight on the fracture. Walking starts with the aid of parallel bars and progresses to the use of a walker or crutches with the return of sufficient strength and endurance.

Heart Disease

Aggressive physical therapy is essential for disorders of the cardiovascular system. During the acute phase when the patient is at bedrest in the hospital, prevention of respiratory complications, stagnation of blood in the veins, and loss of motion and strength are primary concerns. Long term goals of therapy include recovery of endurance and strength, instruction of the patient in energy-conserving techniques, and preservation of respiratory function.

Postural drainage (positioning the patient so that gravity helps mucus to drain from the lungs), vibration, and percussion (for example, striking the body sharply with cupped hands to loosen the mucus and keep it flowing) prevent accumulation of mucus in the lungs and promote proper aeration. Deep breathing exercises help to move the diaphragm and expand the lung more fully to improve the exchange of carbon dioxide and oxygen.

Initially, the heart patient is restricted to isometric exercises and assisted range-of-motion movement of the limbs to prevent muscle atrophy and loss of strength and to increase venous blood flow. As the patient's condition improves, active and resistive exercises are added with a careful watch for signs of shortness of breath or chest pain. Pulse and breathing rates are measured before any change in the exercise program is made. Walking, under close supervision of the therapist, begins as soon as the attending physician gives approval.

Discharge instructions include a physical therapy program. The patient will return to the therapist periodically for checkups and adjustments in the exercise program.

Chronic Obstructive Lung Disease

Bronchitis, emphysema, and asthma can develop into chronic obstructive lung disease, a long-term disorder with symptoms of shortness of breath, excessive sputum formation, cough, and eventual disability. The patient has difficulty coughing up lung secretions and often does not breathe adequately to aerate the lungs. Shortness of breath limits physical activity, which in turn results in loss of strength and endurance. Intensive physical therapy, preventive treatment, and education of the patient are essential to control the disease.

Vigorous postural drainage, percussion, and vibration are necessary during the acute phase of the illness when mucus secretions increase and hinder breathing. Frequency and duration of treatment will vary with the patient's tolerance and degree of lung congestion. Weak and severely debilitated individuals will need short but frequent treatment. Adjustments must be made in drainage positions to accommodate shortness of breath. An effective and productive cough will necessitate frequent rest periods.

Breathing exercises are essential to help ventilate all parts of the lungs and to increase the strength and coordination of the respiratory muscles. Initially, exercises are performed in a semi-reclining or flat position. Gradually, they are coordinated with standing and walking. This is difficult and requires the patience and perserverance of the patient and family.

Physical disability is a consequence of chronic lung disease primarily because of the patient's reluctance to undertake activity that causes shortness of breath. Participation in an exercise program can minimize the loss of strength and endurance. This program begins with active exercises of both arms and legs at a gradually increasing rate of repetition. Use of a stationary bicycle will improve endurance and make it possible to walk longer and longer distances.

Peripheral Vascular Disease

Disorders which impair circulation in the arms and legs include *atherosclerosis* (hardening of the arteries), Buerger's disease (inflammation and clotting of blood vessels), and varicose veins. Atherosclerosis thickens blood vessel walls, reducing the opening and slowing circulation. Buerger's disease is characterized by inflammation, clotting, and eventual obliteration of blood vessels in the limbs. Varicose veins are abnormally wide and winding blood vessels that occur most commonly in the legs.

The most effective means of improving the circulation in an arm or leg is careful and gradually increasing active and resistive exercise. Progressive resistive exercises may be administered initially by a therapist or family member, then continued by the patient alone. Daily walks of gradually increasing length are encouraged.

Heat in any form is inappropriate for circulatory disease because it increases blood flow, which is harmful to a limb with deficient blood vessels. Whirlpool temperatures should not be higher than 35.6°C (96°F).

Ulcers due to poor circulation frequently respond favorably to physical therapy. Massage helps to reduce the swelling responsible for their formation, softens hardened areas, and improves the blood supply to the ulcerated tissue. Ultraviolet light diminishes infection and hastens healing. Cool whirlpools clean the wound and aid healing.

When the ulcer is painful, the patient will tend to hold the foot in the most comfortable position which is usually with the toes pointing downward. The therapist must observe the leg closely to detect development of a deformity. Exercises are essential to maintain mobility and to prevent a deformity which can make walking difficult.

Low Back Pain

Eighty percent of the adult population suffers from low back pain. Its causes include our upright posture, degenerative joint disease of the lumbar spine, and muscle strain and injury. In the elderly, changes brought about by normal "wear and tear" of the intervertebral discs are largely responsible for back problems.

Conservative management of low back pain calls for physical therapy and education in how to use the body properly in daily activities. Hot packs, ultrasound, and massage relieve the pains of muscle spasm and aid relaxation, while an exercise program strengthens abdominal and buttock muscles. The patient is taught the pelvic tilt, and exercise which reduces strain on the back by decreasing the lumbar (lower back) curve. Proper body mechanics, including correct techniques for rising from various positions and for lifting and carrying, help to prevent recurrence of painful episodes.

While there is no cure for the low back pain caused by degenerative joint disease, regular back exercises and the use of proper body mechanics can minimize discomfort and prevent further disability.

Cancer

Physical therapy has an increasingly significant role in the care of cancer patients as new treatment methods and earlier diagnoses result in longer life expectancy. The therapist is often part of a team that also includes a social worker, dietitian, nurse, physician, and psychologist who provide comprehensive services to the patient and assist in establishing realistic goals.

When planning a treatment program, the therapist must first consider the patient's prognosis. In cases where the expected survival period is short, there is insufficient time to develop an extensive program. Therefore, the goal is to help the patient achieve maximum possible independence so that he or she may return home. A long-term outlook permits intensive therapy with the aim of restoring normal strength and independence in walking and other activities of daily life.

Surgery for treatment of cancer is the most effective. Physical therapy objectives are similar to those for a patient undergoing any other type of surgery. Chemotherapy and radiation, often used as adjuncts to surgery, may cause debilitation and increased susceptibility to infection. Physical therapy therefore aims to prevent lung complications and to maintain good joint mobility, muscle strength, and posture. Because many patients are unable to withstand intensive treatments, to keep the lungs and airway clear is usually limited to chest physical therapy vibration, changes in position, and deep breathing exercises. Daily exercises may include passive range-of-motion movements to prevent joint stiffening if weakness precludes more strenous effort. Proper positioning in bed is important to preserve correct posture. Stronger patients, however, benefit from more strenuous exercises which aim to improve endurance and encourage independence in daily activities.

In cases of surgery for breast cancer, the arm on the side of the surgery receives close attention. Some physicians approve active shoulder motion within 24 hours after surgery, while others prefer to keep the shoulder immobilized for several days, permitting only the use of the arm and hand. Exercises usually begin with the fingers, wrist, and hand, and then progress to the shoulder. Muscle tightening is prevented with active shoulder range-of-motion and pendulum exercises.

Lymphodema, or swelling of the arm, is caused by removal of lymph channels during surgery and usually resolves itself. However, intermittent compression is sometimes helpful in relieving extensive swelling and reducing discomfort. The patient places her arm in a large sleeve attached to a pneumatic pump which creates the pressure by inflating the sleeve. This decreases swelling by assisting the movement of lymphatic fluid from the periphery of the arm. The patient may also wear an elastic stocking on the arm to give added support.

Intensive physical therapy is appropriate for patients following surgery for tumors of the brain or spinal cord. Passive range-of-motion exercise, percussion, and positioning to promote lung drainage help to prevent joint muscle tightening and lung complications immediately after surgery. Later treatment will include muscle strengthening exercises, gait training, and other activities.

Persistent weakness and paralysis require intensive physical therapy. The paraplegic (a patient with weakness or paralysis of the legs) strives for proficiency in transferring from a wheelchair to bed, toilet, bathtub, and car. The patient with residual weakness in the legs can be assisted to walk independently with braces, crutches, walkers, and canes.

Crutches, Walkers, and Canes

Illness or injury often compromises an individual's ability to walk. The onset of disability can be sudden or gradual and insidious. Gait training with crutches, walkers, or canes may be needed when independent walking is not possible (Figure 1).

Gaits are frequently classified as non-weight-bearing, partial-weight-bearing, and full-weight-bearing. A non-weight-bearing gait, common in leg fractures, means that the foot may not touch the ground. A partial-weight-bearing, or three-point gait, permits weight bearing to the patient's tolerance. It is frequently used after hip fractures and total joint replacement.

Consideration must be given to the patient's age, physical condition, and disability when selecting the most appropriate mechanical aid. Although crutches are often considered more functional and desirable than walkers, they are less stable and require more energy to use. Therefore, they are not always suitable for the elderly or the patient with heart disease, and a walker may be more satisfactory.

Canes, unlike crutches and walkers, are unstable and offer less support. They should never be used when the physician orders a non-weight-bearing or partial-weight-bearing gait. A quadruped, or "quad," cane, frequently used following a stroke, does provide substantial support, but the support from a straight cane is minimal. However, a straight cane is helpful with balance and in protecting a painful leg joint.

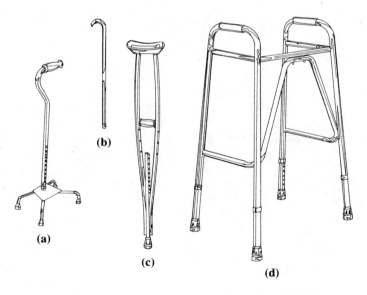

Figure 1. (a) Quad cane, (b) Straight cane, (c) Crutch, (d) Walker.

DIET AND NUTRITION

Laurine C. Simons, R.D.

Registered Dietitian, Pennsylvania Hospital

Food is essential to sustain life, and eating can be one of life's more pleasant experiences. However, the benefits and pleasure depend on good eating habits. This means eating three meals daily, planning menus in advance, and trying—within the limits imposed by income, age, taste, and personal circumstances—to eat a variety of foods.

Besides satisfying nutritional needs, food helps to meet social and emotional needs. Most of us eat in company with others, conversing about daily activities, problems of family, friends, and neighbors, and, of course, personal reactions to the food on the table. Pleasing, wholesome food encourages conversation. Eating in an emotionally satisfying atmosphere contributes significantly to a sense of well-being, digestion, and health.

Our eating habits are determined in large part by national and regional customs, religion, and economics. In addition, the elderly person usually follows set patterns of eating formed over a long period. Some may have few preferences as a result of their lack of exposure to a variety of foods. They may cling to stubborn opinions such as a man's feeling that salads are for women, or an older woman's that milk is only for children. Fortunately, preparing normally rejected food in attractive ways can often overcome habitual aversion.

Because personal preferences affect choices, menu planning should not reflect too closely the likes and dislikes of the planner. A menu planner's narrow preferences may deprive the one being fed of nutritious foods needed to maintain health or to support therapy prescribed for ill-ness. Clearly, what we eat affects us both physically and mentally. There is substantial evidence, for example, that moderately disturbed elderly individuals may show improvement when inadequate nutrition has been corrected with a proper diet.

No single food—not even milk—can supply adequate amounts of all necessary nutrients. For this reason, a healthy diet must include the basic food groups which provide proteins, carbohydrates, fats, and minerals.

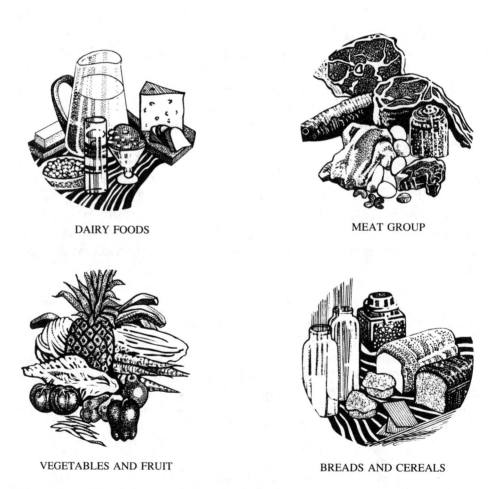

DAIRY FOODS

MEAT GROUP

VEGETABLES AND FRUIT

BREADS AND CEREALS

Figure 1. Build meals around these basic food groups.

While most of us take pleasure in eating a variety of foods, those whose taste is limited to only a few can get by without risk to health by making certain that the preferred foods supply adequate nutrients. It is not necessary to cook if cooking is an unpleasant chore. Cold meals can be both palatable and nutritious. Nor is it always necessary to buy special foods for those on restricted diets. A few precautions taken in the kitchen can allow them to eat almost anything the rest of the family eats. After food is cooked simply, portions for the dieter are removed before sauces, butter, gravy, glazes, or spices are added.

Food has different meanings for different individuals. For most of us, good food is an important aspect of a happy life as well as a necessity for physical well-being.

Eating and Aging

The nutrients we require do not change as we age, but certain requirements do. Men and women in the 55–75 age range need 150 to 200 fewer calories daily than when they were young because of reduced activity and lowered metabolism. Calorie intake can be reduced by decreasing the amounts of sugar, sweets, rich desserts, and fats consumed.

No new diet—especially one that deviates from a normal daily balance—should be attempted without first consulting a physician. Crash diets, injections, and appetite suppressants should be avoided. They are potentially harmful and invariably fail.

When overweight or underweight is a problem, a dietitian can plan meals to fit individual requirements and preferences. The dietitian is trained and experienced in taking into consideration such personal factors as likes and dislikes, income, cooking arrangements, allergies, and similar concerns. Success with a diet depends on making a satisfactory adjustment to a new meal plan that both fulfills dietary objectives and permits the dieter latitude in the choice of foods that accords, to the maximum extent feasible, with personal taste and preference.

When health conditions require a special diet, it must be kept in mind that the diet is a significant part of therapy. Feeling well is not a sufficient reason to abandon the diet. Such action may well aggravate the condition the diet was designed to correct or counteract.

Good nutrition not only contributes to feeling and looking better, but can also reduce the time spent in hospitals because of better response to treatment, faster recovery from surgery, and even more rapid mending of broken bones. Proper diet helps to avoid or relieve medical problems such as obesity, diabetes, high blood pressure, chronic constipation, and heart ailments.

Good Eating Habits

The first essential in establishing good eating habits is to eat no fewer than three meals of moderate size daily. It is best to plan meals well ahead of time and shop with a prepared list of needed items that includes the variety of foods necessary for nutritional balance.

It is important to chew food thoroughly to prevent later discomfort or indigestion, and to drink enough liquid. However, if the appetite is poor, beverages should be taken last. Cooking foods thoroughly will also help to insure comfortable digestion. Grinding or chopping will ease chewing, as will moistening food with sauces, gravies, margarine, or broth. The tough skins of fruits or vegetables should always be removed.

Because their high fat content makes them difficult to digest, creamed foods or foods fried in deep fat should be avoided. Too much concentrated sweets—candy, creamed pies—can cause gastric discomfort by irritating the stomach lining. For the same reason, spices should be used sparingly. Junk foods have little or no nutritive value, and may add to a weight problem or destroy the appetite of the underweight person.

Ways to Cut Food Costs

Care in shopping can help to find bargains, such as day-old baked goods, that will serve as well as more expensive items. Food costs can also be reduced by the use of substitutes that are equally nutritious and differ little in taste, such as margarine in place of butter.

Waste of fruits and vegetables can be minimized by avoiding those that are highly perishable unless they are to be eaten very soon. Ripe fruits last longer if stored in the refrigerator. Fruits such as avocados and tomatoes, often sold before they are ripe, should be allowed to ripen at room temperature. Savings can be realized by selecting lower grade fruits and vegetables, especially for use in stews, soups, salads, or pies, with no loss of nutrient values. Canned or frozen fruits, juices, and vegetables are usually less expensive than fresh varieties, but fresh foods in season, especially if grown locally, may be bargains and also taste better.

Cheaper cuts of meat normally require longer moist cooking than costly chops and roasts but are no less nourishing. The cheapest sources of protein are dried beans, peas, and nuts. Other sources that may be less costly than meat include cheese, eggs, peanut butter, and some fish.

A bargain is no longer a bargain if much of it spoils before it is consumed. Care should be taken in purchasing or storing perishables. Packaged or canned foods should be bought by weight in sizes that suit specific needs without leftover waste.

The following is a summary of helpful hints for cutting food costs:

- Buy smaller packages you can consume in one or two meals.
- Don't buy highly perishable foods you can't eat right away.
- Dried beans, peas, and nuts are the cheapest sources of protein and iron. Cheese, eggs, peanut butter, and some fish cost less than most meats.
- Buy cheaper, tougher cuts of meat and braise, boil, or stew them.
- Watch for sales of day-old baked goods.
- Margarine is a cheaper source of Vitamin A and calories than butter.
- Plan menus around fresh foods in season when they are better and cheaper. (Canned or frozen fruits, juices, and vegetables are often cheaper than fresh.)
- Use cheaper grades (B and C) of fruits and vegetables in casseroles, stews, salads, and pies.
- Powdered milk, especially in larger boxes, costs less than whole milk and can be stored longer.
- No-frills products cost less than brand names.
- Store ripe fruit in the refrigerator. Ripen others at room temperature.
- Freeze variety and ground meats not used within 24 hours. Separate individual portions with waxed paper.
- Never buy cans with bulging ends, rusty seams, or signs of leakage.

- Make bread crumbs by oven drying and grinding stale bread and storing in a jar. Add to scrambled eggs to make them go further and improve flavor.
- Cracked eggs can be boiled safely if one tablespoon of salt is added to each quart of water.

Weight Problems

Reduction of caloric intake is the only safe, inexpensive, and lasting way to lose weight. This means maintaining a balanced diet, adhering to low calorie cooking methods (baking, broiling, roasting, boiling) and omitting foods such as fats, alcohol, and sugar that are high in calories but low in essential nutrients. Success will hinge on the dieter's ability to modify old habits and tastes and adjust to a permanent change that satisfies basic needs.

When the problem is underweight, it must first be determined whether disease is involved by having a physical checkup. In general, gaining weight means temporarily overeating. Liquid meals can be nourishing, and, if properly planned, can furnish all needs except bulk. However, a prolonged liquid diet will cause some loss of intestinal peristalsis, often resulting in constipation when intake of solid food is resumed. For this reason, a combination of solids and liquids is recommended. If malnutrition and anorexia (loss of appetite) persist, the physician may prescribe a balanced pre-digested commercial formula.

Common overweight is caused by consumption of too many calories. Primary calorie sources are protein, carbohydrates, fats, and alcohol. Extra calories not used by the body over a period of time are stored as adipose (fatty) tissue. Individuals 10 pounds above their ideal weight are considered overweight. An excess of 20 or more pounds is considered obesity.

Excess calories from too much good basic food—fish, vegetables, fruit, cereal, milk—are as damaging as the empty calories from such foods as soft drinks, candy, pastries, and alcohol.

Calculating Ideal Weight and Diet

Five factors determine ideal weight: height, gender, body build, basal metabolic rate, and activity level. Women with a medium build should allow 100 pounds for the first five feet of height, and five more pounds for each additional inch. For a small frame, 10% should be subtracted, and, for a large frame, 10% should be added. Males allow 106 pounds for the first five feet of height, and six pounds for each additional inch.

The normal metabolic calorie requirement (with no allowance for activity level) is 10 times the ideal weight. To compensate for activity level, add to this base requirement the ideal weight multiplied by three, if sedentary, by five if moderately active, and by 10 if very active. Thus, for the different activity levels, the calorie requirement is, respectively, 13 times, 15 times, and 20 times the ideal body weight.

Overweight people can usually lose one pound per week by subtracting 500 calories from the calculated requirement.

When a daily diet has been calculated, Exchange Lists can be used to relieve the monotony of dieting. Foods are divided into six groups, and an item in any group can be substituted for any other item in the same group. All exchanges within a group give roughly the same amount of calories, carbohydrate, protein, and fat, and contain similar minerals and vitamins. A balanced diet should include a variety of foods from all the groups.

Low Salt Diet

Individuals who retain fluid or have high blood pressure often benefit from a low salt diet. This restriction should be prescribed by a physician.

In general, no salt should be used in preparing or eating foods. Salt substitutes that contain no sodium are permissible. Because most vegetables are canned with salt, fresh or unsalted vegetables should be used. Similarly, canned, smoked, or salted meats should be avoided. Bouillon cubes and pickles are also salty, and even water may be treated with sodium-containing softeners. Drinking water sources should be checked on travel away from home.

Low Fat Diet (Low Cholesterol)

High blood levels of cholesterol and triglycerides may be related to heart disease. Diet is sometimes effective in controlling such fat abnormalities. If your physician prescribes a diet low in cholesterol and fat, the suggestions in the tables at the end of this chapter can be used as a guide.

Meals on Wheels

First begun in Escambia County, Florida, in 1972, Meals on Wheels is now a popular program in many communities across the country. It is funded through Title III of the Older Americans Act and contributions of cash or services from local sources. Food is provided to the elderly who are unable to obtain a nutritious diet because of physical or other disabilities. Five days a week—Monday through Friday—two meals, one hot and one cold, are delivered at noon by volunteers, and provide 75% of the recommended daily allowance of nutritional elements. Clients are screened for need by public health nurses and are charged according to ability to pay, under Federal Food Stamp guidelines.

FOOD TABLES

The following tables permit the choice of healthy, balanced diets for purposes ranging from losing, maintaining, or gaining weight to restricting salt, cholesterol, or triglycerides. The exchange list divided into six basic food groups is especially useful for diabetics and others who wish to introduce variety without departing from the basic diet.

Quantities are given in the list in terms of unit servings. One serving of any food item in a given group may be substituted for one serving of any other item in the same group with little change in nutritional value. The number of calories and the weights of protein, fat, and carbohydrate in grams in a single serving are given at the beginning of each food group.

SIX BASIC FOOD GROUPS

LIST 1 MILK EXCHANGES

SKIM MILK OR SKIM MILK
PRODUCTS
Each 8 oz = 80 calories, 8 g protein, 12 g
carbohydrate.
 Evaporated .... ½ cup
 Milk, skim or butter, or
  plain yogurt .... 1 cup
 Powdered .... 3 tbsp

MILK OR MILK PRODUCTS WITH 1%
FAT
Each 8 oz = 115 calories, 8 g protein, 3 g
fat, 12 g carbohydrate.
 Buttermilk .... 1 cup
 Milk .... 1 cup
 Yogurt .... 1 cup

MILK OR MILK PRODUCTS WITH 2%
FAT
Each 8 oz = 125 calories, 8 g protein, 5 g
fat, 12 g carbohydrate.
 Buttermilk .... 1 cup
 Milk .... 1 cup
 Yogurt .... 1 cup

WHOLE MILK OR WHOLE MILK
PRODUCTS
Each 8 oz = 170 calories, 8 g protein, 10 g
fat, 12 g carbohydrate.
 Buttermilk or plain yogurt..... 1 cup
 Evaporated .... ½ cup
 Milk .... 1 cup

LIST 2 VEGETABLE EXCHANGES

Each ½ cup serving = approximately 25
calories, 2 g protein and 5 g carbohydrate.

Asparagus	Cucumbers
Bean Sprouts	Eggplant
Beets	Green pepper
Broccoli	Greens:
Brussels sprouts	Beet
Cabbage	Chards
Carrots	Collards
Cauliflower	Dandelion
Celery	Kale

LIST 2 Continued

Greens	Summer squash:
(continued):	Flat scalloped
Mustard	Yellow crookneck
Spinach	& straightneck
Turnip	Zucchini
Mushrooms	Tomatoes and
Okra	tomato juice
Onions	Turnips, yellow
Rhubarb	and white
Rutabaga	Vegetable juice
Sauerkraut	

The following *RAW VEGETABLES* may
be used as desired, referred to as *FREE
VEGETABLES*.

Chicory	Lettuce
Chinese cabbage	Parsley
Endive	Radishes
Escarole	Watercress

LIST 3 FRUIT EXCHANGES
Fruits and Juices, Unsweetened

Each serving = 40 calories, 10 g carbohydrate (canned, fresh, dried, frozen)

Apple....................	1 small
Apple juice	⅓ cup
Applesauce	½ cup
Apricots, fresh...........	2 medium
Apricots, dried	4 halves
Banana..................	½ small
Berries	
Blackberries	½ cup
Blueberries	½ cup
Raspberries	½ cup
Strawberries	¾ cup
Cherries	10 large
Cider	⅓ cup
Dates	2
Figs, fresh	1
Figs, dried	1
Grapefruit	½
Grapefruit juice..........	½ cup
Grapes	12

LIST 3 *Continued*

Grape juice . . . . ¼ cup
Mango . . . . ½ small
Melon
  Cantaloupe. . . . . ¼ small
  Honeydew . . . . ⅛ medium
  Watermelon . . . . 1 cup
Nectarine. . . . . 1 small
Orange. . . . . 1 small
Orange juice . . . . ½ cup
Papaya . . . . ¾ cup
Peach . . . . 1 medium
Pear . . . . 1 small
Persimmon, native . . . . 1 medium
Pineapple. . . . . ½ cup
Pineapple juice . . . . ⅓ cup
Plums. . . . . 2 medium
Prunes. . . . . 2 medium
Prune juice. . . . . ¼ cup
Raisins . . . . 2 tbsp
Tangerine. . . . . 1 medium

Cranberries may be used as desired if no sugar is added.

LIST 4 BREAD EXCHANGES
(Starches) Breads, Cereals, Crackers, Starchy Vegetables

Each serving = approximately 70 calories, 2 g protein, and 15 g carbohydrate.

BREAD

White (including French and
  Italian). . . . . 1 slice
Whole wheat . . . . 1 slice
Rye or pumpernickel . . . . 1 slice
Raisin . . . . 1 slice
Bagel, small . . . . ½
English muffin, small . . . . . . ½
Plain roll, bread 1
Frankfurter roll. . . . . ½
Hamburger bun . . . . ½
Dried bread crumbs . . . . 3 tbsp
Tortilla, 6″ 1

CEREAL

Bran, corn, Grapenut
  Flakes. . . . . ½ cup
Other ready-to-eat
  unsweetened cereal . . . . ¾ cup
Puffed cereal (unfrosted) . . . . 1 cup
Cereal (cooked) . . . . ½ cup
Grits (cooked). . . . . ½ cup

LIST 4 *Continued*

CEREAL *(Continued)*

Rice or barley (cooked) . . . . ½ cup
Pasta (cooked, spaghetti,
  noodles, macaroni . . . . ½ cup
Popcorn (popped, no fat
  added) . . . . 3 cup
Cornmeal (dry) . . . . 2 tbsp
Flour . . . . 2½ tbsp
Wheat germ, Grapenuts. . . . . . ¼ cup

CRACKERS

Arrowroot 3
Graham, 2½″ sq. 2
Matzoth, 4″ x 6″ . . . . ½
Oyster 20
Pretzels, 3⅛″ long x ⅛″
  diameter. 25
Rye wafers, 2″ x 3½″ 3
Saltines 6
Soda, 2½″ sq. 4

DRIED BEANS, PEAS AND LENTILS

Beans, peas, lentils . . . . ½ cup
Baked beans, no pork
  (canned). . . . . ¼ cup

STARCHY VEGETABLES

Corn . . . . ⅓ cup
Corn on cob. . . . . 1 small
Lima beans . . . . ½ cup
Parsnips. . . . . ⅔ cup
Peas, green . . . . ½ cup
Potato, white. . . . . 1 small
Potato (mashed) . . . . ½ cup
Pumpkin . . . . ¾ cup
Winter squash:
  Acorn, butternut,
    Hubbard. . . . . ½ cup
Yam or sweet potato . . . . ¼ cup

LIST 5 MEAT EXCHANGES
(Protein) Meat, Fish, Poultry, Cheese

LEAN MEAT

Each serving = 55 calories, 7 g protein, 3 g fat.

Beef: Baby beef (very lean), chipped beef, chuck, flank steak, tenderloin, plate ribs, plate skirt

LIST **5** *Continued*

LEAN MEAT *(Continued)*

steak, round (bottom, top), all cuts rump, spare ribs, tripe . . . . 1 oz

Lamb: Leg, rib, sirloin, loin (roast and chops), shank, shoulder . . . . 1 oz

Pork: Leg (whole rump, center shank), ham smoked (center slices) . . . . 1 oz

Veal: Leg, loin, rib, shank, shoulder, cutlets . . . . . . 1 oz

Poultry: Meat without skin of chicken, turkey, cornish hen, Guinea hen, pheasant . . . . 1 oz

Fish: Any fresh or
frozen . . . . 1 oz
Canned salmon, tuna, mackerel, crab, and Lobster . . . . ¼ cup
Clams, oysters, scallops, shrimp . . . . . . 5 or 1 oz
Sardines, drained 3

Cheese containing less than 5% butterfat . . . . 1 oz

Cottage cheese, dry and 2% butterfat . . . . ¼ cup

Dried beans and peas (omit 1 Bread Exchange) . . . . ½ cup

MEDIUM-FAT MEAT

Each serving = approximately 80 calories, 7 g protein, 5.5 g fat.

Beef: Ground (15% fat), corned beef (canned), rib eye, round (ground commercial) . . . . 1 oz

Pork: Loin (all cuts tenderloin), shoulder arm (picnic), shoulder blade, Boston butt, Canadian bacon, boiled ham . . . . 1 oz

Liver, heart, kidney, and sweetbreads (these are high in cholesterol) . . . . 1 oz

MEDIUM-FAT MEAT *(Continued)*

Cottage cheese, creamed . . . . ¼ cup

Cheese: Mozzarella, ricotta, farmer's cheese, Neufchatel . . . . 1 oz
Parmesan . . . . 3 tbsp

Egg (high in cholesterol) 1

Peanut butter (omit 2 additional Fat Exchanges) . . . . 2 tbsp

HIGH-FAT MEAT

Each serving = approximately 100 calories, 7 g protein, 8 g fat.

Beef: Brisket, corned beef (brisket), ground beef (more than 20% fat), hamburger (commercial), chuck (ground commercial), roasts (rib), steaks (club and rib) . . . . 1 oz

Lamb: Breast . . . . 1 oz

Pork: Spare ribs, loin (back ribs), pork (ground), country style ham, deviled ham . . . . 1 oz

Poultry: Capon, duck (domestic), goose . . . . 1 oz

Veal: Breast . . . . 1 oz

Cheese: Cheddar types . . . . 1 oz

Chinese cabbage . . . . 1 slice

Cold cuts 4½″ x ⅛″ . . . . 1 slice

Frankfurter . . . . 1 small

LIST **6**   FAT EXCHANGES

Each serving = 45 calories, 5 g fat.
**Margarine . . . . 1 tsp
Avocado (4″ in diameter) . . . . ⅛
**Oil, corn, cottonseed, safflower, soy, sunflower . . . . 1 tsp
Oil, olive . . . . 1 tsp
Oil, peanut . . . . 1 tsp
Olives . . . . 5 small
Almonds . . . . 10 whole
Pecans . . . . 2 lg. whole
Peanuts
Spanish . . . . 20 whole
Virginia . . . . 10 whole
Walnuts . . . . 6 small

LIST 6 *Continued*

Nuts, other . . . . 6 small
Butter . . . . 1 tsp
Bacon fat . . . . 1 tsp
Bacon, crisp . . . . 1 slice
Cream, light . . . . 2 tbsp
Cream, sour . . . . 2 tbsp
Cream, heavy . . . . 1 tbsp
Cream cheese . . . . 1 tbsp
**French dressing . . . . 1 tbsp
**Italian dressing . . . . 1 tbsp
Lard . . . . 1 tsp
Mayonnaise . . . . 1 tsp
**Salad dressing, mayonnaise
   type made with poly-
   unsaturated oil . . . . 2 tsp
Salt pork . . . . ¾ " cube

MISCELLANEOUS FOODS

The following foods may be used in your diet if you wish. They must be figured into the daily diet plan, with the food exchanges allowed as indicated.

Biscuit or corn muffin, 2" diameter (1 Bread, 1 Fat Exchange—115' calories) . . . . 1 small

Peanut butter (1 Meat, 2 ½ Fat Exchange—170 calories) . . . . 2 tbsp

Crackers, found butter type, Ritz, Butterthins, Town House, Snack, etc. (1 Bread, 1 Fat Exchange —115 calories) 5

Ice cream (1 Bread, 2 Fat Exchange—160 calories) . . . . ½ cup

Jello (1 Bread Exchange—70 calories) . . . . ⅓ cup

Muffin, plain 2" diameter (1 Bread, 1 Fat Echange—115 calories) 1

Pancake 5" x ½ " diam. (1 Bread, 1 Fat Exchange—115 calories) 1

Potato or corn chips (1 Bread, 2 Fat Exchange—160 calories) 15

Potatoes, french fried 2-3 ½ " long (1 Bread, 1 Fat Exchange—115 calories) 8

Sausage, beef or pork (1 Meat, 2 Fat Exchange—145 calories) . . . . 2 oz

Sherbet (2 Bread Exchange—140 calories) . . . . ½ cup

Fruit ice (1 Bread, 1 Fruit Exchange—110 calories) . . . . ½ cup

Waffle, 5" x ½ " (1 Bread, 1 Fat Exchange—115 calories) 1

Ginger ale (1 Bread Exchange—70 calories) . . . . 7 oz

French toast (1 Bread, 2 Fat Exchange—160 calories) 1

**high polyunsaturated fat

MEAL PLAN FOR CALORIE-CONTROLLED DIETS BASED ON THREE APPROXIMATELY EQUAL MEALS

Division of Calories: Protein 20% of Total Calories (4 cal = 1 g)
Carbohydrate 60% of Non-Protein Calories (4 cal = 1 g)
Fat 40% of Non-Protein Calories (9 cal = 1 g)

CALORIES

	900	1100	1300	1400	1600	1700	1900	2100

GRAMS

	900	1100	1300	1400	1600	1700	1900	2100
Protein	45	55	65	70	80	85	95	105
Carbohydrate	110	130	155	170	190	205	230	250
Fat	30	40	45	50	60	60	70	75

Servings (see SIX BASIC FOOD GROUPS)

BREAKFAST:

	900	1100	1300	1400	1600	1700	1900	2100
List 1, Skim milk	½	1	½	1	1	1	1	1
List 3, Fruit	1	1	1½	1½	2	1	2	3
List 4, Bread	1½	1½	2	2	2	3	3	3
List 5, Egg	1	1	2	2	2	2	2	3
List 6, Fat	1	1½	1	1	2	2	3	2

LUNCH:

	900	1100	1300	1400	1600	1700	1900	2100
List 1, Skim milk			½	½	½	½	½	½
List 2, Vegetable	1	1	1	1	1	1	1	1
List 3, Fruit	1	1	1	1	2	2	2	2½
List 4, Bread	1½	2	2	2½	2	2½	3	3
List 5, Meat	1½	2	2	2	2½	2½	3	3½
List 6, Fat		½	1	1	1	1	1	1

DINNER:

	900	1100	1300	1400	1600	1700	1900	2100
List 1, Skim milk			½	½	½	½	½	½
List 2, Vegetable	1	1	1	1	1	1	1	1
List 3, Fruit	1	1	1	1	2	2	2	2½
List 4, Bread	1½	2	2	2½	2	2½	3	3
List 5, Meat	1½	2	2	2	2½	2½	3	3½
List 6, Fat		½	1	1	1	1	1	1

CALORIES

	2300	2400	2600	2700	2800	2900	3100	3200	3300	3400

GRAMS

	2300	2400	2600	2700	2800	2900	3100	3200	3300	3400
Protein	115	120	130	135	140	145	155	160	165	170
Carbohydrate	275	290	310	325	335	350	370	380	395	410
Fat	80	85	90	95	100	105	110	115	115	120

Servings (see SIX BASIC FOOD GROUPS)

BREAKFAST:

	2300	2400	2600	2700	2800	2900	3100	3200	3300	3400
List 1, Skim milk	1	1	1	1	1	1	1	1	1	1
List 3, Fruit	2	2½	3	3½	4	3	4	4	3	3½
List 4, Bread	4	4	4	4	4	5	5	5	6	6
List 5, Egg	3	3	4	4	4	4	5	5	5	5
List 6, Fat	2	3	2	2	3	3	2	2	2	2

LUNCH:

	2300	2400	2600	2700	2800	2900	3100	3200	3300	3400
List 1, Skim milk	1	1	1	1	1	1	1	1	1	1
List 2, Vegetable	1	1	1	1	1	1	1	1	1	2
List 3, Fruit	3	2	3	3	3½	2½	3	3½	4	4
List 4, Bread	3	4	4	4	4	5	5	5	5	5
List 5, Meat	3	3	3½	4	4	4	4½	5	5	5
List 6, Fat	2	2	2	2	2	3	2	2	2	2

DINNER:

	2300	2400	2600	2700	2800	2900	3100	3200	3300	3400
List 1, Skim milk	1	1	1	1	1	1	1	1	1	1
List 2, Vegetable	1	1	1	1	1	1	1	1	1	2
List 3, Fruit	3	2	3	3	3½	2½	3	3½	4	4
List 4, Bread	3	4	4	4	4	5	5	5	5	5
List 5, Meat	3	3	3½	4	4	4	4½	5	5	5
List 6, Fat	2	2	2	2	2	3	2	2	2	2

Low Salt Diet (1½–2 g salt)

FOODS ALLOWED:

Soups	Commercial *low sodium* soups, low sodium bouillon, unsalted home made soups.
Meats	Fresh or frozen meat, poultry, liver, fresh water fish, *low sodium* cheese, canned meat, peanut butter, water packed tuna, salmon. 6 oz or servings are allowed per day.
Egg	1 per day.
Cereals	Hot cereal, rice, grits, puffed wheat, puffed rice, shredded wheat.
Breads & Starches	Unsalted commercial bread, rolls, matzo, wafers, crackers, melba toast unsalted home made breads. Eggs and milk used in cooking must be omitted proportionally from the diet. Macaroni, spaghetti, noodles, cowpeas, soybeans, black eye peas, white potatoes, sweet potatoes.
Vegetables	*Low sodium* canned asparagus (green & white), lima beans, green beans, wax beans, carrots, corn (cream style & kernel), green peas, tomatoes, tomato puree. *Fresh vegetables:* all kinds except beet greens, Swiss chard. *Frozen vegetables:* spinach, summer & winter squash, green beans, wax beans, broccoli, Brussels sprouts, cauliflower, collard greens, kale, mustard greens, okra.
Fruits & Juices	All kinds. Unsalted tomato juice.
Fats	*Unsalted* butter, margarine, French dressing, mayonnaise, nuts. Cream 1 oz per day.
Milk	2 cups per day, homogenized, low sodium.
Beverages	Coffee, Sanka, Postum, tea.
Sweets	Granulated sugar, honey, maple syrup, home made syrup of white sugar, gum drops, hard candy, jelly beans, pure jams and jellies that contain no preservatives.
Desserts	Plain gelatin, fruit flavored gelatin. Rice, tapioca, cornstarch puddings. Sherbet, fruit ice. Desserts made with sodium-free baking powder or low sodium commercial cake mixes. Consider the allowance of milk and egg for the day and omit proportionally from the diet when used in baking.
Miscellaneous	*Low sodium* pickles, catsup, chili sauce, mustard, vegetable relish, meat tenderizer.

Low Salt Diet

FOODS AVOIDED:

Meats	Canned, salted or smoked meat, fish, bacon, cold cuts, chipped or corned beef, frankfurters, ham, sausage. Frozen fish fillets, clams, lobster, crabs, oysters, scallops, shrimp. Regular cheese, regular peanut butter.
Cereals	Quick cooking cereals, enriched cereals containing sodium compounds.
Breads & Starches	Regular breads, hot breads & pastries prepared with baking soda or regular baking powder. Regular commercial pies, cakes & mixes.
Vegetables	Frozen green peas, lima beans. Vegetable juice. Sauerkraut & all vegetables not listed under *foods allowed*.
Fruits & Juices	Crystalized or glazed fruit, maraschino cherries, dried or frozen fruit with sodium sulfite or sodium benzoate added. Regular tomato juice.
Fats	Salted butter or margarine, bacon, olives, salted nuts, regular commercial mayonnaise, French dressing, etc.
Milk	Powdered, condensed, evaporated, eggnog, buttermilk.
Beverages	Instant cocoa mixes, ''Dutch Process'' cocoa, mineral water.
Sweets	Brown sugar, molasses, commercial syrups, candies, jams, jellies containing sodium preservatives.
Desserts	Regular baking mixes, rennet tablets, commercial ice cream.
Miscellaneous	Regular commercial bouillon, catsup, mustard, pickles, horseradish, chili sauce, meat extracts, meat tenderizers, meat sauces, relishes, pickles, soy sauce, Accent, monosodium glutamate. Table, celery, garlic, onion salt.

* *

Persons with severe cardiac conditions should *avoid* the following *gas* forming foods: broccoli, cauliflower, cabbage, sauerkraut, Brussels sprouts, cole slaw, green peppers, onions, corn, cucumbers, radishes, lima beans, turnips, sweet potatoes, melon, raw apples. *Avoid* the following stimulating beverages: strong coffee, strong tea.

Low Sodium Salad Dressing — Makes 1 ¼ cups

> 1 can of ready to serve low sodium tomato soup
> ¼ cup salad oil
> 2 tbsp wine vinegar
> 1 tbsp lemon juice
> 1 tbsp finely chopped onion
> 1 tbsp sugar
> 1 large garlic clove, minced
>   dash of pepper

Low Triglyceride Diet

FOODS PERMITTED	DAILY ALLOWANCES
Milk	As desired — skim milk, powdered and skim buttermilk
Meat	6 oz — *lean beef,* lamb, veal, pork, fish, fowl, tuna, salmon (water packed), peanut butter
Egg	3 *per week,* eggwhites as desired, egg substitutes as desired (Eggbeaters, Scramblers, Chono)
Cheese	As desired — plain cottage cheese, skim milk cheese (ricotta, Lite Line, Jarlsberg, Count Down)
Bread and Substitutes	6 servings — sliced baker, muffins, rolls, biscuits, bagels, crackers (made with vegetable shortening), potatoes, spaghetti, macaroni, noodles, rice, corn, limas, green peas, cereal (hot & cold)
Soup	As desired — broth, consomme, bouillon, soups made with skim milk
Fat	As desired — oil (sesame, sunflower, safflower, corn, peanut, soybean), margarine made from these oils, French dressing, walnuts, peanuts
Vegetable	As desired — all kinds, include one yellow or dark green leafy each day
Juice & Fruit	2 servings — UNSWEETENED, any kind, take one citrus
Miscellaneous	As desired — D'Zerta, Tab, Fresca, no-calorie sodas, herbs & spices (except sugar), mustard, coffee, tea, sanka, sliced lemon, vinegar
Desserts	1 serving — sponge or angel cake, jello, junket made with skim milk and sugar substitute

* *

FOODS NOT PERMITTED

sugar	sherbet	alcohol	caviar
candy	fruit ice	chocolate	lox
cake	pie	coconut	liver
jam	pastry	coconut oil	sweetbreads
jelly	doughnut	lard	brains
syrup	condensed milk	butter	kidney
honey	cocoa butter	non-dairy creamer	gizzards
marmalade	cream	fried food	sausage
molasses	sour cream	potato chips	salt pork
soft drinks	mayonnaise		

All foods containing sugar.

Low Cholesterol Diet

FOODS PERMITTED   **DAILY ALLOWANCES**

Milk	As desired — skim milk, powdered skim milk, skim buttermilk
Meat	6 oz lean beef, lamb, veal, pork, fish, fowl
Egg	3 per week, eggwhites as desired
Cheese	As desired — plain cottage cheese, skim milk cheese (ricotta, Lite Line, Jarlsberg, Count Down)
Bread	As desired — sliced baker, muffins, rolls, biscuits, bagels, crackers (made with oil)
Cereal	As desired — all kinds
Soup	As desired — broth, consomme (fat free) soup made with skim milk
Fat	3-4 tsp — oil (safflower, sunflower, corn, soybean), margarine made from the above oils, *or* 4 tbsp French dressing
Vegetable	As desired — all kinds, include at least one yellow or green one daily
Juice	As desired — all kinds except clam
Fruit	As desired — all kinds, take at least one citrus daily
Dessert	As desired — jello, fruit ice, sherbet, sponge and angel cake, junket made with skim milk
Sweets	As desired — jelly, honey, syrup, molasses, marshmallows, hard candy, gum drops
Beverages	As desired — tea, coffee, Sanka, 7-Up, ginger ale
Spices	As desired — all kinds

FOODS NOT PERMITTED

Chocolate, coconut, coconut oil, cocoa butter, sour cream, lard, butter, mayonnaise, palm oil, salt pork, non-dairy cream and milk substitutes

Frankfurters, sausage, kidney, liver, sweetbreads, brain

Lobster, shrimp, clams, crabs

Cheeses high in fat, fried foods, potato chips, fritters, doughnuts, pancakes, pastry, cookies, cake made with hydrogenated fat or butter and eggs

Whole milk, regular evaporated and condensed milk

Avocado

PHYSICAL FITNESS

Jim Thacker

Health Educator, Philadelphia Health Plan

If you look out your window any morning or early evening, you are likely to see a jogger. The magazine on your coffee table may have a jogger on the cover. TV commercials promoting any kind of product, from soap to hardware, may feature the jogger. Concern with fitness has become a national preoccupation, and the reasons are not hard to find. The physically fit have stronger hearts and leaner bodies; numerous studies have shown that those who work at becoming fit feel better both physically and mentally.

But what does the fitness revolution mean to the older individual who may never have been an athlete and who seldom engages in strenuous physical activity? A study conducted for the President's Council on Physical Fitness and Sports in 1972 found that the attitudes of older citizens toward physical activity and fitness were as follows:

- It is believed that the need for physical activity decreases and may actually disappear as individuals age.

- There is a tendency to exaggerate the risks involved in vigorous physical activity after middle age.

- The benefits of light, occasional activity are overrated.

- Older individuals underrate their own abilities and capacities.

Facts About Physical Fitness

What is Physical Fitness?

A typical definition of physical fitness describes it as "the ability to carry out daily tasks with vigor and alertness, without undue fatigue and with ample energy to enjoy leisure-time pursuits and to meet unusual situations and unforeseen emergencies." However, this definition is less than adequate. With few exceptions, our daily tasks require relatively little physical effort. Labor-saving devices such as escalators, power mowers, and the ubiquitous automobile are everywhere in use, and the usual emergency involving running for a bus or up a flight of stairs demands only momentary output of extra effort. When measured by the standards of exercise physiologists, very few of us are physically fit.

The following definition of physical fitness is rather broad, but covers the basic components that must be considered when fitness is measured with some degree of accuracy:

> ...the capability of the heart, blood vessels, lungs and muscles to function at optimal efficiency. Optimal efficiency means the most favorable health needed for enthusiastic and pleasurable participation in daily tasks and recreation activities. Optimal physical fitness makes possible a lifestyle that the unfit cannot enjoy. Developing and maintaining physical fitness require vigorous effort by the total body.

The four components of muscular strength, muscular endurance, flexibility, and cardiovascular endurance are the pillars of physical fitness. Muscular strength is the strength of the muscles in a single maximum effort, as in lifting a heavy weight. Muscular endurance is the ability of the muscles to perform work, which might be measured by the number of pushups an individual can complete. Flexibility is the ability to use a muscle throughout its full range of motion involving the joints, as in bending, stretching, or twisting. Touching the floor without bending the knees indicates good flexibility. Cardiovascular endurance, the ability to use large muscle groups over a period of time, requires the smooth functioning of the heart, lungs, and blood vessels. Such endurance can be improved and strengthened by activities such as brisk walking, jogging, cycling, swimming, and similar exercise.

It is generally agreed that cardiovascular endurance and flexibility, discussed in the following pages, are the most important components of physical fitness.

The Need for Physical Activity

The remarkable health of older individuals in three areas of the world—the Caucasus in the Soviet Union, the village of Vilcabamba in Ecuador, and the Hunza region in Pakistan—has been the subject of numerous articles in books and journals. These regions have no air pollution, the average diet is low in saturated fat, and there is little excessive smoking or drinking and practically no obesity. While each of these factors surely contributes to the health of older inhabitants, an additional major factor is the level of physical activity. Traditional farming and household duties require physical exertion without the benefit of tractors, dishwashers, and similar aids. Everyone is physically active from birth to death; in Caucasus villages, 60 percent of those over 80 still work daily.

It may be objected that most of us do not farm and have no need to do physical work each day, and therefore why shouldn't we take life easy in our later years?

One answer can be found in a recent study of 17,000 Harvard alumni which established a relationship between heart health and physical activity, showing that those who were not active physically were subject to more heart attacks and to earlier death than physically active individuals. Several similar studies have shown that lack of physical activity leads to changes normally associated with aging, including general weakness, shrinking muscles, loss of bone calcium, an increase in total body fat accompanied by a decrease in body muscle, and a reduction in the body's ability to use oxygen. It seems reasonable to deduce from these studies that at least some changes in our bodies and perhaps in our health as we grow older are due as much to inactivity as to aging. Clearly, the need for physical activity remains strong as we age.

The Risks of Physical Activity for the Aging

A sudden run at full tilt to the limit of physical endurance would be a risky endeavor for someone past middle age. But a brisk walk or easy jog until one begins to tire, then slowing to a walk until rested before resuming the faster pace, entails little or no risk.

Roy Shephard, a leading Canadian physician and exercise physiologist, contends that the risk for dying while exercising is extremely remote. He estimates the risk at one in five million for males, and one in seventeen million for females. Minimum risk can be realized by beginning an activity program at a low, easy level and increasing it gradually to a more strenuous level. It is also advisable to have a physical examination before making any major change in the level of physical activity. Any sign of chest pain or unusual dizziness is an indication that the activity should be stopped immediately.

Per Olof Astrand, a Swedish exercise physiologist, has proposed that physical examinations be required for the sedentary individual, who, he says, is in greater need of such attention than the physically active person. As support for such a requirement, Astrand points to the studies showing a connection between inactivity and heart disease, as well as other problems, such as obesity.

The Overrated Benefits of Light Activity

Though many of us enjoy activity such a golf or gardening—and enjoyment is important in choosing a physical activity—these activities are of little or no benefit to the heart. Strengthening the heart requires an activity that stimulates the pulse rate to at least 100 per minute for those of age 55, which is repeated three times a week for periods of fifteen minutes or more. Thus, only a quick run to the first tee on the golf course, or vigorous work with a hoe in the garden will cause the heart to reach the minimum rate necessary to achieve some benefit.

Some years ago Dr. Roy Shephard conducted a study in which he analyzed normal levels of activity among a group of workers in Toronto, Canada, ranging in age from 23 to 65. Each subject in the study was required to wear a device which recorded pulse rates for 24 hours over a period of three days. It was found that, with only few exceptions, the work performed by the subjects did not raise pulse rates high enough to provide heart-strengthening benefit. Shephard therefore concluded that systematic participation in vigorous physical activity is vital to the maintenance of a healthy heart, lungs, and blood vessels.

Underrating Abilities and Capabilities

The average person only rarely engages in sustained physical activity and has not participated in sports in school or college where team membership is typically restricted to the better athletes. In addition, most of us are employed in work that does not demand physical endurance, and our leisure time is largely spent in sedentary activities such as watching TV. Perhaps because of this relative inactivity we assume that our age of 55 or more precludes vigorous exercise to improve our physical fitness level. Happily, this is not so. Age is no bar to engaging in a program to improve fitness.

Dr. Herbert de Vries, a well-known exercise physiologist, is director of the seniors' fitness project at the Laguna Hills, California, Leisure World. Several years ago, he supervised a study involving 41 sedentary male volunteers ranging in age from 50 to 87. Following a careful physical examination, the volunteers took part in one-hour workouts three times a week over a period of six weeks. When the 41 active subjects were compared with 26 control subjects who had not participated in the workouts, dramatic differences were found. The former had reduced their blood pressure and the percentage of body fat, and had improved their arm strength and cardiovascular endurance. The most encouraging finding of the study was that subjects who had been least active in youth and middle age benefitted most from the program.

De Vries pointed to five ways in which his activity program improved participants' health:

- The heart muscle was strengthened.

- Blood pressure was reduced.

- Some subjects experienced reduced tension.

- There was a reduction in the percentage of body fat, in turn reducing the statistical probability of heart attacks.

In older males the ability to breath deeply and efficiently was improved.

A second study by Adams and de Vries involved seventeen women aged 52 to 79 who participated in a physical activity program similar to that of the men in the earlier study. Again there was an improvement in physical fitness, but not to the degree shown by the men.

A third study was designed to analyze the effect of physical activity on certain physiologic characteristics of 22 men aged 49 to 65. The group participated in 30-minute periods of walking and jogging three times a week for 20 weeks. Results included significant increases in maximal oxygen uptake—a measure of heart and lung efficiency—decreases in resting heart rate, diastolic blood pressure, body weight, total body fat, and waist measurement. It was concluded that men in this age group respond well to endurance activity, with beneficial changes similar to those in studies involving younger subjects.

Training the Heart

It should be kept in mind that the heart is a muscle, and like any muscle in the body, must be trained by systematic use over a period of time. Thus, effective training for the heart requires activity vigorous enough to reach a heart beat of at least 115 for not less than 20 minutes a day, three or more times a week, at age 55. At age 60, the heart beat should be at least 112, 109 at 65, and 105 at 70. These rates are percentages of maximum heart rates—the fastest the heart will beat under the stimulus of intensive exercise.

The maximum heart rate for any individual can be estimated by either of the methods as follows:

- By subtracting chronological age from 220

- By means of an exercise stress test

It has been determined by exercise physiologists that a pulse rate of 70 to 85 percent of the maximum heart rate is required to achieve improvement in the heart itself.

How to Count the Pulse

Place the index and middle fingers on the groove at the side of the neck, or below the thumb on the underside of the wrist. A strong beat should be felt at both positions. When measuring the pulse at rest, make the count in the morning before arising. When measuring the pulse following activity, count the beats for ten seconds and multiply by six. It is important to find the pulse quickly, as the heart slows rapidly when activity ends (Figure 1).

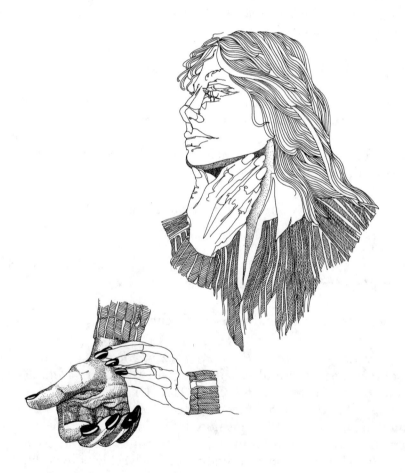

Figure 1. The Pulse Can be Measured at the Side of the Neck or on the Wrist.

To test the pulse to see if it is within normal range, count it for 60 seconds. If the rate exceeds 80 beats per minute, take a second reading before arising in the morning, and if the rate remains over 80, consult a physician. In most cases, a high pulse rate is a sign of poor physical fitness, excessive smoking or consumption of caffeine, or stress from overwork or other causes. Because smoking narrows blood vessels and requires the heart to work harder, the smoker may have a pulse rate 20 beats higher than it would otherwise be for his or her age.

As the heart is exercised, it will become larger and stronger, doing its work with fewer beats as each beat is able to pump more blood than before. The success of an exercise program can be gauged by measuring the resting pulse before arising; as the heart becomes stronger, the resting pulse rate will decrease.

Activities for Strengthening the Heart

The most effective activities for strengthening the heart are those that are continuous and rhythmic: brisk walking or jogging, swimming, cycling, rowing, jumping rope, and so on. In choosing the activity best suited for particular individuals, the following questions should be considered:

- Is the activity one that can be done at any age?

- Can it be done alone?

- Is it convenient and enjoyable?

- Does it fit personal tastes and inclinations?

The Cooper Aerobic Point Program   One of the better guidebooks for developing a physical activity program is *The Aerobics Way,* by Dr. Kenneth Cooper (M. Evans & Co., 1977). Dr. Cooper offers recommendations and has designed tables based on "aerobic points." These are presented in an easy-to-follow fashion to facilitate setting up an effective activity program. The tables include point values for a variety of activities, allowing a choice of one or several to reach a weekly point goal.

There is a close relationship between aerobic points and the improvement of cardiovascular fitness level. Table 1 illustrates how fitness categories and weekly points are related.

Table 1. The Cooper Aerobic Point Program

Fitness level	Women	Men
Very poor	Less than 1 point	Less than 1 point
Poor	1–9	1–14
Fair	10–23	15–29
Good	24–40	30–50
Excellent	More than 40	More than 50

Adapted from K. Cooper, *The Aerobics Way*, M. Evans and Co., 1977.

For those in the 50–59 age range, Cooper offers progressive exercise programs for the following activities:

cycling	stationary cycling
skipping rope	running in place
running	swimming
stair climbing	walking
handball	racquetball
squash	basketball
soccer	lacrosse
hockey	

For individuals in their 60's, Cooper's programs include cycling, stationary cycling, swimming, and walking. The walking programs for both age groups are included in Tables 2 and 3.

Cooper's program requires working toward a fixed number of points each week, and his studies have shown that those who average more than 34 points have a lower risk of heart attack than individuals with lower averages.

Pollock Heart Rate Program   For those who may feel that a heart rate program better suits their needs and preferences, the following recommendations developed by Michael Pollock, an exercise physiologist at the Institute for Aerobic Research, will serve as guides to a level of fitness:

Table 2. Walking Exercise Program
   (50–59 years of age)

Week	Distance (miles)	Time goal (min)	Freq/Wk	Points/Wk
1	1.5	29:30	4	8
2	1.5	28:00	4	8
3	1.5	26:00	4	8
4	2.0	36:00	4	12
5	2.0	35:00	4	12
6	2.0	34:00	4	12
7	2.0	32:00	4	12
8	2.0	31:00	4	12
9	2.5	38:00	4	16
10	2.5	37:45	4	16
11	2.5	37:00	3	19.5
12	2.5	37:00	4	26
13	3.0	44:00	4	32
14	3.0	43:00	4	32
15	3.0	43:00	4	32
16	3.0 or 2.5	42:30 36:00	4 5	32 32.5

Adapted from K. Cooper, *The Aerobics Way*, M. Evans and Co., 1977.

Table 3. Walking Exercise Program
   (age 60 and over)

Week	Distance (miles)	Time goal (min)	Freq/Wk	Points/Wk
1	1.0	20:00	4	4
2	1.0	19:00	4	4
3	1.0	18:00	4	4
4	1.5	29:00	4	8
5	1.5	28:00	4	8
6	1.5	27:00	4	8
7	2.0	38:00	4	12
8	2.0	36:00	4	12
9	2.0	34:00	4	12
10	2.5	42:30	4	16
11	2.5	41:30	4	16
12	2.5	40:00	4	16
13	3.0	55:00	4	20
14	3.0	52:30	4	20
15	3.0	50:00	4	20
16	3.0	48:00	5	25
17	3.5	56:00	4	24
18	3.5	55:00	5	30

Adapted from K. Cooper, *The Aerobics Way*, M. Evans & Co., 1977

Frequency: 3 to 5 days per week, evenly spaced

Intensity: About 75 percent of maximum heart rate

Duration: 15 to 60 minutes—can be continuous or with short rest periods

Type of activity: Run, jog, walk, bicycle, swim, row, arm crank, or endurance sport activities

It is essential when starting an activity program for the first time to exercise at a level that is both safe and comfortable. This can be assured by taking care to exercise at 60 percent of your maximum heart rate for at least eight weeks.

The pulse rate should be checked after the first three minutes of exercise, and the activity slowed or speeded up to reach the correct heart training rate. This should not be necessary after initial trials, when familiarity with the interaction between exercise and heart rate makes the adjustment more or less automatic.

The Half-as-Much Approach The "half-as-much" program, developed by the Department of Health for the Canadian province of British Columbia, is based on the simple principle that activity at the beginning of a program is limited to half of what the individual believes he or she can do. A capacity for 20 laps in the swimming pool is cut to 10, or 10 sit-ups to 5, and so on. It is recommended that half-as-much be continued for a period of two weeks for those in their 20's, three weeks for the 30's, four for the 40's, five for the 50's, and six for the 60's, before increasing the activity.

Half-as-much activity recommendations are similar to those outlined by Michael Pollock:

Frequency: 3 to 5 days per week,

Intensity: Work up to and sustain the cor-
             rect target heart rate dor your age

Time: When the body adjusts to the new
        activity, keep moving for at least
        15 minutes, slowing if necessary

Type: Any endurance activity: walking,
        jogging, swimming, etc.

Flexibility

As noted before, flexibility is an essential component of fitness. Joints not in regular use may become stiff, restricting the range of motion. The importance of flexibility is underlined by the fact that some types of arthritis can be prevented by regular, gentle stretching. Such stretching differs from exercise like walking or jogging in that the pulse does not increase. Slow, easy stretching releases energy, but care should be taken not to exceed the body's capabilities.

In addition to improving the spine's elasticity and strengthening stomach muscles, stretching helps to remove body tension and tends to correct poor posture. Stretching will also firm up the skin, reduce the potential for a double chin, and improve the tone of flabby arm muscles. Combining a stretching program with heart fitness exercise should bring beneficial results almost immediately.

Practical Suggestions

Things to Do and to Avoid

The following list of do's and dont's, taken from Casey Conrad of the President's Council on Physical Fitness and Sports, should be studied before beginning any kind of activity program.

DOs

DO Listen to your body. It will tell you when you're doing too much. Switch to a less demanding activity, or rest, if you are overdoing it.

DO Warm up for several minutes before beginning more difficult activity. Start easy to help avoid injuries. Also, taper finish to let your heartbeat return to a normal level.

DO Participate in activity at least 3 times a week. Make it part of your normal routine.

DO Strive for a balance between flexibility and endurance activities. Don't neglect either.

DO Gradually increase your workload. You need to do this to increase your fitness level.

DO Take ten deep breaths four or five times a day to help increase your lung capacity.

DON'Ts

DON'T Compete with others to see who can do the most. Work at your own level and gradually increase your level.

DON'T Engage in activities that require quick, jerky movements while undergoing a long period of conditioning. Sudden exertion can lead to injury and strain.

DON'T Be a weekend athlete. It's risky. You will be much better off to space your activities throughout the week.

DON'T Push yourself to the point of exhaustion. You want to increase your pulse rate into a zone which improves your fitness, but stop short of being winded and weak.

DON'T Take a sauna bath after your activity is completed for the day. This places an additional burden on your heart. If you want a sauna or steam bath, do it before your activity (and follow the sauna or steam bath with a cool shower).

DON'T Sell yourself short. Many people—particularly older ones—underestimate their physical capabilities.

Exercise Program

The following exercise program is recommended for the older person who wants to increase flexibility and improve cardiovascular fitness.

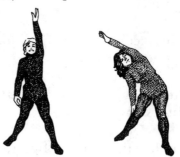

Flexibility exercise 1: stand with your legs spread comfortably. Reach up with left arm, bend from the waist to the right, and let your right hand slide down your leg toward your ankle. Hold for 15 seconds and come up slowly to starting position. Do the same using the other arm.

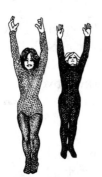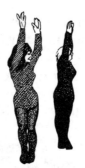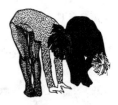

Flexibility exercise 2: stand comfortably with feet together. Stretch your arms up, then twist so that your chest faces left but your hips face forward. Bend from the waist as far as you can — don't force it. Hold the position for 15 seconds, then come back up slowly, twist to your original position, and let your arms hang down. Do the same on the other side.

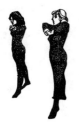 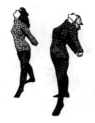

Flexibility exercise 3: stand with your left foot slightly ahead of your right. With your fingers touching, put the back of your hands on your chest. Circle your arms back until you can interlock your fingers behind you. Straighten your arms and lift them upward as you bend backwards. Hold for five seconds, then bend forward in the direction of your left knee and hold for 10 seconds. Return slowly to the starting position and repeat starting with your right foot slightly forward.

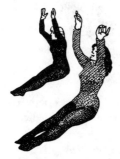

Flexibility exercise 4: sit with your legs extended and raise your arms above your head. Lean back slightly and hold for 5 seconds. Then bend forward and reach the farthest point on your legs that you can hold without straining. As your elbows move out, pull yourself toward your knees. Hold the position for 30 seconds.

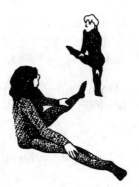 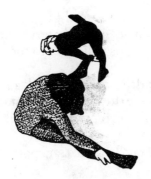

Flexibility exercise 5: still sitting on the floor, spread your legs in a straddle position. Bend forward as far as you can (comfortably), then hold your legs to keep the position and stay for 30 seconds.

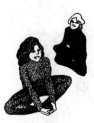

Flexibility exercise 6: stay sitting on the floor in the position for exercise 5. Put the soles of your feet together, clasp your hands around your feet, and pull them to your body as far as possible — don't strain. Then push your knees toward the floor. Push as far as you can with straining and hold for 15 seconds.

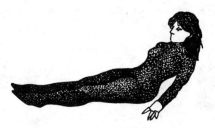

Flexibility exercise 7: lie on the floor and slowly raise your legs between 6 and 12 inches off the floor. At the same time raise your shoulders so that your head and feet are the same distance from the floor. Hold for 15 seconds.

Additional Suggestions

For those who would like to start a physical activity program, but are unable to do so immediately, the following suggestions for changes in habits or customs will serve to increase daily physical activity.

- If you drive to work, park a half mile from your destination and walk the rest of the distance. A brisk one-mile walk each day will burn up seven pounds in a year.

- If you take public transportation, get off a few stops earlier.

- Cover all short distances on foot, if possible.

- Eat a light lunch and take a walk of at least fifteen minutes.

- Walk, jog, or ride a bike before breakfast.

- Trade coffee for activity when there is a break.

- Walk up and down stairs once each hour during the day.

- Try stretching exercises when watching TV.

- Replace some power tools with manually operated devices.

- When at the beach, walk or jog as well as sunbathe.

PLASTIC SURGERY

R. Barrett Noone, M.D., F.A.C.S.

Assistant Professor of Surgery
University of Pennsylvania School of Medicine

Lawrence P. Kerr, M.D.

Assistant Professor
State University of New York, Binghamton

The plastic surgeon is now called upon more frequently than ever by people over 55 for reconstructive surgery. Although plastic surgery for deformities caused by accidents is still common among older people, the majority seek assistance with problems related to aging or malignancy (either the disease or consequences of treatment). For example, deformities due to malignancies of the skin, breast, and mouth can be reconstructed by plastic surgery.

The Aging Face

Aging of skin usually parallels the aging of other body organs. However, many factors sometimes prematurely age the skin so that its appearance is inconsistent with the general good health and well-being of the rest of the body. Although individuals differ, the main causes of apparently premature skin aging are heredity, past illnesses, particular lifestyles and habits, and environment such as prolonged exposure to sunlight.

Whatever the cause of the disparity between "old skin" and otherwise youthful good health, a growing number of individuals are unwilling to allow their appearance to "age gracefully." In years past, the appearance of aging implied wisdom. This association no longer holds in a society that values most a youthful, dynamic appearance. Preoccupation with youth, beauty and success causes more and more people to seek ways

425

to obliterate the physical signs of aging, and plastic surgeons have responded with appropriate surgical techniques. "Sagging skin" and wrinkling develop earlier in some individuals than in others. For this reason, the timing of surgery to control the process also varies, but most aesthetic facial procedures are done between the ages of 50 and 60 years.

These procedures moderate the effects of aging on the forehead and eyebrows (brow lift), the eyelids (eyelid plasty), the lower face and neck (facelift), and the fine skin wrinkles (chemical peel, or dermabrasion). Many of these operations have been developed and popularized only in the past three or four decades, and are constantly being improved and refined as long-term effects are observed and better understood.

Preparing for Surgery

Both the patient who undergoes aesthetic face surgery and the surgeon who performs it desire a pleasing change. To achieve success, certain preparations must first be completed. Since major aesthetic surgery of the face involves a degree of physical trauma for the patient, a thorough medical examination is essential to disclose any serious contraindications to the operation. In addition, the patient must be emotionally healthy, psychologically evaluated and prepared by the operating surgeon, and adequately informed about possible outcomes so that expectations are realistic.

Considerations vary with the individual and must sometimes take into account complications of the surgical procedure. The anticipated result should be clearly understood before aesthetic surgery is performed. If the patient has not been fully informed, especially about possible complications, the operation may cause unhappiness and even pyschological disturbance. Fortunately, this is rare, because the competent plastic surgeon spends the time and effort needed to adequately prepare the patient before surgery.

How the Operation is Done

Surgery to improve jowl lines or sagging folds of the face and neck is generally referred to as a facelift (*rhytidectomy*). Eyelid surgery, to remove excess skin and reduce upper or lower eyelid sag is termed a *blepharoplasty*. The operations may be done simultaneously with one anesthetizing and hospitalization, or in separate procedures, depending upon the patient's desires. Some patients are concerned only with the eyelids, others more with the lower face. Most desire surgery for both areas. Occasionally, the eyebrows and forehead skin are tightened in combination with eyelid or facelift surgery.

Hospitalization ranges from one to three days, depending upon the extent of the operation and the wishes of the patient and surgeon. Comfortable intravenous anesthesia and local facial anesthesia are normally used. General anesthesia is applied only in unusual circumstances. Photographs before the operation are routinely entered into a permanent record.

The facelift incision (Figure 1) begins in the hairline at the temple, passes downward in front of the ear and around the earlobe, and ends in the scalp behind the ear. Excess skin is removed after the facial skin is lifted away from underlying fat and muscles. In many instances, fat is removed from beneath the skin, and tightening procedures are done in the muscles. The surgical wounds are sutured under tension and covered with a dressing.

Eyelid surgery may be performed alone or in combination with a facelift. It is usually done to remove excess eyelid skin (which can be so extreme in some older people that it falls over the eyelashes and obstructs vision), or to reduce protruding fat around the eyeball caused by relaxation of the eyelid lining with aging. This fat is usually most prominent over the inner corner of the eyelids near the nose. In the eyelid operation, incisions are made in the upper lid (Figure 2) in the normal fold, and excess skin and fat are removed. The lower lid incision (Figure 3) is made along the margin of the eyelashes, the skin is lifted from the eyelid, and the excess skin and protruding fat are reduced to lessen the "baggy" look.

In some individuals, eyebrow tissue may overhang and block the upper eyelids. This is often hereditary and longstanding, and may not be related at all to aging. Also, the attachment of the forehead muscles to the skin can produce horizontal grooves which aging may accentuate. These abnormalities can be helped by a combined forehead and eyebrow lift involving an incision extending behind the hairline of the scalp and near the upper portion of the ears. The skin of the forehead and eyebrow is then undermined and lifted, and excess skin is removed at the upper scalp and above the ears. This procedure can give a more youthful ap-

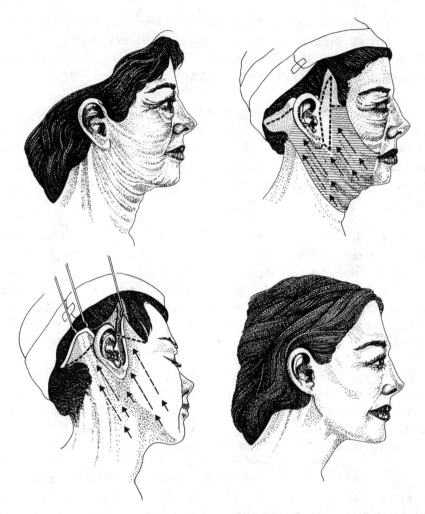

Figure 1. The facelift tightens aging skin of the cheek, jowl, and neck. Excess skin is removed through a surgical incision in the scalp, in front of and behind the ear.

pearance to the eyebrows and forehead, but will not totally eliminate wrinkling caused by the forehead muscles that express a frown.

The chemical face peel (*chemosurgery*) has limited usefulness in treating problems of aging tissue because it only slightly tightens loose skin. However, as an adjunct to a facelift, it helps to eliminate fine wrinkles and skin blemishes such as keratoses. Chemosurgery can occasionally by itself minimize fine wrinkling that is not or only minimally

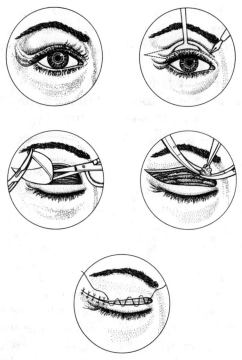

Figure 2. Upper lid blepharoplasty involves removal of excess skin and protruding fat.

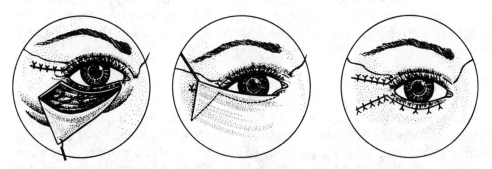

Figure 3. The lower eyelid incision is made along the lash margin, the skin is raised, and excess tissue is removed.

associated with sagging of facial tissues. People who benefit most from a chemical peel are women with fair skin, fine wrinkling, and minimally sagging facial tissue. Those with olive complexions are often less satisfied with the result because the peel may change skin pigmentation. This technique produces the most satisfactory results on the forehead, lips, and chin.

The chemical contains phenol mixed with croton oil and liquid soap. Although the procedure can effectively eliminate many of the fine wrinkles of aging skin, it can also involve complications. After peeling, skin color changes from red back to pink, usually over a period of two or three months. However, the fading may sometimes take longer, and the change in skin color may also become a permanent problem. Fortunately, this aberration is rare, as are permanent scarring by the chemical peel and small whiteheads or pimples called *milia*.

If a chemical peel is combined with facelift surgery, the two procedures are not performed on the same area of skin. Coupling a peel with a facelift may extend hospitalization by one or two days.

What to Expect After Surgery

There is some discomfort and occasional pain for 24 to 48 hours following surgery, but pain medication is rarely needed after 48 hours. Bandages are usually removed before discharge from the hospital, and the patient then visits the physician's office at frequent intervals for wound examination and suture removal. Washing the hair with mild soap and combing it with a large-toothed comb are permitted three days after surgery, but tinting and coloring should be postponed for three weeks. Eye makeup (mascara, eyeshadow, false eyelashes) may be applied after final removal of the sutures in the eyelids. Face makeup may be used about the 10th day after surgery, but must be carefully removed at the end of each day.

Before the expected improvement is apparent, the patient goes through a postoperative period with a bruised appearance, followed by another period of feeling strange on self-examination. Most healing takes place during the first three weeks, but scars will continue to fade for as long as a year. Some oozing from the incisions can be expected for a few weeks, usually behind the ears, which can be effectively camouflaged with makeup. The plastic surgeon strives to place scars in natural lines in the face and eyelids where they are least noticeable and more easily hidden by cosmetics or hairstyle. While such scars are permanent, they are rarely prominent or troublesome.

Facelift or eyelid surgery can be expected to significantly improve the appearance, and patients are usually pleased with results. Improvement is most pronounced in the eyelids, jowls, and neck skin, but the surgery has little effect after the first few months on the creases running from the nose to the corners of the lips, and does not reduce crowsfeet or fine lip wrinkles. Although improvement is permanent in some patients, about 75 percent of aging lines and skin looseness return in six or seven years.

As with any surgical procedure, unfavorable aftereffects are possible, but fortunately infrequent. Collections of blood (*hematoma*) beneath the skin may need evacuation. Rare loss of skin or scalp hair and damage to the nerves controlling facial muscles have been reported. The skin may darken, especially where severely bruised. Occasionally, the wound may become infected, requiring suture removal and drainage. Scarring and loss of earlobe sensation may cause minor annoyances. Occasionally, a scar on the lower eyelid will temporarily tend to pull the eyelid down, but this usually lasts only a few months. Very small cysts may appear along the eyelid incisions, but these are also temporary and usually disappear spontaneously.

Cost

Except for certain plans, the cost of cosmetic, as opposed to reconstructive, surgery is not covered by most medical insurance programs such as Blue Cross/Blue Shield, Medicare, and those of most major insurance companies. Therefore, it is normal practice for plastic surgeons and hospitals to request payment in advance for this type of surgery. Surgical fees and hospital costs vary widely with the procedure to be done and geographical location. For these reasons, a clear financial arrangement should be agreed on before the operation is scheduled.

The Breast

Because much can be done to correct breast deformities (whether congenital or due to cancer treatment) and to remedy over-or underdevelopment, the plastic surgeon is justifiably enthusiastic about breast surgery. This enthusiasm is often shared by affected patients (generally, but not all, women), many of whom are the happiest beneficiaries of the plastic surgeon's skill.

This has not always been so. Modern surgical techniques evolved slowly. Improvement in technique is likely to continue, but many abnormalities can now be treated satisfactorily, especially if the objective is a normal clothed appearance. Although plastic surgery may fall short of creating the idealized nude breast long pictured in paintings, ideal anatomy is rare among real women and men, as can be seen in any private or public dressing room.

The normal breast starts out in childhood as merely a nipple of differently colored skin. Through puberty, it becomes cone-shaped, fuller below than above, and the nipple lies just above the midline. During pregnancy, the cone fills and becomes more globular. A slackening of muscles with age or an increase in weight due to obesity or pregnancy can cause the breast to droop so that the nipple points down rather than forward. The downward pull elongates the breast and its center falls lower on the chest wall (*ptosis*, or fallen breast). After pregnancy and breast feeding, the breast may lose substance and elasticity, an aging process that accelerates after menopause. Some observers think that ptosis is appearing at a younger age in the "bra-less generation."

The left and right breasts are rarely identical. Some loss of symmetry is apparent in all paired parts of the body. A significant mismatch is an obvious abnormality which may result from unequal development or a defect in the chest wall remaining from surgical treatment of cancer.

Breasts may fail to develop to a reasonable size (*hypoplasia* or *micromastia*) or grow too large (*hyperplasia* or *macromastia*). Although what constitutes "too small" and "too big" is mostly a matter of personal preference, there are some objective criteria. Clothing is usually designed for people whose dimensions do not range far from the average, so that a woman who needs special dresses or tops is aware of being different. Very large breasts may cause back and neck pain, aggravate arthritis, produce rashes in overlapping folds of flesh, and make brassiere straps cut into the shoulders.

Augmentation Mammoplasty (Breast Enlargement)

Breasts are enlarged by insertion of a permanent prosthesis behind the existing breast. The prosthesis consists of a thin-walled silicone plastic bag filled with either salt water or a silicone gel. It is not detectable to the touch and requires only a few weeks to get used to. This technique can be used to restore youthfulness to a minimally fallen and shrunken breast.

The major drawback of this operation is the chance that the body will develop an envelope of scar tissue around the prosthesis. As the scar tissue shrinks, it forms a firm capsule which can be felt beneath the breast and which also causes the breast to fall unnaturally on the chest. Infection may also necessitate removal of the prosthesis. However, the operation can be repeated.

Reduction Mammoplasty

While breast enlargement is defined as cosmetic surgery, reduction mammoplasty is considered reconstructive and is covered by most medical insurance plans. Indications for breast reduction are back and neck pain, bra straps cutting into the shoulders, and difficulty in keeping the skin under the breasts clean, dry, and free of irritation, particularly in hot weather.

The objectives of the operation are reduction of the bulk of breast tissue, restoring the nipple to a normal position, and establishing structural support for breast weight by, in effect, creating a skin brassiere. Surgical corrections actually follow clothing industry patterns.

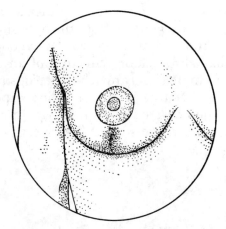

Figure 4. Scars from reduction mammoplasty form an inverted T. The wide vertical scar runs downward from the minor scar around the nipple to join a horizontal scar hidden in the fold beneath the breast.

The incision involves a large area of the chest and leaves extensive scars. Viewed from the front (Figure 4), they appear as a circle around the nipple and a vertical scar running down to the fold beneath the breast where it meets a horizontal scar concealed in the fold. Patients are usually happy to accept the scars as the price of being able to engage in athletics (often for the first time since puberty), to wear better fitting clothes, and to be relieved of pain and discomfort. The operation also often relieves the feeling of heaviness and aching of large breasts, but this alone may not be considered enough to justify surgery.

Drooping breasts are corrected by the same technique except that little or no breast tissue is removed.

Post-Mastectomy Reconstruction

Breast reconstruction after a mastectomy involves a silicone prosthesis like that used to enlarge the breasts. However, radical mastectomy does not leave enough tissue so that more skin is needed and a smooth cover of muscle must be placed over the prosthetic bag to give the chest a natural contour. This problem is now solved by transferring the *latissimus dorsi* muscle of the back and arm to the front of the chest (sometimes wth extra skin) so that the muscle fibers fan out across the chest wall (Figure 5). This causes only one additional scar, six to nine inches long, on the back in the area normally covered by the bra.

A second procedure is needed to construct a natural-looking but non-functional nipple. Skin grafting from the opposite breast, the inside of the thigh, or the entrance to the vagina allows a good color match. The second procedure may also include reduction of an oversize remaining breast, if necessary, to more closely match the reconstructed breast. A reconstructed breast is obviously abnormal when exposed, but appears completely normal when covered, even if only by a bathing suit. It is a satisfying alternative to a tissue-stuffed bra or externally-worn artificial breast.

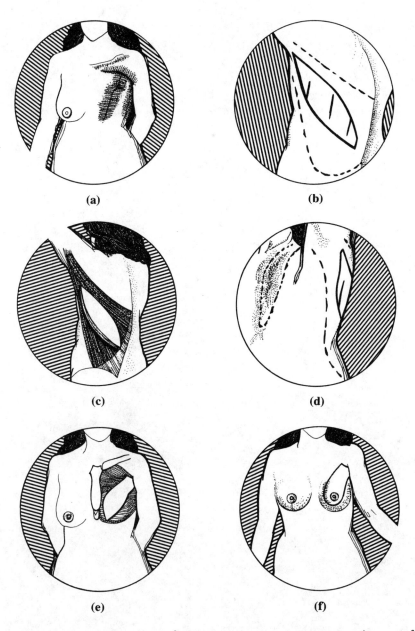

(a)

(b)

(c)

(d)

(e)

(f)

Figure 5. Breast reconstruction after a mastectomy (a) may require transfer of skin and muscle from the back to the front of the chest (b). The fan-shaped *latissimus dorsi* muscle (c) is moved into the mastectomy defect (d), and the resulting island of skin and muscle (e) is used to cover a breast implant. A nipple is then formed and the opposite breast reshaped (f).

SEX AFTER 55

Edward T. Auer, M.D.

Clinical Professor of Psychiatry,
Institute of the Pennsylvania Hospital

The steadily increasing number of men and women living beyond the age of 55 has been accompanied by a burgeoning interest in their life styles. And as their awareness of this focus of interest grows, the aging tend to seek standards of behavior to compare with their own experience. Whether motivated by scientific or commercial interest many professionals and others are prepared to offer lists of items such as weight, blood pressure, bowel function, sleep, special diets, food supplements, health foods, drugs, vitamins, minerals, and so on.

That a variety of special interests should develop to serve the social, psychological, and recreational needs of this growing population seemed inevitable. Few anticipated these needs or foresaw the political issues that have arisen. This was to be expected in a society that has traditionally organized effectively to deal with current problems, while cultivating a strong work ethic which denigrated the abilities of the over-55 group. But there have also been constructive responses, often actively supported by the aging themselves. The American Association of Retired Persons, Catholic Golden Age Club, Gray Panthers, and a growing number of community and church-related groups have mobilized to support older individuals' needs for socialization, education, political action, and recreation.

While many of these activities have gradually developed over the past 50 years, curiosity about the sexual behavior of the population over 55 is relatively recent. The cultural taboos imposed on the sexuality of parents and grandparents have inhibited both young investigators and their older subjects, but there have been some efforts to study sexual behavior of the aging population. In his reports, *Sexual Behavior in the Human Male* (1948) and *Sexual Behavior in the Human Female* (1953), Kinsey included males from age 56–80 and females from age 56–90. Although he found a decline in sexual activity in the aging, his samples also reported sexual activity in male and female octogenarians.

A helpful rule in diagnosis and treatment of any ailment is that an individual whose capabilities may be limited by physiologic (e.g., age) or pathologic (disease) changes also has inherent abilities to cope which must not be overlooked. Unfortunately, our society tends to ignore the fact that sexual feelings, desires, and activities do not disintegrate as we age. The medical history of an older person which fails to take his or her sexual life into account is simply incomplete. If the person is suffering from an acute physical illness, the doctor may appropriately defer seeking a sexual history. However, many such patients affected by an acute episode, such as coronary thrombosis, need advice about their sexual activity and whether it should be moderated during recovery.

A few years ago, Dr. William Masters told of a study involving a number of men who had been hospitalized and treated for coronary occlusion. In follow-up interviews, he found that neither the patients nor the physicians had raised the question or discussed their post-coronary sexual behavior, yet it was an issue of concern to most patients shortly after their return home.

Dr. Masters' story brings to mind an incident in which a patient was about to leave the hospital following a severe attack of hepatitis. His internist, a competent young man, carefully advised him about diet and the strict need to limit his physical activity. The patient inquired, "What about sex?" "Oh, you can go right ahead with that," responded the embarrassed physician, leaving the room with the roar of the patient's laughter ringing in his ears. The internist was young enough to be the patient's son, and the older man's query about sexual behavior apparently damaged his self-assurance. Nevertheless, although the internist warned against climbing stairs more than once a day and against living heavy objects, he gave the green light to sex which might also involve strenuous physical activity.

Our current knowledge of the limits on sexual functioning imposed by physiologic change is scant, as reflected in the exchange between the internist and his aging patient. This lack of knowledge has stimulated a continuing study at the Marriage Council of Philadelphia "seeking to determine how hormone levels, personality traits and social interactive ability of a group of older couples, who have recently remarried after widowhood or divorce, relate to their sexual adjustment." To obtain a significant number of subjects for the study, couples are paid $500 for their participation in 26 interviews.

It is generally accepted today that the potential for sexual pleasure appears to begin at birth and need not end until death. However, the intensity and quality of the sexual response may vary considerably in different individuals and at different ages.

Masters and Johnson's studies revealed that the male ejaculatory response is most vulnerable to the effects of aging. Some capabilities and vigor decline after peaking in adolescence, but the erection remains relatively unaffected. Though the aging males in the study no longer experienced the intense multiple orgasms of their youth, some 80-year-olds had occasional orgasms and sustained erections when effectively stimulated.

After 50, the sexual effects of aging appear most in the frequency of ejaculation (it decreases) and in the time required before another erection can be achieved (it takes longer). Men between 50 and 60 are commonly satisfied with one or two orgasms per week. Based on interviews with 212 men, of whom 33 were directly observed, Masters and Johnson reported that many normal men in their fifties are unable to repeat an erection for 12 to 24 hours after an ejaculation. Clearly, longer and more intense stimulation is required to achieve an erection and ejaculation.

This implies that the touch of the woman's body, an embrace or a kiss during love play may not produce an immediate erection. Direct stimulation of the partner may be required. Masters and Johnson also reported that some elderly men may lose an erection with orgasm, perhaps during prolonged love play, and be unable to achieve another for 12 to 24 hours. Ejaculation is less forceful when it occurs and the erection is rapidly lost afterward.

Does a male menopause exist? There is some evidence that male hormone production decreases at the same time that men in their fifties begin to suffer from increases in depression, irritability, easy tiring, and sexual changes. However, controlled studies of hormone replacement have not yet been done. Certainly no abrupt age-related changes in men's reproductive organs occur to match the changes in women when menopause rapidly stops ovarian activity. However, if psychologic effects are included, it is reasonable to suppose that a kind of male menopause exists. Both men and women experience wide variations in their responses to psychological, social, and biological forces at this time of life.

Female sex after 50 varies appreciably from woman to woman. While it is affected by the cessation of ovarian activity, it also depends on the previous personality, psychological state, and relationships with the sexual partner and others important in a woman's life. The sharp drop in circulating hormones (estrogen and progesterone) is often accompanied by feelings of irritability, depression, emotional instability, and aggressive outbursts.

The effect of menopause on the erotic drives of women also varies. In some, depression and irritability diminish interest in sex, while others report strengthened sexual desire. These differences appear to depend on many factors, some preceding the menopause. Others, such as physiologic changes, changes in sexual opportunity, and diminished inhibitions, are associated with the menopause itself. Biologically, an increase in sexual drive and interest might be expected when estrogen no longer opposes the action of androgens and the woman is freed of anxieties about pregnancy. Some women do experience such an increase. However, if her male partner's sex interest wanes, the woman may misinterpret his difficulties as an adverse judgment of her physical attractiveness. She may then avoid sex, fearing disapproval, and feel frustrated and rejected.

Today, women continue to vary widely in sexual desires and responsiveness. The relative decline of sexual interest among older men reduces the number of available partners. Women who have regular opportunities for sexual activity tend to remain sexually responsive, but without opportunity, their sexual drive declines. After 65, women tend to be less preoccupied with sex, but remain capable of seeking and responding to sexual opportunities. Erotic involvements are not uncommon, and masturbation and erotic dreams are reported. According to Masters and Johnson, vaginal lubrication tends to occur more slowly, and orgasmic contractions are less vigorous and less frequent, but continue to occur, together with the capacity for multiple orgasms. Although many older women cease to have intercourse, some studies report that 25 percent of 70-year-old women continue to masturbate.

Replacement hormone therapy is still controversial, especially because of its possible contribution to cancer of the uterus. Also, difficulties older men and women may have in enjoying sex are not necessarily due to reduced hormone production by sex glands, but may be related to previous longstanding problems. Complaints may now be voiced for the first time because they are perceived as age-appropriate, and thus more acceptable.

Although there are no supporting data, it seems likely that many men and women are able to adapt to sexual age-related changes in ways that are compatible with their new status while others suffer stress and a crisis with which they are unable to cope.

Impotence and retreat from sex interest may characterize many older persons resigned to the loss as a natural and inevitable consequence of aging. However, those who resist passive surrender should be heartened by the fact that a couple should be able to enjoy sexual pleasure throughout their lives so long as their general health is good. The majority of sexual complaints after 55 stem from adverse psychological reactions to normal changes in the sexual response. It is essential that an adviser be thoroughly acquainted with the facts to be able to deal adequately with intimate questions and to keep sex limitations and capabilities of older people in rational perspective. Particularly, partners should be taught to perceive and understand changes occurring in each other, and to use this knowledge practically to retain a healthy pleasure in sex.

Because of certain personalities, some men are especially vulnerable to the effects of middle age. Some behavior is a defensive response to neurotic needs. Among the more successful defenses are placation, compulsive work patterns that achieve job success, and excessive independence. They defend against the fear of rejection and mistreatment created by inner feelings of helplessness and worthlessness. Sexually, such individuals may sublimate their own needs to satisfy the demands of a partner. The sexual act may also be seen as a strenuous effort to conquer and manipulate women, rather than a means to achieve an intimate relationship and mutual sexual pleasure. Although such defensive patterns may keep neurotic symptoms under control, the cost is often neglect of the man's own needs and the risk that others will take advantage of him by imposition and mistreatment. The result may be physical and psychological stresses which accelerate the normal consequences of aging.

Premature loss of physical strength and sexual stamina can also cause problems with work and careers. Vulnerable individuals are also more sensitive to an aging physical appearance that forecasts the loss of youthful drive and sex appeal. First to be lost are the defensive habits which have weakened the ability to cope openly with the normal problems of aging. The result is usually a form of physical or psychological decompensation that is difficult for the individual and his close associates to understand because it seems to be an overreaction to relatively moderate signs of aging. Such individuals often develop physical symptoms, assuming sickness as a defense against their basic problems.

This process may also cause some men to become sexually hyperactive. A middle-aged man may pursue younger women who promise a greater challenge and enhanced self-esteem, or he may take up with prostitutes. In others, decompensation may lead to impotence, masturbation, exhibitionism, or even homosexual pairing.

For example, a highly successful businessman in his late fifties began to develop anxiety prior to situations he had previously handled easily. He eventually suffered a coronary occlusion, and, on recovery, returned to work with heightened anxiety about his ability to perform as before. He began to drink heavily, and on one drunken occasion submitted to a homosexual seduction. This compounded anxiety with guilt, which increased his drinking, impaired his work performance, caused him to be fired, and resulted in protracted psychiatric hospitalization. His own inner strength and the support of an understanding wife contributed to a fortunate outcome. But this required learning to give up compulsive living patterns which he could no longer support mainly because of his forced retirement from a high-pressure job.

Certain psychiatric illnesses of older age groups are frequently accompanied by sexual symptoms. Depressions often bring withdrawal from interpersonal relations, impotence in men, and loss of interest in sex by women. Many respond well to antidepressant medication, psychotherapy, and occasionally electroconvulsive treatment, and regain their sex drive and activity.

However, some drugs used to treat psychiatric disorders impair sexual ability, especially in men. Candid recognition of this fact and reassurance that normal function will return when the medication is stopped can be therapeutic.

Older patients who develop organic brain disorders may regress in behavior. They sometimes become exhibitionistic and may masturbate openly.

Alcohol can also deter sex. Many men first experience impotence after excessive drinking. One failure generates a self-defeating anxiety about repeated failure, and drinking to relieve anxiety only increases the likelihood of further failure. The cycle can be broken only with an awareness of the detrimental effect of alcohol. Absence of understanding not only stands in the way of the man's success but also harms the woman who sees the failure and drinking as signs of rejection by her partner.

Individuals over 55 are also more prone to physical illnesses which can affect all behavior including the sexual. Some illnesses may diminish the ability or desire for sex, sometimes as psychological side effects of the primary disorder. For example, male impotence is often one of the earliest symptoms of diabetes, or may be associated with kidney or liver diseases which interfere with the detoxification and excretion of estrogen and other metabolic products.

Surgical procedures may cause functional as well as physiologic changes which interfere with sexual functioning. Of special concern in the male are such procedures as prostatic surgery, and estrogen administration or even castration in the treatment of prostatic cancer. In the female, hysterectomy and mastectomy often make a women feel less attractive and desirable. In such cases, a frank discussion of sexual reactions to treatment is imperative. A physician who feels uncomfortable or unprepared to offer such assistance should refer the patient to a more capable colleague.

Colostomy often causes considerable distress and anxiety about loss of physical attractiveness. Those strongly affected can be helped by skilled psychological assistance. Others need to talk out their feelings with a knowledgeable person who can help them to restore vitally important closeness with a spouse or loved one.

Paraplegic patients need special assistance in learning to accept the limitations of their affliction and to develop the ability to retain normal sexual outlets or find new ones to bring pleasurable relief to their heavily burdened lives. In one case of surgery for a spinal cord tumor, a young female patient was told that she might regain control of her lower extremities, but would not be able to control her bladder function, have a normal sexual life, marry, and have children. She was understandably despondent, but psychotherapy and a great effort to succeed helped her to defy prediction. She learned to control her bladder, did marry, and had children. Few cases can be so dramatically successful, but these can inspire the efforts of others to reach their optimal potential as human beings despite handicaps.

Treatment of sexual dysfunction associated with aging or its common maladies, whether biological or psychological, starts with a comprehensive diagnostic evaluation. A careful review of the past history of sexual adjustment must often involve the sexual partner, who may need guidance to appreciate the patient's changing needs, responses, and sensitivities. It is necessary to learn about those aspects of sexual intimacy that can serve as building blocks to strengthen a relationship, rather than to dwell on the pathology that impedes healing.

Based on current knowledge, hormonal therapy is questionable in the treatment of sexual dysfunction. Replacement therapy should be considered only after deficiency has been clearly demonstrated, and should be closely monitored for possible adverse effects. This is especially true for estrogen therapy, frequently used for menopausal distress in women.

In summary, it is important to bear in mind that aging may bring physiologic changes that influence sexual activity. People in general should be prepared to meet such changes with a rational response, and guidance professionals should keep up to date with advancing information in the field, including helpful resources available within the community. It is inappropriate to blame aging for any problems when other possible causes remain unexplored. The pessimism expressed by the clinician who advises, "You ought to expect certain things at your age," is often a cop-out. Patients and health professionals too often take refuge in old age. Older people have adaptive capacities and potentials to offset their limitations. These can be developed by nurturing the special potential in each individual.

PSYCHIATRIC PROBLEMS

J. Martin Myers, M.D.

Psychiatrist-in-Chief, Pennsylvania Hospital

Psychiatric problems do not inevitably accompany aging. Also, properly diagnosed and appropriately treated psychiatric illness is often reversible.

Each person is truly an experiment of nature, an individual with a unique hereditary background, physical and psychosocial history, physiological and interpersonal means of adapting to the environment, and expectations of the future. Problems in living can be caused by many factors, but their alleviation may require modification of only one or a few sources of distress, or strengthening of the ability to cope.

Because older people are longer-term experiments of nature, their lives are usually more complex than those of younger people and demand deeper understanding. Standard psychological formulas may not apply, and individual consideration of difficulties is more likely to be appropriate than generalizations.

What are Psychiatric Problems?

Health problems have several basic components: biological, physiological (functioning of the body), psychological, and social (interaction of the individual with others). Thus, understanding and alleviating illness require a bio-psycho-social approach. Although disease is often narrowly considered as purely organic (a malfunction of body organs), the feelings and attitudes toward the illness of the victim, family, friends, and acquaintances can have an aggravating or mitigating effect.

The biopsychosocial approach rejects attempts to separate the physical body from either the psyche or society. The interconnections are significant in illness at any age, but are especially so after 55. For psychiatric problems in particular, whether construed narrowly as psychosis (major dysfunction of thinking, feeling, or behaving) or broadly as any personal distress, a prejudiced view that is overly biological, physical, medical, or social is a barrier to understanding.

Distinguishing illness from normal development is especially important for the aging because it is often difficult to tell if a particular complaint is a disease to be treated or simply the toll of passing years. In childhood and adolescence, psychological and somatic changes are more varied and rapid, and therefore more distinct.

Determination of the prevalence of a disease in any population entails defining the disease and clarifying what we mean by average, normal, and optimal health. In our culture, the definition of ill health is steadily broadening. One reason is that advanced technology now enables the detection and measurement of more subtle abnormalities. However, this is largely true only in non-psychiatric areas.

In psychiatry, the emphasis has been on trying to understand human personality and observing individual behavior. A half century ago, the only persons generally considered psychiatrically sick had major disabilities or obvious signs of illness such as delusions or wildly disorganized behavior. Some severe neuroses, for example, an incapacitating compulsion such as continual handwashing, or blindness due to hysteria rather than an organic defect, would also have been recognized as psychiatric problems, but a tremendous range of behavior was considered within average limits and therefore healthy. Later, more and more significant variations were identified, and the concept of health was raised to the "normal," which might be defined as the average after eliminating known pathology.

In recent years, this trend has been extended to classify anything less than optimal health as illness, and to expect that optimal health can be achieved by all. Mental health practitioners strongly tend to view all "disease" as disease.

Statistically, men and women over 55 face an increasing probability of acquiring some chronic disease. A psychiatric symptom such as poor memory may be related to organic illness, for example, a brain disorder, or represent a psychological aspect of an illness, for example, depression. If memory lapses are intrinsic to aging itself, then questions of definition and classification arise. Current scientific opinion tends to regard many disabilities previously attributed to aging as actually part of a pathological process.

How Common Are They?

Individuals over 55 have a disproportionately high amount of psychiatric illness. This is due in large part to a corresponding increase in physical problems and depression. A study by the National Institute of Mental Health found ten times as many reported new cases of psychiatric illnesses per 100,000 population in those over 65 (236.1) as in those under 15 (2.3).

About 5 percent of the adult population needs psychiatric treatment to maintain health. The rate rises with age so that by 65, 15 percent could benefit from such help. The proportion of moderate-to-severe psychiatric illness increases from about 10 percent at age 65 to approximately 30 percent at age 80.

Depression is the most frequent incapacitating psychiatric problem throughout life. More than half the victims of a serious depression have their first episode after 60, and estimates are that careful clinical examinaton would confirm depression in 10 to 30 percent of those over 65.

Suicide is the most tragic outcome of depression. The rate increases with age and is highest for elderly white males—especially the widowed, divorced, and alcoholic. In the 70–74 age group, white men commit suicide at a rate three times that of non-whites and five times that of females. The increase in the suicide rate for aging white men is so high that it more than balances the decrease from a peak in middle adult years for white females and all non-whites. However, the rates for elderly white females and non-whites have recently begun to climb.

Because depression is one of the most treatable psychiatric illnesses, early identification can prevent many tragedies. The public must be better informed about the signs of depression and suicidal tendency, especially in the elderly. While only one out of seven suicidal attempts by an adolescent results in death, one out of two in the elderly succeeds. The elderly can also commit suicide in ways that escape conclusive detection, such as not taking prescribed medication, so that the attributed rate is probably lower than it really is.

Because the number of older people is increasing so rapidly—from 4 percent of the U.S. population in 1900 to 10 percent today, and a probable 20 percent in 2010—the number of older mentally ill has also increased. Studies indicate that more than 50 (some say 70) percent of all residents of nursing homes show signs of moderate or severe psychiatric illness. Fortunately, a large proportion of this illness is of a treatable behavioral type, usually depression. Others with clearly organic disease can also often be helped.

It should be noted that while 5 percent of the over-65 population live in nursing homes, 15 percent have been in nursing homes at one time or another, indicating that the condition of many improved so that they were able to leave. It should also be noted that 95 percent are not so incapacitated as to need institutionalization. As many as 75 percent are intellectually and socially able, mentally vigorous, interested in their surroundings, and eager to participate in the life of their families and communities. Given the opportunity, they are apt to be productive. The goal for the elderly is to be integrated and living comfortably within the society with which they are familiar. Impairment is not the result of aging alone.

What Causes Them?

Problems develop when an individual's equilibrium is upset by stress beyond the capacity to recover. The tolerable limit varies with the person and is based on both genetic inheritance and physical and psychological development in a particular social environment. Thus, numerous factors affect the capacity of an individual to deal with stress. They can be grouped into three categories: physical (biological, organic, or cellular), psychological, and social. The three categories constantly interact with each other because the individual in action is greater than the sum of his or her parts.

Stress in later life is more likely to arise from losses than from new roles and responsibilities. In contrast to adolescence when new functions are assumed—having children, earning an independent living—the years beyond 55 are experienced by most as a period of loss of strength, loss of friends, and loss of financial independence. One study of the attitudes of those in their 60's and 70's revealed frequent surprise that poor health was their most severe problem. They had feared it, but had expected it to rank far below financial problems and loneliness resulting from the loss of friends.

Physical Factors

Our physical bodies are biochemical factories engaged in processes that result in feeling, thinking, and interactions with others. Our bodies change over time, but not due to an isolated series of steps called aging. Hereditary factors established at the time of fertilization of the egg, and subsequent life events (the physical traumas and diseases suffered by the individual) all influence the aging process.

Each individual is programmed at birth for certain changes in cellular function, some of which may occasionally produce well-defined psychiatric illness late in life. Examples are Huntington's chorea, a progressive disease with symptoms of erratic movements and mental deterioration, which usually first appears in middle or late life, and Alzheimer's disease, degeneration of brain cells in middle age, which also has an hereditary basis.

Certain physical changes associated with aging, such as wrinkling and age spots, appear at varying rates or times in different individuals. For some persons, the appearance of spots and wrinkles in their own skins before those of contemporary friends or spouses may be a source of stress. Other common changes of age are diminishing height and gray hair. Breast changes may strongly affect some women or their sexual partners. Psychological reactions, such as the conflict between the body's present condition and the old self-image, can be more significant than the physical changes which may actually impose little organic stress. Conscious and unconscious fears of aging and death may stimulate defensive reactions of denial and withdrawal. Yielding to anxiety may also provoke rejection by a spouse and the desire for a younger partner.

Chronic disease is one of the most severe stresses to which those over 55 must adjust. An individual who reaches 65 has an 80 percent chance of suffering from a chronic disease such as hypertension, arteriosclerosis, arthritis, respiratory difficulties, and kidney problems. Twenty-five to 30 percent will have arteriosclerotic heart disease; 30–40 percent will have arthritis. Impaired eyesight and hearing will affect 30–40 percent. The conscious and unconscious emotional reactions to illness are often more incapacitating than the physical impairment.

Many illnesses of the aging are accompanied by a loss of appetite which can lead to malnutrition. The lack of a rounded diet with adequate vitamins and minerals is a particular threat in the development of psychiatric problems. Chronic diseases and resulting deficiencies of the blood, heart, lung, and kidneys may decrease the nutrients such as oxygen and increase the toxic substances transported to the brain. Although decreases in both visual and auditory acuity are common in older persons, poor hearing causes greater emotional problems. Impairment of these senses increasingly isolates a person from others and the environment.

Use of multiple medications can significantly contribute to the development of psychiatric problems. Harmful interaction of drugs may occur when a patient sees several physicians, each of whom prescribes for a different illness without knowing which other drugs are being taken, including over-the-counter preparations. Drugs are far more potent today than they were several decades ago.

Except for the central nervous system, all organs of the body are capable of cell regeneration. Thus, liver or heart muscle cells may die and be replaced, but dead brain cells are lost forever. Although we have many more brain cells than we need, they deteriorate, expecially if deprived of sufficient oxygen and proper nutrition. Eighty percent of those with severe psychiatric problems in late life have lost some brain tissue, a condition which can now be measured with new X-ray techniques.

The health of elderly persons distinctly correlates with their relationship with their adult children. A good relationship tends to accompany better health and fewer problems. One possible reason is that parents in poor health impose heavier demands on the children, which leads to difficulties that strain relationships. Poor physical health also closely correlates with adverse personal attitudes toward aging and a lowering of self-esteem.

Psychological Factors

It is commonly said that as persons grow older they become more like themselves. There is some truth in this assertion, but also some distortion. It is perhaps an extreme way of stating that previously developed personality patterns and coping mechanisms are not apt to change markedly, that personality persists over time, and that characteristics and cherished values become more apparent. However, it erroneously implies that adult experience does not change character at all.

Various psychological schools (Freud, Jung, Erikson, Levinson) have speculated about the effects of aging and present a variety of viewpoints. A general assumption holds that aging brings a progressive decline in psychological reserves, and that the accumulated stress of many losses retards recovery to the status before stress. However, research has destroyed some formerly widely held beliefs, for example, that aging decreases the ability to remember and to comprehend. Although the elderly do tend to react more slowly to certain test stimuli and have some difficulty counting numbers backward, memory lapses seem due to diminished motivation rather than inability to learn and retain, and might more appropriately be considered abnormal rather than a natural consequence of age.

Healthy coping mechanisms, by definition, are those which help one to deal with the real world and to find socially acceptable ways of gratifying desires and achieving goals. They may include short periods of withdrawal to replenish the energy needed to continue the fray. On the other hand, coping mechanisms which deny personal needs, depend on others for approval, or blame others for one's own lack of achievement, only make the elderly person more vulnerable to severe stress. However, generalizations do not always apply. In special circumstances, some relatively unhealthy responses may deal with stress more effectively than more wholesome ones. For example, troubled individuals who are perpetually unhappy in a family and job situation that demands many interpersonal encounters may find relief and comfort after retirement by exercising their habit of withdrawal to an isolated haven with only books for company.

In addition to physiological losses, aging individuals experience the loss through death of those around them, loss of employment, and loss of illusions. Increasing evidence that unrealistic goals set in young adulthood will never be achieved can become overwhelming and induce depression and other pathologic reactions.

For those over 55, the greatest psychological stress is the loss of a spouse. A woman is more likely to become a widow than a man a widower because she is usually younger than her spouse. Even if their ages are the same, her life expectancy will be eight years greater than his. A middle-aged woman who is more than five years younger than her husband has three chances in four of outliving her spouse.

Widows are better able to deal psychologically with the death of their husbands, than widowers are with the death of their wives and are less prone to suicide. A suggested reason is that women, who are more likely to have spent most of their lives at home, develop closer and more supportive personal relationships than men do at work. Men are also more apt to remarry to replace their loss, and can do so more easily because there are nearly three elderly women to every two elderly men.

Social Factors

Modern social attitudes incline us to reject the older person. Constantly encountered, such rejection diminishes self-esteem and is harmful to mental health.

The dominant American view has been that psychological and personal maturity is reached in the early or middle adult years, and that life is downhill from then on. If middle-class, middle-aged people who are raising a family, working regularly, and enjoying good health, are normal, then older people who don't do these things are obviously not. This encourages a belief that the older person's different behavior reflects an altered ability to meet the expectations of earlier years, reduced motivation to do so, or both. It demands that the disapproved behavior be corrected or, if not corrected, at least isolated. And it denies the older age groups psychological support and a sense of belonging.

This set of negative attitudes has been titled ''Ageism'' by Robert N. Butler, Director, National Institute on Aging. It is more detrimental than regarding age as sickness. Genuine sickness often evokes compassion, while old age classifed as a feigned illness meets with hostile tolerance.

Our modern industrial and technological society prefers young workers. Because of rapid changes, the older worker occupies a precarious position. The pool of skills which improve over time without extensive retraining and reeducation grows smaller. Yet people are most commonly identified in our society by their occupation. The first question asked a new acquaintance is, "What do you do?" Loss of job thus threatens loss of identify.

Retirement, even when self-imposed, brings a job (and possible identity) loss, a reduced income, and an uncertain social role. These are problems which seem to trouble the professional and white-collar worker more than the blue-collar worker. The professional who retains an identifying title has the least difficulty in this respect. The blue-collar worker may have been engaged in routine, impersonal tasks, often as part of a work crew, and minimally absorbing, so that retirement appears as an opportunity to seek more personally satisfying pursuits. The white-collar worker, in an intermediate position, may not have such compensations.

The reduction or loss of income with retirement may require adaptation to diminished circumstances, even departure from the community in which adult years were spent. Relocation, which may also be required by ill health, can be the occasion for disruption of personal relationships with old friends and neighbors, and a difficult period of isolation until new friends can be made.

Changing family patterns add to the difficulties of adjustment. Earlier marriages and greater longevity have increased the number of four-generation families. People of late middle age now often have grandchildren at the same time they are faced with problems of caring for their own parents. About 25 percent of people just under 60 have a surviving parent, and about 10 percent have both parents living. Stress can be great if ill health or financial problems require the generations to live together. The smaller nuclear family and the high percentage of women who work do not provide the maiden aunts formerly available to care for surviving grandmothers at home. The difficulties of caring for aged parents may interfere with the healthy growth of members of younger families. Unfortunately, many such families fail to make use of community support facilities either because of guilt feelings or ignorance of their availability.

Social psychologists have argued for almost two decades about the decreasing interaction between the elderly and society. The Activity Theory has blamed society for withdrawing from the elderly against the personal desire of most older people. The alternative Disengagement Theory, offered in 1961, held that older individuals and society withdrew voluntarily from each other. It is often held that the individual initiates the withdrawal because of diminished expectations and the desire for more leisure. The controversy is not yet settled, but much evidence disputes the Disengagement Theory, at least as a valid description of optimal aging.

Evaluation and Diagnosis

Diagnosis and appropriate treatment of a psychiatric problem depend on a rational assessment of numerous contributing factors and the strengths and weaknesses of the individual. Ideally, each should receive a thorough biopsychosocial evaluation including a physical examination, laboratory tests, a detailed medical and social history of both the patient and family, and a psychiatric history of previous events, feelings, habits, relationships, and means of coping with emotional difficulties.

The investigation must often be intimately personal and probe into abnormal thoughts and impulses, morbid preoccupations, notions of suicide, perceived sights and sounds that others do not seem to sense, hopes and fears, successes and failures, religious beliefs, and memory lapses. Formal psychological tests may be used to obtain objective evidence of mental disorders, especially when these are relatively minor. Since the questions must be comprehensive to be most useful, the troubled person being questioned should try not to be embarrassed or angry. Contrary to the whimsical notion that psychiatrists can read minds, they actually depend more than other medical practitioners on the trust, honesty, and candor of the patient.

Evaluation and diagnosis may require varied knowledge and skills, especially with older people whose apparently psychiatric problems may contain intertwined physical and functional components that are difficult to distinguish or separate. A team of practitioners is often necessary, representing various disciplines such as internal medicine, psychiatry, psychology, social work, nursing, and religion.

Diagnosis involves classification of psychiatric conditions according to similarities so that accumulated experience can be brought to bear on a particular case. Although accurate diagnosis is necessary to indicate the most effective treatment, diagnostic classification must not be allowed to mask the particularity of each individual as a unique "experiment of nature."

Psychiatric conditions are broadly sorted into two groups: *Organic Brain Syndromes* (OBS), which are disorders of thinking, feeling, and behavior due to malfunctioning brain tissues, and *Functional Disorders,* those which have no detectable physical basis. The two may coexist, but assessment of the contribution of each is valuable for planning appropriate treatment.

Organic Brain Syndromes

These are further separated into *chronic* and *acute* brain syndromes, largely on the basis of whether brain cells have died or only malfunctioned. Because brain cells do not regenerate, conditions arising from cell death are chronic and not reversible. If the cells are alive but temporarily not functioning properly for whatever reason, they may potentially return to a normal state. This condition is called acute.

Although OBS may present a wide variety of psychiatric symptoms, special hallmarks are disorientation as to time, place, and person (usually in that order), loss of memory (particularly of recent events), and rapidly changing emotions. Unfortunately, when disturbed behavior occurs in an elderly person, it is apt to be attributed to ''senility''—an improper term for a condition believed to be caused by deterioration of brain substance and which inevitably worsens. The term should be discarded, and, more importantly, the attitude it encourages should be denounced. It is a superficial diagnosis which implies that no therapy is possible and has led to many avoidable deaths.

The term *dementia* is used for the loss of cognitive brain function and behavior caused by cell damage. Reversible dementia is equivalent to Acute Brain Syndrome and irreversible dementia to Chronic Brain Syndrome. Neurologists and psychiatrists lay heavy claim to this area of organic brain disease, emphasizing the importance of distinguishing it from non-organic illnesses it may occasionally resemble. For example, a severe depression may look like an OBS. As many as 35 to 40 percent of patients believed to have dementia also have some treatable psychiatric disorder.

Chronic Brain Syndromes (CBS). Brain cell death which brings about CBS may be due to a primary disease of the brain cell itself or secondary to a process elsewhere in the body. The most important primary diseases of brain cells are senile and pre-senile (Alzheimer's and

Pick's) dementias. Evidence is accumulating that cell damage is similar in all three, though the cause is unknown. The onset of pre-senile symptoms is earlier (before 60) and their course more rapid. Orientation and memory difficulties are common.

Case: A very successful stockbroker, aged 53, was forced to see his doctor by fellow brokers after a short period of failing to place orders and trading the wrong stocks. He would not admit the errors even when confronted with factual evidence. His wife had recognized for six months that he had shown personality changes and had become increasingly forgetful, argumentative, and sensitive. Examination revealed gross memory defects and disorientation about time but not about people. He had to stop work and stay home where the family was very protective of his increasing difficulties (wandering from home and getting lost). After attacking his wife several times, he had to be hospitalized and died at the age of 57. The autopsy showed gross brain atrophy with widened surface grooves, and microscopic examination disclosed degeneration typical of Alzheimer's disease.

Brain cell degeneration can be secondary to arteriosclerosis, which can impair the blood supply to the cells. However, although many people have cerebral arteriosclerosis, physicians are less likely than formerly to attribute all cell damage to this mechanism. Present medical belief is that a co-existing primary cause or multiple blockages of small blood vessels are often at fault.

Acute Brain Syndromes. The significant aspect of these brain dysfunctions is that they can be treated and possibly reversed. Brain function can be altered by infections, toxins, metabolic disorders, injury, and tumor. If slow in onset, it may be mistaken for chronic brain syndrome and given no treatment. If sudden, it may be considered a functional psychosis such as schizophrenia and given improper treatment. Proper and prompt diagnosis can be life saving. This points up why every emergency psychiatric problem must receive medical as well as psychological evaluation. Correct treatment must focus on the underlying disease.

The elderly person often has a physical disease which can produce symptoms of acute organic brain syndrome such as confusion, disorientation, and sensory illusions. Poor kidney function, congestive heart failure, thyroid disease, chronic lung disease, blood loss, anemia, dehydration, malnutrition, and indeed, almost any debilitating condition, can affect the activity of brain cells and produce psychiatric symptoms. Since borderline equilibrium can be thrown off balance by disturbing circumstances such as darkness and dread of loneliness at night, the first symptoms most often occur after dark. The patient with this syndrome is usually excessively fearful and may develop paranoid delusions. Nurses and other hospital personnel on night duty have often been unjustly suspected of mistreating patients because the patients' tenuous hold on reality during the day is lost at night.

Drugs and medications are a very common cause of psychiatric problems in the older person, including both drugs given by physicians and those taken on the patient's own initiative. A study of a population over age 60 revealed that 70 percent were taking prescription drugs, 54 percent over-the-counter drugs, 20 percent home remedies, and almost half were also using alcohol, so that 25 percent were taking four or more drugs at once. Drugs taken together frequently produce symptoms that they do not cause separately at the same dosage. With today's specialized medical care, it is essential that each physician be informed of all medications a patient may be taking. Sedatives and hypnotics such as barbiturates may paradoxically cause excitement instead of sedation in the elderly, even when taken alone.

In dealing with the victim of delirium or acute brain syndrome, it is helpful to continually voice as many bits of information as possible to help the patient stay oriented: names (yours, the patient's, other's), dates, and names of places. Identification should be in a fashion previously familiar to the patient, for example, the use of last names when appropriate.

Case: The children of a 76-year-old man called to say their father, who had disappeared, had been found in a distant motel in Ohio claiming that he was going to be killed. Because he had known me for some years and had seemed to trust me, I was asked to contact him. He answered the phone and told me that a gang, headed by Mr. Weak Knees, was going to kill him by five o'clock. He was unable to tell me how he had gotten to Ohio or the name of the town he was in. Although he had refused any communication with his children, he agreed that if his favorite grandson would come for him he would return to see me even though he was convinced it was an utter waste of time since he would be dead by then.

Eighteen hours later he arrived at my office unkempt, with swollen ankles due to heart failure and local infection, the odor of urine on his breath, very dehydrated, and breathing with difficulty. He clutched to his chest a briefcase stuffed with both valuable papers and trash. He recognized me by name, knew his own name, and knew the hospital where my office was, but did not know the day, date, and year, and denied that he knew where he had been. He elaborated on Weak Knee's plot against his life and his fortune. All of his family except the grandson were conspirators in the plot.

With a great deal of persuasion, he consented to enter the hospital. Examinations revealed he was suffering from heart and kidney failure and an infected foot. Initially, he refused food and medication except those given personally by or in the presence of the physician. He then began to eat and took medications when shown by the nurse that the doctor had ordered them. Treatment was aimed at the heart failure and the infection.

After five days of treatment, throughout which he was disoriented and delusionally concerned about his life, his symptoms disappeared rapidly one morning. Mr. Weak Knees was identified as his name for a disapproved suitor of his favorite daughter.

Case: A 57-year-old woman was brought to the Emergency Room by her brother and uncle, who reported that for one week she had been belligerent, violent, and confused. She had accused her family of trying to kill her and threw furniture at them. This was a sudden personality change for her.

On examination, she knew the time and place and could name people but could not recall several recent events. She was alternately hostile and euphoric, and had grandiose delusions with both auditory and visual hallucinations. Her skin was dry and scaly. Laboratory tests disclosed suspected hypothyroidism. A major tranquilizer was given initially to alleviate the erratic behavior but was no longer needed after synthetic thyroid medication effectively relieved the underlying condition.

Alcohol abuse, occurring in two different groups, accounts for about 5 percent of observed organic brain syndromes. One group has habitually used alcohol for a long time, while the other group did not drink excessively until late in life and then did so to assuage feelings loss and depression. Prolonged use of alcohol accompanied by poor nutritional habits results in Korzakoff's psychosis, marked by gaps in memory which are filled with pseudo-recollections that have no basis in truth. This disease is reversible in its early stages, but becomes permanent if chronic drinking and poor eating continue.

Functional Psychiatric Disorders

Most psychiatrists believe that psychiatric disorders without a detectable organic cause are psychogenic (emotional in origin), even though heredity may play a role. They include a spectrum of problems ranging from psychoses to disorders called Transient Situational Reactions, with the neuroses, neurotic personalities, and other personality trait disorders falling between the extremes.

As the term indicates, Transient Situational Reactions are short-lived responses to severe stress. They are seen more frequently in late life than in adulthood, often following a severe or tragic stress such as death, fire and loss of home, and moving to a different residence. If the symptoms persist longer than a few weeks, they are not considered transient.

Affective Disorders. The most common reaction to loss is sadness or depression. Life over 55 is frequently filled with such events as deaths of friends or spouse, the loss of a job, and other traumatic changes. Physical ability and stamina may decrease, causing a loss of body image. Feelings of sadness or grief following such events are of course normal. The problem becomes psychiatric only if the depression is prolonged and profound.

To avoid or deny normal grief after the death of a loved one may lead to psychiatric difficulties later. Crying and talking about the deceased may pain the survivor, but some of this is necessary to make it possible to give up the lost one. Friends should not avoid reference to the deceased for fear of distressing the survivor, but should encourage talking out and sharing of the regret to help prevent unhealthy suppression. Aided by catharsis, the survivor can refocus on living and the future. Customs which tend to deny that tragedy has occurred are poor mental hygiene and sometimes result in later depression.

Case: A single, 55-year-old woman sought help a year after the death of her father to whom she had been closely attached. His death at 74 had been very difficult for her because he had been an active man who had had to cope with a leg amputation near the end of his life. Everybody praised her nobility and strength through the funeral and ensuing months during which she managed just as "he would have wanted her to." She came for help because she was experiencing crying spells "without cause" at work, severe trembling when she got a little angry, and some weight loss. She denied any feelings of depression, but spoke of how wonderful her father had been and how much she missed him. In the first interview, she regularly referred to her father as if he were alive and used the pronoun "we." She had done a superb job in settling the estate, but at home everything was as he left it. Treatment consisted essentially of helping her work out her grief.

This case is classifiable as a neurotic depressive reaction—a mild depression. Severe depressions may occur repeatedly, beginning in early adulthood, or as a single episode late in life after an apparently successful adjustment. Its symptoms include feelings of hopelessness and despair, morbid and suicidal thoughts, difficulty in concentration, retarded thinking, sleep difficulties characterized by early morning awakening, loss of appetite for food and sex, constipation, and weight loss. Since difficulty in concentration and an attitude of despair cause incorrect answers on examination to questions on orientation and memory, the examiner may mistake the depression for an organic brain syndrome.

In late middle age, many severe depressions are accompanied by agitation and delusions about the body, especially the gastrointestinal tract. Feelings of emptiness may become the supposed absence of any insides. Because they appear later in life, such depressions were formerly known as involutional melancholia. The woman who develops this illness frequently has a history of having been a meticulous housewife and sacrificing mother whose children have grown and left the family. The feelings may include a deep sense of unworthiness, guilt, sinfulness, suicidal thoughts and acts, agitation, poor sleep, and loss of appetite, even a refusal to eat which may be life-threatening dispite the absence of an overt suicidal intent. Such people are occasionally not only suicidal but homicidal in their delusional state; the world becomes such a terrible place in which to live that they may kill their children to spare them the suffering of living.

Case: A woman in her fifties came to the hospital after a suicide attempt. She had been active in her community and church and had raised three children who had married. Two daughters had moved out of town. Her son lived in town, but the birth of a grandchild had brought increasing friction with her daughter-in-law. At the urging of her husband, she had consented to sell their home of twenty years to "spare the hardship of keeping such a big house" and they moved to an apartment in center city more convenient to the husband's successful business. The woman became depressed after the move, had severe insomnia, and lost weight. Her general appearance, which had always been tidy, deteriorated as did her housekeeping. She became hopeless about life and tried to kill herself with gas. After psychotherapy and antidepressants failed to modify her depression, electroconvulsive therapy was used. She then received psychotherapy and counseling, together with her husband, and was helped to find a volunteer job working with children in an orphanage near her apartment. The depression vanished and never reappeared.

One group of recurring major depressions commonly begins in the 20's and 30's but may also first appear in the 50's, and is more likely to be accompanied by slowness of movement than agitation. In some instances, episodes of depression alternate with episodes of elation (mania), which may include overactivity, dancing, singing, extravagant spending of money, and exceptionally high spirits. This is manic-depressive illness. It is called bipolar if both manic and depressive episodes occur, unipolar if episodes are all of the same kind. The illness has a strong familial trait. Since the mid-1950's, lithium carbonate has been used very successfully to treat the manic attacks and to prevent recurrent alternation of mania and depression. Depressive attacks may need additional treatment with one of the antidepressants. Many attacks do not seem to be related to a personal loss, but rather occur without apparent cause. Also, they tend to become less intense with age. In this respect, the following case is atypical.

Case: A 58-year-old man was hospitalized because he was wildly excited. He had became overactive and unable to sleep after his mother's death. At her funeral, he had stood up and sung a lullaby, and that night had taken his wife to the local taproom to dance. He later became too busy to eat, could not rest, and was constantly in motion. He finally agreed to hospitalization, but in the hospital refused to wear clothes or eat. He had had a similar but milder episode eight years before when his father died, but had not needed hospitalization and recovered in about six weeks. Since this was before tranquilizers, he had been heavily sedated, wrapped in sheet pack, and fed through a gastric tube. He recovered in two months and returned to work.

Hospitalization for severe depression may be essential to protect the victim's life. Fortunately, effective antidepressants are now available, and with outpatient psychotherapy, hospitalization is generally avoided. The small percentage of depressed patients who fail to respond to other treatment and are suicide risks even in the hospital, may benefit from electroconvulsive therapy which can be life-saving.

The prognosis for severe depressions is very favorable. Only a small number of patients fail to recover or succeed at suicide. For the aging patient, it is not a life-threatening illness like a coronary attack or broken hip, so the risk of not surviving hospitalization is minimal.

Less severe depressive reactions may follow any loss: job, body injury, or loss of freedom and independence due to illness. The reaction is usually accompanied by loss of appetite and weight which may then upset the body's already tenuous balance. This can bring on a vicious cycle of physical illness, depression, and worsening physical condition.

Case: The severe psychosis described above of the disoriented 76-year-old man who irrationally feared he was to be killed, had the following onset. Because of his poor eyesight and physical disabilities, his car was taken away from him after he had several accidents. When he rented another car, his family appealed to the rental agencies to refuse him. His independence gone, symptoms of depression appeared: poor sleep, decreased appetite, and expressions of a wish to die. Ensuing malnutrition undoubtedly contributed to the development of his brain syndrome. When his confusion increased and he lost touch with reality, he became more frightened and paranoid.

Paranoid Disorders. The predominant symptom of paranoia is the belief that a malevolent person or force intends harm to the patient, contrary to all rational evidence. Paranoid individuals are frequently highly intelligent, competitive, and rather autocratic in dealing with others. They are sensitive to slights that the normal person might disregard. Losses they find especially stressful tend to be decreases of prestige and power or failures to gain authority, in contrast to the loss of love and caring for others that evoke depressive reactions in other personality types. Paranoid delusions and the self-accusatory delusions of the depressive do not occur simultaneously, but rapid alternation of the two may be possible. The paranoid attributes failures and wrongs to another, thus escaping the pain of feeling personally inadequate, whereas the depressive finds the pain of personal fault more tolerable than anger at another whose love is desired.

Paranoid reactions are common in late life, ranging from mild suspicions to full-blown psychoses. An adult who loses a promotion to a younger person may feel that the choice was devious rather than justifiable.

Psychiatrists disagree as to whether the functional paranoid psychoses of late life are the same as adult paranoid schizophrenia. There seems to be little reason to classify them separately. Treatment of both frequently includes use of one of the major tranquilizers: phenothiazines or butyrophenones.

Case: A 61-year-old engineer was forced into early retirement. He developed the belief that his company fired him to keep him from reaping the benefit of an idea he had for a new product, even though his incompetence on the job was obvious to many fellow workers, and his product idea was poorly conceived. He became more withdrawn and delusional, believing his telephone was tapped and that he was monitored by hidden TV. On examination, he was well oriented, had a good memory, but was broadly suspicious and delusional. His agreement to take medication was finally obtained and his symptoms moderated.

Paranoid beliefs may also appear in organic brain syndromes. For example, the elderly person with a poor memory loses things and always blames the loss on somebody else.

Special note should be made of the frequency of paranoid reactions in those who develop hearing difficulties in late life. As deafness increases the difficulty of communicating with others, suspicion of others' motives builds until it becomes a conviction that harm is intended.

Case: A 63-year-old man was brought to the hospital because he had been bothering the sheriff with claims that his neighbors were trying to force him to move by poisoning his spring. A simple examination showed that he was very hard of hearing, and a poorly functioning hearing aid was found among his belongings. It was sent out to be repaired, and after the man wore the repaired device for a few days, his suspiciousness immediately decreased, and his delusions soon disappeared. A review of the case revealed that his paranoid ideas developed about a week after he stopped wearing his hearing aid.

Paranoid individuals are usually proud and sensitive types for whom saving face is very important. In dealing with such persons, it is best to avoid confrontations and conflicts. This applies equally to paranoid reactions resulting from brain syndromes, for example, accusations of theft when forgetful people mislay or hide objects and then cannot find them.

Hypochondriasis. Hypochondriacs who demand attention by persistently complaining of ailments with no discernible physical basis present a difficult problem for the physician. The suffering may be obviously genuine and may dominate the individual's life.

Hypochondriasis is occasionally part of a larger depression, and tendencies appear in many elderly persons. Preoccupation with the condition and functions of the body is common. When lives are narrowed by increasing isolation and diminishing social relationships, a physical complaint may summon attention and care not otherwise forthcoming. However obvious the cause, it cannot be dealt with by confrontation which only intensifies the problem because the motivation is not conscious. Effective treatment includes considerate support and psychotherapeutic techniques that gradually help the hypochondriac to find more wholesome ways to gratify personal needs. Family or marital counseling may also be important.

Psychiatric Therapy

Treatment of psychiatric problems is of three types: biological or somatic, psychological or interpersonal, and social or environmental. Rarely can one type of therapy be totally isolated from the others. For example, even if biological treatment consists merely of the administration of pills, the patient responds to the personality and moods of the administering physician, nurse, and family members, senses their hopes and anxieties, and is influenced by variations in their expectations. A special difficulty in treating psychiatric as opposed to other disorders is that the patient, because of delusions, may be unaware of the predominant symptom of the illness—the delusions themselves.

Somatic Therapies

Drugs and medications: Since 1950, there have been extraordinary improvements in the pharmacological treatment of psychiatric illnesses. Within one decade, the major tranquilizers, new groups of antidepressants, lithium carbonate, and a class of new minor tranquilizers were introduced to the physician's armamentarium.

Prior to 1950, drug treatment consisted of hypnotics for severe insomnia, and stimulants such as amphetamine for loss of appetite and morning depression. Electroconvulsive treatment was widely and successfully used to terminate depressions. The amphetamines were greatly abused and now have little or no legitimate use.

Antidepressants now in use are of two classes: tricyclics and mono-amine oxidase inhibitors (MAOI's). They are highly effective, but do not produce euphoria and so are not habituating. Unlike the stimulants which produce prompt and artificial elation, these antidepressants generally take at least a week to effect a lifting of the spirits. They are potent medications which must be taken under medical supervision because of cardiovascular side effects. Individuals taking MAOI's must avoid tyramine-containing foods such as beer, wine, and cheese, which may dangerously raise the blood pressure.

The major tranquilizers such as the phenothiazines, butyrophenones, and thioxanthenes are antipsychotic medications. They promptly calm patients disturbed by schizophrenic, paranoid, or organic brain syndrome delusions, but do not affect the basic condition. An undesirable side effect in a small number of cases, primarily older women, is tardive dyskinesia, erratic mouth and tongue movements. The symptoms are unpredictable and do not disappear with discontinuation of the major tranquilizer.

Lithium carbonate, used to prevent manic-depressive illness and to treat the manic phase, is a toxic drug. Dosage must be adjusted by careful monitoring of blood levels of lithium.

The minor tranquilizers include the benzodiazepines, Valium and Librium, which are among the most often prescribed drugs in the country. Like the hypnotics and sedatives before them, they are used excessively. They should rarely be used longer than a week or two to relieve tension, anxiety, or sleeplessness. They are less frequently prescribed by psychiatrists than by other physicians, and use by older persons requires careful supervision.

Electroconvulsive therapy (ECT): ECT is effective for severe depressions that fail to respond to antidepressants, or when the wait for a drug to take effect involves too great a risk. Indeed, under some circumstances, ECT may sometimes be the safest therapy and the first treatment of choice, especially among the elderly.

Psychotherapy

Psychotherapies appropriate for younger persons are also useful for older ones. Contrary to earlier reservations, psychoanalysis can benefit those with personality disorders or neuroses who are motivated to seek help even after they pass the age of 60 or 70. The most prevalent problems, depression, memory lapses due to chronic organic brain syndromes, and continuing attempts to sustain personal integrity and self-esteem, favor a psychotherapeutic approach that involves active life-review. This means deliberate encouragement of talk about the past to help retrieve a healthier perspective on life and to balance a justified respect for personal accomplishments against the despair over failure to achieve adolescent and early-adult fantasy goals. Retrospection can disclose important clues to special personal assets and interests that can be valuable elements in therapy. Reminiscing about the past is not pathological, but, if used properly, can contribute to means of coping with the present and future.

Group and couple therapy are useful when appropriate family involvement is essential, especially when the members must collectively decide if institutionalization of an elderly relative is desirable or necessary. Family therapy involving several generations, and more direct family counseling may both be useful. Many studies show that families tend to care for elderly members too long before seeking professional help.

Social Support Systems

Community services developed in the last two decades by government and community agencies can provide for basic needs in or near the patient's home and help to avoid institutionalization. Some of these services are:

Home help—homemakers who visit the home.

Meals—group dining at a place to which the diner is transported. This is preferable to Meals-on-Wheels because it reduces isolation.

Escort and transportation—one of the most important needs of the elderly.

Friendly visitors—volunteers who visit or regularly telephone housebound persons. They are trained to recognize problems as well as to be supportive.

Group housing—a residential facility with minimal kitchen and central food service.

Respite services—poorly developed in this country, but effective in England and Scandinavia, they provide care for an elderly person while the family takes a vacation.

Geriatric day hospitals—professionally organized and managed centers were the elderly spend the day while living at home at night.

Psychiatric Hospitalization

Hospitalization of psychiatrically ill patients not only requires a medical institution (part of a general hospital or a separate psychiatric facility), but must comply with laws and regulations which vary from state to state. The psychiatric patient who is voluntarily hospitalized has to complete formalities not required of other medical patients. If family or friends initiate the hospitalization, they are subject to procedures modeled after the adversary proceedings found in criminal courts. The emphasis on civil liberty within recent years has brought laws which make it very difficult to medically treat a person who is unable to comprehend the fact of illness. A recent Supreme Court decision requires proof of an overwhelming need for "deprivation of liberty" and hospitalization. In many states, acts of violence toward the self or others must be proven before hospitalization can be arranged. Abuses were formerly common, especially in hospitals which had inadequate staff and resources to give even minimal treatment. Now, the consensus of psychiatric practitioners who administer primary care to the mentally disturbed is that many states must have more flexible laws to allow the psychiatrically ill to obtain the treatment they need.

How to Prevent Problems

Primary prevention is the taking of action early enough to forestall the development of symptoms. One example is the prevention of dementia due to the vitamin-deficiency disease pellagra by providing a sufficient amount of nicotinic acid in the diet. Secondary prevention is prompt treatment of the first symptom before an illness can become severe or chronic, for example, early treatment of syphilis to prevent progression to the final stage of brain infection and psychosis (general paresis). Tertiary prevention is the effort to reduce the incapacitating effects of a chronic illness, for example, giving lithium carbonate regularly to manic-depressives to decrease the likelihood of recurrence.

As more is learned about the contribution of heredity to psychiatric and other illnesses, genetic counseling as a specialty in its own right can be useful in prevention. It can provide information to help in family planning, consideration of adoption, choice of a marital partner, and alerting susceptible people to detect and seek early treatment for familial diseases.

Good health practices and good health care are basic to all levels of prevention. All adults, and especially those over 55, should have access to a primary physician in whom they have confidence, and who will manage other medical contacts. Just as previously established credit is especially valuable when funds are suddenly needed, so are previous examinations and knowledge of one's personal medical history by a primary physician especially useful when sudden medical problems must be evaluated. The availability of medical care of high quality should be taken into account in choosing a residence.

A change of residence can be a trying experience for older persons and should be well planned in advance with full consideration given to their needs and desires. As many tokens and symbols of more familiar surroundings as possible should be taken along to ease the transition. Even a change of circumstances without relocation, for example, retirement and the pre-retirement period, can be the occasion for great stress.

Social activities and living near others help to minimize feelings of isolation and neglect. Although several generations of the same family should probably not live together in the same dwelling because of unavoidable friction, visits and other frequent contacts are desirable. The relationship between parent and son or daughter is especially important. Adult offspring are a continuing focus of interest for their elders and can give in return their own interest, support, appreciation, and respect. Even if the family is widely scattered, the telephone, automobile, and airplane make gatherings or conversations as attainable as in earlier, more closely-knit generations.

The best preparation for later years is the development of genuine selfconfidence. Such development indicates an ability to solve problems at work, at home, and in the world at large, and implies productivity in spare time, hobbies, and interests that can continue into retirement. However, regardless of how well equipped an aging person is to meet unavoidable problems, outside resources should not be neglected. Middle class people in particular are often poorly informed about available assistance from community resources. Lower-income groups are sometimes more skillful in seeking help and less embarrassed to use it. Although the quantity and distribution of services are inadequate for the needs, great improvements in the last decade have made help more available than ever before. Concerned people should consult the physician, the hospital, the family service agency, or the local community mental health center for information.

COPING WITH CRISIS

Lynn Hubschman, M.S.W.

Director of Social Service,
Pennsylvania Hospital

An attractive 59-year-old woman, in distress that her husband had recently left her, sought counseling. To the best of her knowledge, her husband was living with another woman. She was not handling the situation very well, and her depression was threatening to embitter her. With counseling and time, her crisis was resolved, permitting her to move on to a new and better understanding of herself and her personal relationships.

Crises like this happen to most of us at one time or another. Unfortunately, the word crisis has a bad reputation because it is usually associated with disasters such as floods, hurricanes, plane crashes, sudden illness, and death. These are newsworthy because they are essentially dramatic accidents and death. But many other types of crises that do not reach the newspapers happen to all of us as part of daily living.

What is Crisis?

A simple definition of crisis might be, "an upset in a steady state." We all strive to maintain a state of equilibrium, using various maneuvers and problem-solving tactics to help us fulfill our basic needs. However, disturbing situations may catch us off guard so that we are unable to function in familiar patterns. In a state of crisis, methods that solved problems in the past are not adequate to re-establish equilibrium, and new solutions must be found.

A misconception about crisis is the widely held belief that it is caused only by negative circumstances. In fact, good things may also represent an unsettling change. Events as normally harmless as vacations or job promotions can upset one's life style, routine, and responsibilities and occasionally develop into full blown crises.

Accidental or random events are only one type of crisis. Another type results from normal development, such as passing through adolescence, becoming an adult, or reaching old age. A third type involves changing roles, such as becoming a husband, wife, mother, or boss. If we are unprepared for the change, the situation appears threatening and we fear losing control. Because of this fear and efforts to evade crises, we are unable to deal with them constructively when they come.

Whether a situation is perceived as a crisis depends on several factors. An event that may throw one person off balance may have little effect on another. Reactions depend on individual backgrounds, life experiences, strengths, coping abilities, available sources of support, and readiness for change. When our vulnerabilities are touched, crises may result. We may be able to handle one situation well up to a point, but further changes may cause a loss of control.

Returning to the example of the woman deserted by her husband, we can see that she was caught in several crises beyond the role change from married life to living alone. Her ego and her emotional and financial security were threatened by a change from the life style that had become customary and comfortable over a period of many years. Her self-concept changed as did her role within her family and community. While this was clearly a role-change crisis, a developmental crisis was going on at the same time. The woman was into her middle years, experiencing menopause, and beginning to see herself as a different person. In such a demanding situation, a characteristic pattern of responses usually emerges.

Stages of Response

These responses arise from an inability to cope adequately with a threat, loss, or challenge. If one feels emotionally threatened, intense anxiety usually appears. An emotional or physical loss brings mourning or depression. A challenging crisis may also evoke anxiety, but often with hope that the challenge can be met and successfully handled.

Shock

The most common first reaction to crisis is shock. The psychological impact freezes the ability to function. Some individuals become docile and react automatically; others panic or become confused. The shock period may be very short or persist, depending on the intensity of the crisis for the particular individual. The intensity of a crisis is measured by the degree of reorganization required to cope with it. Thus, loss of a leg in a car accident requires more time for emotional adjustment than returning to a burglarized home.

Defensive Retreat

A defensive retreat often follows the shock period, and consists of attempts to diminish the implications of the crisis, to avoid chaos, and to control the threat. Wishful thinking is common, such as the delusion that the dreaded event did not really happen, and reflects a yearning to feel safe again. Someone who has lost a leg in a car accident may deny the loss and even feel pain in the missing foot.

During this stage, an outsider offering help is fought off as another threat. Attempts to present less dismal facts about the situation will often be interpreted as unwarranted interference. A change of life style, values, or goals cannot yet be contemplated. So much energy is directed at keeping matters under control that little remains for the real problems.

Acknowledgment

The third stage of reaction to crisis is acknowledgment, a confronting of reality. Defenses have been shattered, the individual realizes that return to a former state is impossible, and awareness reaches a level at which reorganization for recovery can begin. Perceptions change, making it possible to plan a course of action. However, this stage may be characterized by extreme agitation, feelings of worthlessness, occasionally deep depression, and even suicidal thoughts or attempts.

An individual who is naturally apathetic may tend to withdraw or feel embittered and bereft. However, desirable alternatives may be perceived, and a willingness to cope actively with the situation may emerge. Help will be most effective at this stage, as the individual permits the true situation to be discussed and explored. Communicating with another person brings the comfort and support needed to restore a more receptive attitude. Focusing on past strengths and stressing retained positive values are helpful.

Adaptation

The fourth stage is adaptation, active coping with the difficulties in a constructive new manner. Abraham Maslow has described this stage as growth-oriented, in contrast to the first three stages which are primarily concerned with safety. During this stage, the individual is ready for change. A different self-image may develop, with a renewed sense of worth, a new ability to experience satisfactions, and a lessening of anxiety and depression. Thinking and planning become organized in terms of present resources and future potentials. The crisis is seen in a positive light, even as a path to greater understanding and a preparation for future crises.

The first three stages are prerequisites for the fourth. Those who are unable to progress this far remain blocked in one of the earlier stages. An example illustrates this.

> CASE 1: A woman whose husband died after a long illness was in a state of shock, unable to accept the fact of his death. After a short period of counseling, she advanced to the defensive retreat stage, pretending that her husband would return. She kept his clothes in the closet, cooked things that he liked to eat, and talked to him as if he were nearby. After six months, she moved on to the next stage, acknowledgement. She realized her husband had died and would not return. She began to show interest in new activity, donated her husband's clothes to a thrift shop, and only rarely attempted to talk with him. However, life seemed empty, and she gradually fell into depression, drinking alone and rejecting suggestions that she develop new interests or friends. A year later she was still unable to advance beyond this stage.

Individuals are unable to reach the fourth stage for many reasons. Some refuse to give up a "learned helplessness," using the situation as an excuse for not growing. Others remain locked in a defensive retreat, fantasizing that nothing has changed. Some are severely depressed and unable to recover. As Maslow states, the need for safety takes precedence over the need to grow because safety is closely related to basic survival, to needs such as food, physical health, and a predictable environment. Growth needs, such as independence and achievement, can come only after safety needs are met.

Shock demands all of one's resources to preserve psychological stability. Defensive retreat keeps the ego from disintegrating, provides a period of suspension, and permits realities to become clearer and the individual to call on remaining resources. Before the crisis is acknowledged, communication with others is both difficult and limited. Eventually, however, most individuals realize that evasion does not bring safety, and growth needs become more pressing. When defense mechanisms no longer satisfy, the individual is motivated to move forward.

Temporary setbacks often cause a relapse to a defensive attitude but need not preclude ever reaching the adaptation phase. With positive reinforcement of behavior, the individual can be remotivated, helped to take risks and to move from a safety orientation to a more satisfying growth-oriented life. The optimum period for this growth and change is when defenses have failed and given way to genuine self-examination.

Crisis rarely remains static. Either a solution is found which helps to restore equilibrium, or the situation becomes worse. Some people live in a state of ever mounting crisis—drowning in debt, on the verge of divorce, or anticipating being fired. They drift from crisis to crisis in their lives, some even preferring uncomfortable or unpleasant circumstances, such as a poor marriage relationship, to the risks inherent in grasping an opportunity to grow and develop natural abilities.

Most of us fall somewhere between the two extremes. We face crises in our lives, solve some and grow richer for the experience, and also develop new ways to deal with future problems and a better sense of our control over events. We move at our own emotional paces from childhood to adolescence and on to adulthood and old age.

Developmental Crises

Erik Erickson has proposed eight stages of life, with associated key problems and strengths to be gained from constructive resolution of the problems. Each stage can incur a developmental crisis.

Stage of Life	Dilemma to be Resolved	Psychosocial Strength To Be Derived
Infancy	Basic Trust vs Mistrust	Home
Early childhood	Autonomy vs Shame and Doubt	Will-power
Play age	Initiative vs Guilt	Purpose
School age	Industry vs Inferiority	Competence
Adolescence	Identity vs Confusion	Fidelity
Young adult	Intimacy vs Isolation	Love
Adulthood	Generativity vs Stagnation	Maturity
Old age	Integrity vs Despair	Wisdom

These eight stages neatly divide the life span. Dilemmas, such as Intimacy vs Isolation, are rarely either-or issues; most of us are more or less intimate with others while cherishing some privacy but not extreme isolation. Some individuals fail to work through particular stages successfully, leaving them with vulnerable areas throughout life. Some families fail to assist children to feel good about themselves when their egos are being formed. We do not all reach old age with wisdom and without despair.

Swiftly changing social views of aging and family relationships contribute to crises by casting doubt on long-established and comforting customs. Older people may find it particularly difficult to accommodate to new circumstances as the following example illustrates.

CASE 2: A couple reported having a good marriage until the husband retired. The wife remained busy with friends, organization work, and running her household. However, the husband, who was now home most of the time, had few friends for company except for infrequent visits from previous coworkers, and he became increasingly lonely. He had had no hobbies before his retirement and was unable to develop them now. He was also a diabetic and needed meals prepared on a strict schedule. As he became more demanding of his wife's time, she began to resent the required changes in her life. They were considering divorce because of continual conflict over minor matters such as the preparation of a cup of coffee or the choice of a TV program. With counseling, the couple was able to develop a more positive relationship and a recognition of the true cause of their difficulty.

Marriage and Crisis

The institution of marriage is in a state of crisis. Four out of ten marriages in the United States now end in divorce, and breakup carries little stigma. A third of all divorces take place within the first three years of marriage, about half after eight years, and the remainder after 15 years. Two-thirds of divorced women and three-fourths of divorced men remarry, usually within two to three years, and one-fifth of the remarriages end in another divorce.

Conventional marriage is also endangered by alternatives that were not freely available to earlier generations. These include remaining single, homosexual pairings, swinging or group marriages, and communes. In the last eight years, the number of people in the 25–30 age group who have never married has increased 50 percent, and the number 24–54 years of age who have separated or divorced and not remarried rose 30 percent.

Although three out of five broken marriages are childless, over one million children are the offspring of divorced parents, twice as many as in 1965. Families headed by women alone increased 30 percent in the last eight years and include one of every six U.S. children. Four out of 10 children born in the 1970's will spend part of their childhood in single-parent families, usually with the mother, and 17 percent now under 18 live with one parent.

Remarriages make 18 million American youngsters stepchildren. Also, 15 percent of American births are illegitimate and about half these infants are born to teenagers.

As a consequence, older people who used to enjoy frequent contact with children and grandchildren, and often received their support, must now face the fact that there are few three-generation families under one roof and fewer extended families living in the same neighborhood. The family's role in education, religious training, and entertainment has greatly weakened under the influence of modern technology. The result is increasing alienation as social stress makes successful management of personal crises more difficult.

CASE 3: A woman in the midst of divorce proceedings found it necessary to return to work to support herself and a young daughter. To save the expense of child care, she asked her mother to look after the child. Differences arose when the grandmother found that the task required more time and effort than she felt able to give, and expressed her resentment by commenting that she wished the divorce had never happened. Repeated disagreements about how to raise the child made matters worse. The crisis was resolved when the divorcee decided to hire an outsider to care for the child during the day, freeing the grandmother to resume her normal life.

Not only have modern alternatives weakened the institution of marriage, but some psychiatric theorists have encouraged experimentation in behavior and the seeking of pleasure without guilt. Our changing society is characterized by extraordinary changes in concepts of family living. People live much longer than previous generations, and strings of marriages have become so common that one of every four weddings is the second for at least one partner. Also, as more people are unable to sustain marital love and intimacy for long periods, extramarital relationships seem less forbidden.

Women's roles are changing. As greater emphasis is placed on education and careers, many women decide to delay having children or to have none at all. Today, 44 percent of all married women are employed, and 52 percent of this number have children between the ages of 6 and 17. Because they earn one-fourth of an average family's total income, most women work because they feel they have no choice; to do otherwise means a reduced standard of living. Crises may arise as the pressures of being a wife, mother, and homemaker conflict with those of the workplace.

In a 1972 study, *The Future of Marriage,* sociologist Jessie Bernard noted that the happiest people were single or newly married women without children. Married men came next, and were both happier and healthier than their unmarried counterparts. Married women had more mental health problems, and widowers had very high death rates. Men felt that marriage brought a heavy burden of economic responsibility and sexual restrictions. Women felt that the duties imposed by marriage and the low status of a housewife were a high price for love.

Another sociological study points out the difficulties of achieving success in a career as opposed to success in marriage. People often do not have enough time and energy to succeed in both, and must make critical choices from which marriage or career may suffer. An important element of success in marriage is the resolution of potential conflicts in decision-making, emotional and financial dependence, and division of duties and responsibilities, by bringing to bear on such questions all the resources of mutual affection and trust, maturity of judgment, sharing of common goals, sexual attraction, education, and (not least) a sense of humor.

Stress

Any significant change in circumstances can create stress. Robert Holmes has listed some of these and assigned numbers (points) that estimate their contribution to overall stress (see Table 1). A study indicated that a total of 150 points or more in a year represented severe stress that could result in mental or health problems.

Frequently, stress from various sources accumulates for weeks or months and remains controlled until an otherwise trivial incident triggers the brewing crisis.

CASE 4: A formerly well-behaved hospital patient in his sixties caused a commotion when he threw a tray of food at a nurse. His history revealed that he was frustrated by physical signs of aging, had business problems, financial difficulties, a stressful marriage, and troubles with a grown son, and a heart condition had brought him to the hospital. When a careless nurse spilled food on him, she became the target for suppressed anger and anxiety.

Defenses

A variety of mechanisms are commonly employed, often unconsciously, to defend against daily stress and a fear of vulnerability:

Rationalization:	Giving an acceptable rather than the true reason for an action.
Projection:	Attributing responsibility to others.
Displacement:	Shifting one's own reactions to another person.
Repression:	Submerging guilt and forgetting.

Table 1. Stress Indications

Rank	Life Event	Mean Value	Rank	Life Event	Mean Value
1	Death of spouse	100	23	Son or daughter leaving home	29
2	Divorce	73	24	Trouble with in-laws	29
3	Marital separation	65	25	Outstanding personal achievement	28
4	Jail term	63	26	Wife beginning or stopping work	26
5	Death of close family member	63	27	Beginning or ending school	26
6	Personal injury or illness	53	28	Change in living conditions	25
7	Marriage	50	29	Revision of personal habits	24
8	Fired at work	47	30	Trouble with boss	23
9	Marital reconciliation	45	31	Change in work hours or conditions	20
10	Retirement	45	32	Change in residence	20
11	Change in health of family member	44	33	Change in schools	20
12	Pregnancy	40	34	Change in recreation	19
13	Sex difficulties	39	35	Change in church activities	19
14	Gain of new family member	39	36	Change in social activities	18
15	Business readjustment	39	37	Mortgage or loan less than $10,000	17
16	Change in financial state	38	38	Change in sleeping habits	16
17	Death of close friend	37	39	Change in number of family get-togethers	15
18	Change to different line of work	36	40	Change in eating habits	15
19	Change in number of arguments with spouse	35	41	Vacation	13
20	Mortgage over $10,000	31	42	Christmas	12
21	Foreclosure of mortgage or loan	30	43	Minor violations of the law	11
22	Change in responsibilities at work	29			

50 points: Can be handled by most individuals
100 points: Generates moderate stress
150 or more: Severe stress, need for special aid

Suppression: Deliberate removal from one's mind of the offensive or objectionable reality.

Compensation: Failure in one area, success in another.

Substitution: Changing from a difficult goal to an easier one.

Reaction formation: Relieving guilt by expressing a feeling opposite to the appropriate one.

Sublimation: Channeling aggression into acceptable activity.

Avoidance: Withdrawal (may lead to guilt).

Fantasy: Indulging in make-believe.

Regression: Reversion to an earlier stage.

Growing Old in America

Growing old in a society that places a premium on youth inevitably makes aging more difficult than it need be. The enormous sums spent on skin creams, cosmetics, preparations to prevent baldness, health spas, and attempts to preserve a youthful appearance make it clear that Americans do not value old age. This is ironic in light of the fact that throughout history the old have traditionally been the educators of the young. Instead, in today's America, oldsters emulate youth—grandmas wear miniskirts and grandpas wear blue jeans.

The last seven years have brought an 18 percent increase in the aged, so that one out of nine Americans is now 65 years of age or older. In the same period, the general population grew only 5 percent. While only 40 percent of Americans at the turn of the century could expect to reach 65, the proportion is now 75 percent, due mainly to the elimination of diseases like diphtheria that had long been killers of the young. Increases in life expectancy have been more modest at advanced age levels at which chronic diseases remain major causes of death. Nine percent of the elderly are functionally illiterate, while eight percent are college graduates. Approximately 50 percent of older Americans have not completed a year of high school. Nevertheless, this large group must contend with a society that values most the young, independent, healthy, and attractive.

Most suicides in the United States are committed by men between the ages of 60 and 70. The principal causes are depression over the loss of a spouse, friends, or relatives, the absence of meaningful acitivity after retirement, and reduced opportunities for personal satisfaction because of medical problems. The fear of death, however, is not a major source of depression since elderly individuals often see death as a release from the suffering that accompanies illness. The fear of becoming senile is a greater cause of anxiety for the aging and is intensified if family support is lacking.

While the aging man may be distressed that he is no longer doing productive work, the aging woman may feel concern that she is no longer attractive or desirable. These dissatisfactions in an aging couple can lead to divorce or changes in behavior. The boredom that comes from feeling uninteresting and unproductive can defeat attempts to adopt hobbies and new interests that might keep mind and body alert and morale high.

The mature aging individual is aware that life is a series of choices, and that control over choices helps to make crises manageable. A degree of vulnerability is unavoidable, especially during a crisis, but perseverance to eventual success is a creative act which restores growth and strengthens the ability to cope with future crises.

LIVING TOGETHER AND LIVING APART

Martin Goldberg, M.D.

*Director of Marital Therapy Training and Research
Institute of the Pennsylvania Hospital*

*Clinical Associate Professor of Psychiatry
University of Pennsylvania School of Medicine*

Note: All case histories used to illustrate the following text are fictional. While true to life, they do not refer to real persons.

Living Together

"It would all be much simpler if one could beget one's children after being pensioned."

This quotation from a Swedish sociologist brings into focus a basic dilemma of living together after 55. What is the central purpose and/or task around which a couple can organize their cohabitation? For young married couples, the purposes and/or tasks are usually to start and to further their working lives, to form their own family unit, and to begin having children. For couples in their thirties or forties, life is apt to revolve around the further development of careers and the raising and education of the children. But as the table below shows, the average American woman can now anticipate living more than 30 years after her last child has been "married off." About half those years will be spent with her husband, barring separation or divorce. (The chances of her being separated or divorced are considerable, of course. If the current U.S. divorce rate continues, nearly half the existing marriages will end in divorce and many others will end in permanent separation.)

Census Data on the Average American Woman

	1890	1966
Age at leaving school	14	18
Age at marriage	22	20
First born child	24–25	21
Last born child	32	26
Age when all children are in school	38	32
Age at death of spouse	53	64
Age when last child is married	55	48
Age at death	68	80

Now consider more closely the 15 or more years many couples live together after their children have been raised. Much has been said about the "empty nest syndrome," the purposelessness, meaninglessness, loneliness, and emptiness a parent may feel after the offspring have left home. There is some question, however, as to the validity of this concept. Specifically, although many couples do experience these symptoms, it is not clear that the symptoms are really caused by the departure of the children. Indeed, for many husbands and wives, that departure is liberating and frees time and energy that can then be used for personal concerns and for each other. It is likely that whether a given couple has an empty nest or feels liberated and energized depends on the nature of the relationships that existed within the family. Consider the following two cases.

> *CASE 1:* Mr. and Mrs. A. have been married for over 30 years and raised four children. The three older children are married and the youngest has moved to a city 2,000 miles from the family home.
>
> Since the last child moved away, Mrs. A. has lost her energy, appetite, mental alertness, and enthusiasm for living, and doesn't sleep well. Mr. A. has become increasingly preoccupied with business (he owns a small automobile

agency) and has decided to expand his shop. The more Mr. A. devotes time and energy to business, the more lonely and empty Mrs. A. feels; the more depressed she becomes, the more deeply he is driven into his work. It is a vicious circle.

The circle is not new. Very early in the marriage, the couple developed a pattern in which the husband was absorbed in building his business while the wife threw herself into the role of mother, investing virtually all her energies in nourishing, raising, disciplining, and loving her four children. It would be impossible to determine whose behavior came first since both developed simultaneously. Now Mrs. A. suffers from an empty nest because she has no place to put the love and attention she formerly gave her children. Her husband is not really a candidate to receive it; he did without it so long that he now neither needs nor wants it. Mr. A. is not indifferent to the departure of his children whom he loved and enjoyed in his own way. However, he reacts to the empty nest as he has always reacted to emotional deprivation: by applying himself more to the non-emotional, "safe" world of business.

CASE 2: For contrast, let us look at Mr. and Mr. B., also married over 30 years, with four children now out of the home. Neither is depressed or disturbed. On the contrary, they have just realized a long-held ambition by selling their home, moving into a small apartment, and using the money to purchase a lovely second home on a wooded lake in a resort area two hours away. As an insurance salesman, Mr. B. never attained a very large income, but with the children gone and expenses reduced, that income is more satisfactory and has enabled him to achieve another ambition, reducing his work week to four days. Now he and Mrs. B. routinely spend pleasant, relaxing, 3-day weekends at the lake. Their life has been quite rewarding since their children have left, but this is not surprising since it is a natural consequence of their previous marital and family relationship.

Both Mr. and Mrs. B. placed their marriage first over the years. Even career, so important to most men, came second for Mr. B., and neither he nor his wife was so child-centered as to devote more love and energy to their children than to each other.

These contrasting examples indicate that couples who had a satisfying, reasonably intimate mutual relationship when they were younger are apt to live together gracefully and happily after 55. These later years may also be relatively free of conflict for couples who have not been particularly intimate with each other, but who individually developed continuing interests such as a career or major hobby outside the family. This leaves many couples like Mr. and Mrs. A. who had not been very close and one or both of whom failed to keep and/or develop outside interests. Although such couples may never separate or divorce, the years after 55 are apt to be increasingly unhappy and lacking in harmony.

It is possible to avoid or minimize such unhappiness if a couple can develop the flexibility to work out new and more satisfactory ways of interacting. Authorities on marital problems have pointed out that every marriage involves a *marital contract*. The contract is not a written document, but consists of unspoken assumptions and agreements arrived at in some fashion, consciously or unconsciously accepted. For example: It is agreed that husband and wife will be loyal to each other and have one or more children; that she will bear the main responsibility for rearing the children, and that the husband will bear the main responsibility for financial support of the family. (In addition to these basic elements, a contract will include many items special to the individual couple.) This is obviously a traditional sort of contract which may be viewed as sexist in nature, but it is one that millions of couples enter into, more often by default than by decision. They do not usually discuss these matters and come to an agreement. Rather they assume that this is the way their marriage will be.

A contract like the above may prove unsatisfactory, for example, if the couple cannot bear children, if the husband is an inadequate wage earner, or if the wife becomes a feminist and insists that her husband share more equally in the privilege and duties of child-rearing. Or the contract may work well for 15 years or even 25 years, but then, as we have seen, the circumstances of the marriage may change. A new agreement is needed, and marital counselors and therapists speak of "renegotiating the contract." Flexibility and willingness to change can then help a couple to revitalize a marriage that is becoming stagnant.

Negotiation or renegotiation of a marital contract may include the following areas of possible conflict:

1) Power or Control. This important area encompasses financial and social as well as psychological/emotional control. In some marriages, power is shared, while in others it rests largely or entirely with one spouse. Perhaps the commonest pattern is for one spouse to prevail in certain areas, such as finances, and the other spouse in other areas, such as child rearing. Since "he who pays the piper calls the tune," the spouse who earns or owns more money than the other generally tends to predominate. However, there are many exceptions. We all know wealthy individuals dominated by their less wealthy spouses.

Another generalization (again true with many exceptions) is that men are accorded more power than are women in American society. Although most men *seem* to have more power than their wives, the true state of affairs may be less obvious and vary with the individuals.

It is also worth noting that power may be exercised actively or passively, and the passive exercise is often more overwhelming. Consider Mr. C., a dynamic, successful corporation executive with a forceful, outgoing personality, who loves to have his own way and generally does so in his business career. His wife, a quiet, introverted woman, is "a bit sickly" and suffers from phobias which make her shun travel and social activity. As a result, they have not entertained at home or gone out to movies, theaters, or parties in 10 years, nor has Mr. C. attended the numerous conventions and business meetings to which he would dearly love to go. Obviously, the "strong" partner does not control this marriage.

Conflicts over power or control are very common in marriage as in all human relationships.

2) Nurture or Dependency. If power is the issue of who tells whom what to do, nurture or dependency is the issue of who takes care of whom. Again, various patterns are possible. The husband or wife may do most of the caretaking, or the two may take care of each other in differing ways. Trouble arises when both have an overwhelming need to be nurtured and little or no ability to nurture the other, or when either one neglects the other because of preoccupation with nurturing the children. Many doctors' wives will readily attest to a comparable problem in which the husband devotedly tends to patients but pays little attention to his family.

3) Trust. This involves a good deal more than sexual fidelity. Husbands and wives need to trust each other's loyalty in a much broader sense. Any time one spouse puts someone or something ahead of the other spouse, it may well be felt as an act of infidelity. However, people's needs vary, and some couples may not need fidelity to trust each other. For most of us, however, trust and fidelity are closely interdependent.

4) Intimacy. This refers to psychological/emotional closeness and, in a lesser degree, to physical closeness. There is a marked tendency for those who write or lecture on mental health to treat intimacy as an unqualified blessing. Consequently, we are often told about the merits of being "open," "close," and "frank and honest" with each other. Indeed, intimacy is a quality that can enliven any relationship, but it has another side. Privacy also has merit, and not every person desires or is capable of intense and/or prolonged intimacy. The important factor in marital interaction is not so much the presence or degree of intimacy, but whether both partners feel the same about it. If both cherish it or both would like to hold it to a relative minimum, their marital contract will reflect this and harmony should ensue. However, if one partner longs for intimacy while the other wants little or none of it, conflict is inevitable.

5) Life Style. This category includes inborn temperament as well as personality traits developed in response to environmental forces. For example, consider the contrast between active and passive natures. An active person may relax after a hard day's work by jogging for an hour or two, then take a quick shower and be off to a party or other social event. A passive person may relax after work by curling up in a favorite chair to read a book or watch television. When a passive person is married to an active one, conflict is obviously likely about what they are going to do together and how they will lead their lives.

Other habits that may clash are order and punctuality. Some people are comfortable only in an orderly environment. They need neat, well-arranged homes and cannot tolerate dirty ashtrays, strewn-about clothes, piled-up newspapers, and other clutter. Other people thrive on informality, never notice disorder, and are even uncomfortable in overly tidy surroundings. People with a taste for order often also tend to be unusually punctual about appointments. They are most at ease when they arrive ahead of schedule at an airport, a business meeting, or a social event. Other, more casual people are almost never on time and seem to delight in catching an airplane at the last moment or arriving late for a meeting or party. Marital conflict is common between spouses who differ greatly in their attitude toward order.

These examples by no means exhaust the subject. Many other inherently conflicting personal characteristics could be added.

Changing Needs and Desires

How do marital relationships and conflicts fare after the partners pass 55? Usually, a couple's needs and desires for trust and a particular life style are not apt to change greatly over the years. A husband and wife who got along well in these two areas before 55 are likely to continue to do so afterwards. However, in the areas of power, nurture, and intimacy, the situation may be quite different. New needs and desires often surface, requiring a conscious or unconscious renegotiation of the marital contract and development of a new equilibrium if marital harmony is to be preserved or regained.

With regard to power, the most common change is the woman's gradual development of an awareness of her desire for power and the readiness to assume it. Needless to say, the woman who has a rewarding career or business is in the strongest position to fulfill such a desire. Often, the husband coincidentally has less need for power or, at least, less ability to wield it. A man who retires early at 62 while his wife in her late fifties remains actively employed may well find that the power balance changes in the marriage. Moreover, women in general have recently tended to assume more overt power. This social phenomenon makes it wise for many couples to reconsider their marital power agreements.

Many a man who has repeatedly insisted, "My wife will never work," now finds that she is doing just that. Very often, the reason is not a liberalization of her husband's or society's attitude but rather the desire of the couple to maintain a life style that requires a second income to cope with inflation and increasing expenses.

Changes in the balance between nurturing and being nurtured are also likely to occur. In particular, chronic illness may so affect one spouse that the other must assume more of the nurturing role. However, illness is not the only cause of a shift in the balance. A case in point is Mr. D. who is 59 years old and has worked for most of his adult life as a salesman for a large chemical company. He has been married for 28 years and his wife and he have raised two children. Over the years, Mr. D. was cast in the role of taking care of Mrs. D., a shy, quiet woman with few interests or social contacts of her own, who enjoyed her husband's steady attention and reassurance. Late last year, however, Mr. D. was suddenly laid off by his company because of a reorganization. To date, after months of job-seeking, he is still unemployed. Mr. and Mrs. D. are not in severe financial crisis, since they had considerable savings. But Mr. D. is the one who now needs tender, loving care. He feels crushed and defeated and has lost self-confidence. Fortunately, Mrs. D. has been able to meet the challenge and gives her husband some of the emotional support and reassurance he now needs so strongly. In other words, the contract on nurture has been happily renegotiated. However, other couples do not manage a shift in the nurturance balance so smoothly under similar circumstances. Hostility and recriminations may develop with neither spouse being aware of the real cause of the difficulties.

Needs for intimacy may also change, as already indicated in the example of Mr. and Mrs. A. In that situation, Mrs. A. clearly needed more intimacy with her husband after the children left home, but Mr. A.'s lack of a corresponding need contributed to the development of her depression. Another common, sometimes amusing, sign of the need to renegotiate contracts on intimacy is the complaint by many women that "My husband is retired now and I just can't get used to having him around the house and under foot all the time." Many of these women try to resolve the problem by pushing the husband back out of the house into new hobbies or outside interests. Such attempts really aim to maintain the old contract of not-too-much intimacy. If the husband cooperates, a balance may indeed be restored.

Living Apart

Thus far we have considered people whose marriages survive and who live together after 55. There remain those others who live apart after 55 because of a long-standing or more recent divorce or separation.

Statistics are not totally reliable and can be misleading, but it seems quite evident from clinical practice and experience that the divorce rate in the U.S. has increased for the over-55 age group in the last 10–15 years. Marital breakups are still more common in other age groups: teenage marriages are notoriously fragile, and marital failures in the thirties and forties are so numerous as to be almost fashionable. However, separation or divorce after 55 is no longer the great rarity it once was and is likely to become more common as long as our society remains relatively affluent.

At any age, separation and divorce are devastating experiences for most people. Studies suggest that any great change in living patterns produces stress and that divorce ranks as the second most stressful life change, second only to the death of a spouse. Marital separation is a close third, and both separation and divorce outrank such major disruptions as the death of a close family member (other than a spouse), personal injury or illness, loss of employment, and retirement. (When the death of a spouse was arbitrarily assigned a value of 100 points in these studies, divorce had a value of 73 points and marital separation 65 points. If the stresses within one year total more than 300 points, trouble generally develops. Eighty percent of such people in this study became seriously depressed, had heart attacks, or developed other serious physical ailments).

The finding that divorce is a personal trauma second only to the death of a spouse clearly indicates that it must be a major stress factor for those over 55. Moreover, this finding is important and enlightening for other reasons. We have long recognized that people who experience the death of a spouse or other close relative go through a number of psychological stages in reacting to and resolving their loss. This is also true for those who experience marital separation and divorce. The stages of reaction to divorce usually follow the sequence:

- Denial

- Depression

- Anger

- Resignation

- Acceptance and Proceedance

1) Denial. When faced with an extremely unpleasant and undesirable situation, the human mind often tends to protect itself by *denying* the unpleasant reality and reacting as if it were just not so. Consequently, denial is usually the first reaction to the reality of a marital breakup.

Case Example: Mrs. F., a 56-year-old housewife with three grown children, was referred by her family physician to a psychiatrist because of "family problems." She informed the psychiatrist that these problems centered around her husband who was "terribly depressed and confused" and "badly in need of psychiatric treatment." Mrs. F. had come to these conclusions after her husband told her he had been romantically involved for some years with another woman, that he wanted a divorce, and that he intended to leave home at once. This seemed incredible to Mrs. F., even though she readily admitted that her 30-year marital relationship had been unsatisfactory and full of conflict and that she and her husband had become increasingly estranged. She felt that her husband did not really want a divorce, but must be mentally ill— depressed—and needed help to clear up his thinking.

Mr. F. was subsequently interviewed by the psychiatrist and presented quite a different version of the matter. He stated categorically that he was going to divorce his wife and was delaying leaving home for a few weeks only to give her a chance to get used to the situation. He went on to say that he was amazed that his wife doubted his intentions, since she had talked about divorcing him for many years and had clearly recognized the emotional poverty of their marriage. For the past seven years he had found affection and sexual gratification with another woman, but delayed taking the step to divorce only until all three children finished college and left home. Clearly, Mr. F. was neither depressed nor confused, but was carrying out a well-considered plan which he had developed over the years, albeit he was doing so in a rather cold-blooded manner.

In subsequent interviews, in which the psychiatrist saw Mr. and Mrs. F. together, the couple repeated their stories: Mr. F. insisted that he knew his own mind and wanted a divorce, and Mrs. F. insisted that this wasn't so and he was emotionally ill. Then, Mr. F. made his move and left home, telling his wife he would file for divorce in a month if she did not do so first. Even then, Mrs. F. continued to deny reality. She was certain he would come back; he was only bluffing; he only wanted her to be more affectionate; maybe he *was* mentally ill even though the psychiatrist could not recognize it, and so on.

With continued counseling from the psychiatrist, Mrs. F. gradually became able to progress beyond denial and to accept the obvious fact that her marriage was over.

In another example, sixty-year-old Mrs. G. has not been so fortunate. She has been separated from her husband for four years but still clings to the idea that he will come back to her, that it is somehow all a mistake, and that there will be no divorce. Indeed, because of the laws in her home state, she is able to prevent a legal divorce although clearly a *de facto* divorce has long since taken place. Her husband has offered her the most generous financial settlement possible and her lawyers have urged her to accept it. Friends and family have repeatedly told her that her husband is living with another woman and obviously has no plans for return or reconciliation. Still, she persists in her position, for she is stalled—perhaps permanently—in an attempt to manage her unhappiness by denying that it exists. Meanwhile, she suffers from many psychosomatic symptoms, including migraine headaches, severe insomnia, colitis, and chronic low back pain.

In most divorces, of course, the denial phase is neither as prolonged as Mrs. F.'s nor as permanent as Mrs. G.'s. Rather, it is a transient phenomenon that passes in a few weeks or months. But, not rarely, and particularly after 55, it may persist with devastating effects. In some cases, denial may also be shared by both spouses. In such instances, even though the marriage is clearly breaking up and the couple separates, both husband and wife continue to act, for a while at least, as if it were not so. Separated couples may even continue to have sexual intercourse with each other and talk of reconciliation while legal steps toward divorce are being vigorously pursued.

2) Depression. As denial begins to disappear and reality is faced, depression sets in. This occurs not only in the abandoned spouse, but also in the one who actually initiates the break. Depression generally involves a feeling of profound loss, but also often represents the turning of angry feelings inward on the self instead of outward at another person. Depression due to loss of a marriage may manifest itself in a variety of ways—mild or severe, transient or enduring.

Case Example: Mr. H., a 62-year-old salesman with two grown children, generally believed that he had a rather happy marriage despite repeated quarrels with his wife and many areas of conflict, including a sexual relationship that had never been satisfactory. On his many business trips away from home, he frequently engaged in extra-marital sexual relationships, but regarded these as insignificant dalliances. Sanguine as he was about the state of the marriage, Mr. H. was shocked when his wife told him one day that she wanted a divorce. She revealed that she had fallen in love with another man with whom she was having a highly gratifying sexual relationship. Despite Mr. H's assurances that he would "forgive and forget" her infidelity and his protestation that he wanted their marriage to continue, Mrs. H. remained adamant in demanding a divorce. Finally, and most reluctantly, Mr. H. moved out of their home and rented a furnished room.

Mrs. H. then proceeded to obtain a divorce in the shortest possible time. Meanwhile, Mr. H. underwent marked changes. Formerly aggressive and outgoing, he became quiet and reserved and let his sales work slip badly. His sleep was severely disturbed by early-morning awakenings, and his appetite was so poor that he lost 20 pounds in six weeks. Worst of all, in his view, he became sexually impotent and was unable to find consolation for his hurts in another woman's arms.

These symptoms reflected the depression Mr. H. was suffering from. His difficulties continued until he sought medical help and was successfully treated with a combination of counseling, reassurance, and antidepressant medication.

Most people going through a marital breakup experience a milder depression than that which beset Mr. H. However, this phase is apt to be fairly prolonged, lasting for many weeks or even months. Undoubtedly, the social disapproval and rejection by family and friends, which many people still encounter in divorce, serve to prolong and enhance the depression phase and so does the separation from home and familiar surroundings. Even more apt to promote depression is the incredibly false and malignant legal process surrounding separation and divorce in many states, with its emphasis on an adversary proceeding and the inevitable battles over financial and other matters. Indeed, all the circumstances surrounding divorce are calculated to load the participants with tremendous guilt, a profound feeling of failure, a deep sense of loss, and intense anger.

3) Anger. Quite naturally then, to get through the depression phase, people often begin by externalizing their anger, turning it outward, generally against the spouse or ex-spouse, rather than inward against the self. It is extremely important for this shift to occur. If it does not, or if the depressive thinking is not corrected in some manner, the individual may remain mired in a deep and persistent rut of depression. This is a grave danger and is particularly apt to occur in the mild sort of person who has always had trouble expressing anger or even admitting its existence.

Once the anger has emerged, this phase may be most unpleasant. All the nastiness and hostility that two people are capable of directing against each other are likely to develop. Attacks and counterattacks and furious attempts to fix the blame for the marital failure are almost inevitable. If there are children or other relatives in the family, they are often unfortunately drawn into the fighting. Each spouse tries to make allies of children, other relatives, and friends and may use them against the other spouse. All the pre-existing conflict areas in the marriage, such as differences over children, money, in-laws, sexual behavior, drinking, etc., will now be exaggerated and may cause furious clashes. The picture is not pretty, but may well represent a phase that must be gone through in the final dissolution of the marital bond. Attempts to minimize or completely circumvent the hostility may only prolong the unpleasantness. Indeed, there is very likely a cathartic value in the otherwise ugly expression of anger.

> *Case Example:* Mrs. I., a 63-year-old suburban housewife with three grown children, first consulted a psychiatrist because her marriage was obviously dissolving.

She had gone through a stage of denial, disbelieving her husband's announcement that he was in love with another woman and wanted a divorce, and felt that he would quickly change his mind. When he did not do so, she gradually sank into a profound and persistent depression. She blamed herself for most of the difficulties in the marriage, feeling that she had failed to appreciate her husband and had taken him for granted. Moreover, she was convinced that she could never marry again. Since she must be unattractive, physically and emotionally, to have earned her husband's rejection, she felt, no other man could possibly want her. (Mrs. I. actually was reasonably attractive both in person and personality.)

In counseling Mrs. I., the psychiatrist recognized the dangers that accompanied the persistence of her depression. As weeks went by, she became more and more negative about herself and unfortunately suffered another loss when her 85-year-old father had a stroke and soon died. This deepened Mrs. I.'s depression to such an extent that the psychiatrist felt she was potentially suicidal.

The psychiatrist had also occasionally been seeing Mr. I. who considered the visits only a means to help his wife accept the divorce. Despite guidance from the psychiatrist, he consistently treated his wife in a polite but patronizing manner, refusing to discuss anything with her, but offering vague and ill-defined "help." In other words, he persisted in maintaining his image as a "nice guy" although inwardly full of anger against his wife which he had nursed for years and which had led him to seek divorce in the first place.

As depression deepened in Mrs. I. and the danger of suicide became more evident, the psychiatrist strongly encouraged Mr. I. to undertake more confrontations with his wife, in the hope that this would enable her to mobilize and express her angry feelings. The husband proved evasive. He would agree with the idea, but then continue to completely avoid any facing of emotions with his wife. At this point, the therapist strongly urged Mrs. I., more than ever before, to verbalize her anger at Mr. I. and the world. With this reinforcement, Mrs. I. was at last able to begin to voice her stored-up fury and resentment. As she did so, her depression melted away. The outcome was a happy one, as she was then able to face parting from her husband who promptly obtained the divorce and married his new love. Mrs. I. found that she could survive very well and discovered many advantages in living without her husband. (Ironically, but typically, the husband resented the psychiatrist afterward, claiming that Mrs. I.'s condition had been worsened rather than helped. He expressed the thought that when his wife had been depressed, at least she was "sweet and reasonable" in her dealings with him!)

4) Resignation. After denial, depression, and anger have run their course, resignation sets in. In this condition, the person is not particularly happy or optimistic, but is reconciled to the breakup and ceases to struggle psychologically with or against it. While much of the depression and anger has abated, the individual is emotionally drained and unlikely to embark on new living patterns, new adjustments, and new ventures. This is a sort of "holding pattern" in which little personal growth is accomplished, but the individual is at least able to function at work and in everyday life with reasonable ease. It is probably just as well if the ease is not too great, because the person may otherwise remain permanently at this stage instead of moving on.

5) Acceptance and Proceedance. This final stage is marked by a genuine return of psychic energy, sufficient not only for the tasks of everyday living but also for new experiences. New acquaintances are sought out and significant new relationships may be established. The term "proceedance" was originally coined by Kenneth Mark Colby in 1958 in a different context, but is adopted here because its sound describes very well the central characteristic so desirable for the divorced person to attain. This is the readiness and ability to *proceed* with life, to leave the past behind, and to advance to new situations and new experiences.

(Note that in all the case examples cited above, the spouse initiating the break-up of the marriage already had other involvements and plans for a second marriage. This is often but not invariably true. Most people do not leave something for nothing, so to speak, even when the something is grossly unsatisfactory and unhappy. In any case, it is a reliable rule of thumb that virtually all men who leave long-established marriages are already involved in another relationship. Women are more inclined, on occasion, to leave a marriage simply because it is poor and destructive and to strike out on their own. This may indicate that women, in our society at least, are basically better equipped than men to care for themselves and to live alone for an extended time.)

The five phases of reaction to divorce do not necessarily always occur in the same order. In some people, depression may precede denial, or anger may come first, and so forth, and one or another phase may even seem to be absent. But most often, careful observation will reveal the presence of the five phases in the indicated sequence.

Younger people, particularly those who have been married for only a short period and have a relatively slight emotional investment in their marriage, may in many cases pass through these phases very quickly and smoothly. At times, such people may seem to have virtually no emotional reaction to the breakup. On the other hand, older couples, couples with children who have been married longer, and men and women around the age of the climacteric, are all particularly prone to a very slow and prolonged reaction, with much pain and suffering along the way. For these couples, divorce is often compounded by other concurrent losses such as the loss of vigor, loss of health, loss of employment, or loss of another relative(as was the case with Mrs. I.).

Pre-existing personality and marital patterns often determine which phase will be most devastating or pronounced. For example, if a marriage has been fraught with extreme hostility and constant battles, both spouses are likely to react to divorce with prolonged depression and/or anger. (Bear in mind that depression can result from anger turned inward.) On the other hand, many people who have habitually reacted to emotional problems by denying them will persist in the denial phase during a divorce. A person who felt strongly rejected in childhood is very apt to carry such feelings into a marital breakup, even if he or she is the one who initiates the divorce. The rejected feelings and low self-image then contribute to a particularly intense or prolonged depression.

The stages of emotional reaction to separation and divorce have been described at some length partly to provide easy recognition for those who may be undergoing such a reaction. The knowledge that such feelings are appropriate to the circumstances is often immensely helpful and anxiety-relieving. Certain physical manifestations often accompany some of the emotional phases of reaction. Thus, in the depressed phase, loss of appetite, sleep disturbances, lack of energy, chronic back pain, and loss of libido are all common. Anger may bring on such symptoms as persistent headaches, recurrent bouts of diarrhea and colitis, variable high blood pressure, and various aches, pains, and other symptoms produced by extreme tension in the muscles of the face and/or body. Finally, in the stage of resignation, people may unconsciously use various psychogenic or actual organic difficulties as an excuse for not going forward and facing the world once more. Here again, there is value in being able to recognize the significance of the physical reactions.

Remarriages

In addition to couples whose marriages endure after 55 or break up, there are those who remarry after 55. Their number is not minute, inasmuch as Americans not only have the highest marriage and divorce rates, but also the highest rate of remarriage. It is thus evident that the institution of marriage is still extremely popular in our society, and that the large majority of people prefer the married to the single state at almost any age.

Second marriages after 55 are apt to be conceived in rather different circumstances than first marriages. When bride and groom are both over 55, their manner is likely to be less romantic and idealistic and more practical and realistic. Values such as companionship and security will be more important than sexual passion or infatuation. The marriage contract may well reflect this.

People entering second marriages tend more to discuss and spell out terms of their marital contract. Not infrequently, a written prenuptial agreement is very specific about how finances are to be managed, how much is to be shared, and what protection is to be given to the interests of children by previous marriages. When the husband in a second marriage is over 55 and the wife is much younger, the question of having children will arise. It is always wise for the couple to have an understanding in advance as to whether or not they desire offspring. Raising a second family is no mean trick for a man of this age, and the outlook for children born to such a marriage must also be considered. Is it fair to bring a child into the world if the father will be in his sixties or seventies when the child is a toddler and the father runs a strong statistical risk of dying before the child reaches adolescence? The answer, of course, depends almost totally on the kind of man the father is. Some men both desire this kind of parental role and can carry it off in a way that is more than fair to any child.

The term *blended* family has been used to describe a second marriage grouping that unites not only the husband and wife but children of previous marriages (''his, hers, and theirs''). Blended families fall heir to all the same blessings and ills that characterize families in general, and are apt to show these characteristics even more intensely. For example, sibling rivalry is likely to be more marked in the blended family because the natural inclination of children to compete with each other is accentuated by the anxiety of the parents that *his* daughter or *her* son should not be neglected or receive less attention than the others. Similarly, one may encounter Oedipal conflicts, rebellion against parental authority, overprotection and overdependence, etc., in the blended family. These situations can be handled if the husband and wife are patient and understanding and realize that the formation of a new family does not occur instantaneously but requires time and energy.

The areas of conflict described for marriages in general (power, nurture, trust, intimacy, and life style) apply equally to remarriages. If any one of the five areas is apt to be especially important in remarriages over 55, it is nurture. Unquestionably, many people in this age group remarry to have someone to take care of them. Where the ''fit'' of the couple is good, and either one spouse adequately takes care of the other or both are good at being mutually attentive, then the marriage can be reasonably happy. But if both expect the new partner to do the caretaking and neither is psychologically and/or physically equipped to do so, then the result is a difficult if not chaotic mismatch.

Married life after 55 exemplifies what Neville Vines in 1979 called adult unfolding. Whether the marriage continues or breaks up, the unfolding itself is neither pathological nor healthy but a fact of adult experience. It is possible, as Vines hypothesizes, ''that the developing adult is best understood'' from ''the subtle internal dialogue of change and self-consistency across a 40–50 year span of time.''

POPULATION TRENDS
OF OLDER AMERICANS

David J. Kolasky, M.H.A.

Vice President, Memorial Hospital, Roxborough

Sally Hoover, M.A.

*Statistical Analyst, Center for
Demographic Studies, US Bureau of the Census*

The older population—those 65 or over—is the most rapidly expanding group in the United States. While adults vary widely in physical, social, and psychological attributes, the image of this group as generally sick, frail, and institutionalized is inaccurate and without statistical support. Nor is there statistical evidence that the elderly commonly migrate to warm climates, but those who do move often go south.

Every day, approximately 5000 individuals reach their 65th birthday, and about 3600 this age or older die. The new surviving elderly tend to be healthier, better educated, and more independent than their predecessors.

Since the most advanced age groups suffer the more significant physical deterioration and loss of energy, our analysis will more accurately reflect current trends if we divide the population into two groups: *aging* 60 to 74, and *elderly*—75 and older. Each group presents different problems. The aging tend to be relatively healthy and vigorous and need more outlets for their interests and talents, while the elderly may need more supportive and rehabilitative health care and social services. Moreover, the elderly often have depleted savings and are more likely to need financial support from families and community.

Who are the elderly? What are their distinguishing traits? They are not only significantly different from the aging in economic, social, and health characteristics, but each generation is also distinct in other ways. It is therefore important to assess the characteristics of today's and tomorrow's elderly without prejudgment.

Population Trends

Since the turn of the century there have been dramatic increases in America's older population. This extraordinary growth has resulted in large part from advances in medical care, including the elimination of life-threatening diseases, better nutrition, development of a network of social services, and a sharp reduction in infant mortality. Fewer infant deaths, longer adult lives, and fluctuations in fertility have altered the nation's age distribution. There are now more older people and an increasing proportion over 65.

In 1900, approximately 3 million adults, or one person in 25, was 65 or older. In 1980, there were 25.5 million older Americans, or approximately one in ten, and a ratio of one in eight, or approximately 30.6 million older citizens, is projected for the year 2000. The elderly (75 and older) have not only increased seven-fold in this century, but at a greater rate than the aging (60 to 74). In 1900, individuals 75 or older represented 29 percent of the total over 65, while in 1980, this proportion had grown to 39 percent. This trend is expected to level off at 36-37 percent after 2020. Two factors are significant. A sharp decline in the senior population is predicted for 1990, reflecting the low birth rates of the Depression and early World War II years. However, the post-World War II baby boom will produce an equally dramatic increase by the year 2010.

Since 1900, life expectancy from birth has increased 25 years. Thus, in 1900, a newborn baby could expect to live to the age of 47, while by 1977 life expectancy had increased to 73 years. It should be noted, however, that the major portion of this gain stems from increased expectancy at birth and in childhood rather than after 65. A 65-year-old could expect to live another 12 years in 1900 and only 4 years more than that by 1974. The diseases of old age have seen few breakthroughs.

Race and Sex Differences in Life Expectancy

Although life expectancy at birth is greater for whites than for blacks and other races, most of this difference is due to fewer deaths of whites at ages under 65. Through 1977, death rates for whites 65–74 continued to be lower, but for those 75–79, reported rates were equal for all races, and at age 80, the death rate for blacks appeared to be lower than for whites, tending to unexpectedly increase the proportion of elderly blacks.

Life expectancies for males and females also show variations. In 1980, the difference in life expectancy at birth was 7.6 years, 70.5 for males and 78.1 for females. This contrasts with the difference of only 4.3 years back in 1940. Much of the difference between male and female rates can be attributed to social and environmental factors; one study blamed men's smoking for their poorer showing. However, as more women smoke, it is likely that the death rates will converge. A second factor expected to affect the rates is the increasing proportion of women who work.

Ratio of Males to Females

The ratio of men to women at all ages, but especially the more advanced, has steadily declined for over a hundred years. The preponderance of women increases after 75. Thus, in 1980 at age 65 or older, there were only 68 men for every 100 women, projected to drop even further by the year 2010, and the 85-year-old group had only 44 men to 100 women. The cause of the increasing disparity with age is complex, but a significant factor is the higher male death rate at all ages, especially due to heart disease and cancer, a pattern which is not expected to change.

Living Arrangements and Marital Status

Possibly one of the most enduring misconceptions concerning older persons is the belief that most are institutionalized. In fact, the opposite is true, for 95 percent of the older population live in family settings or alone. While only 5 percent of those 65 or older resided in institutions in 1975, the proportion increased with age to 7.4 percent for men and 10 percent for women 75 or older.

In the decade 1965–75, the number and proportion of older persons living alone and maintaining their own household increased; this corresponded with a decline in the number of those living with relatives. The increase was found to be attributable largely to more older women choosing to live alone.

In addition to living arrangements, the marital status of older men and women also differed significantly. In 1980, almost 74 percent of all men but only 40 percent of all women 65 or older were married. Slightly more than half the older women were widows, while only 13.6 percent of the men were widowers. Factors contributing to these differences included the higher male mortality rate, the tendency of men to marry women younger than themselves, and the high remarriage rate for widowers.

Racial and Ethnic characteristics

In 1980, whites, 65 and older, represented 11.2 of all whites; blacks, 65 and older, represented 7.8 of the total. The difference results from a combination of a higher black fertility rate, a heavy immigration of whites prior to World War I, a sharper decline in mortality at young age for blacks, and differences in mortality rates under age 65.

In 1980, the population 65 and over contained only 4.5 percent of Spanish origin, but this included the relatively high sex ratio of 84 men to 100 women, and the number of older Spanish-speaking Americans is expected to increase dramatically in the future. From 1970–77, older Spanish-speaking persons increased from 382,272 to 462,029, and those 45–54 increased from 729,246 (7.9 percent of the total) to 924,058 (8.2 percent). In 1977, 11 percent were 35–44, about the same proportion as this age group in the general U.S. population.

Educational Attainment

In general, today's older people have had less schooling than the remainder of the adult population. In 1980, only a little over two-fifths of the elderly had completed high school. Of all high school graduates at least 25 years old, only 60 percent were 65 or older. Age had a reverse correlation with education so that those at the upper end of the age scale were less well educated than those at the lower end. As the elderly die, their replacements will have had more years of schooling. In 1980, the median number of completed school years was 12.5 for the 55-59 age group (half had more and half had less).

Labor Force Participation

Since 1950, the number of men 65 or older in the labor force has steadily declined as a result of more stringent retirement rules, increases in social security payments, a drop in self-employment, and more early retirements. The decline was much less for women. In fact, although the proportion of women 65 and over in the labor force declined from 9.7 percent in 1950 to 8.0 percent in 1980, the 55-64 proportion actually increased.

Between 1950 and 1980, an increasing number of older persons retired at 65, a trend that is projected to continue at least until 1990. While this increase could strain the resources of the working population that must support their retired elders, the strain will be partially offset by increases in the total number of workers. By 1990, 100 workers will support only 111 non-workers compared with 131 in 1980.

Income Levels

Partly because of the higher proportion of retired persons in this group, the income level of older individuals tends to be significantly lower than that of the general population. In 1980, the median income was $21,023 for all families; $12,674 for all black families, $12,881 for all families headed by a woman, and $8777 if the woman was elderly.

The 1980 median income for individuals living alone was lower than for families: $8295 for all individuals, $5095 for older persons.

The proportion of the total population 65 and older living under the poverty level decreased from 35 percent in 1959 to 15 percent in 1980, but stayed higher than the 12.6 percent figure for the impoverished population younger than 65. Sorted by race, 38.1 percent of older blacks lived below the poverty level in 1980.

Geographic Distribution

Geographic distribution of the older population parallels that of the general population, with the largest numbers resident in the largest states, notably New York, California, Pennsylvania, Florida, Illinois, and Texas. The greatest increases, over 70 percent, in numbers of older persons in recent years are found in Arizona, Florida, and Nevada. The migration reflects movement from Northeast, mid-Atlantic, and East North Central states to the warmer climates of South Atlantic, Pacific, and West South Central states.

Since the 1950's, the older population located in the central cities has been increasing more than twice as fast as the total population. Although a large proportion of older persons will remain in central cities in future years, changes in residential patterns in non-metropolitan areas should be noted. Thus, between 1970 and 1975, the growth of the suburban older population far exceeded that of the central city, so that by 1975 the suburbs and cities each held 32 percent of this group. In the same period, the suburban older population also increased faster than the under-65 group in the suburbs, in part because of the tendency of the middle-aged to stay in place.

BOARDING AND NURSING HOMES

Kathleen McGrann

Reba Pollock

Ellen Kirsch

Sheila Fox

Social Service Staff, Pennsylvania Hospital,

The Nursing Home

The decision to enter a nursing home can be difficult for the aging individual and the family. Nursing home placement may be desirable for someone who has been living alone, but whose health will no longer permit a solitary life, especially if family members are unavailable or unwilling to provide home care. Similarly, someone who has been living with family and whose health has so deteriorated that care has become a heavy burden, may be a candidate for a nursing home.

The uprooting from a long-familiar environment is a disruptive and distressing experience especially for the one who is ill and aging. The degree of distress depends on how life has been lived, the quality of relationships with family and friends, and the individual's psychological makeup. A major factor bearing on the ability to cope and to adapt to a new environment is impairment by illness and deteriorating physical and mental powers. Thus, the decision to enter a nursing home can put a heavy strain on coping patterns.

Because family relationships form the core of our lives, their importance cannot be exaggerated. Feelings about parents, how we were raised, the expectations of parenthood, and caring for one's own family—all play a significant role that affects our later years. These factors also help to shape attitudes toward authority, dependency, aggression, control, and the degree of need for perfection and self-esteem. Thus, the person who has generally been self-sufficient may have a strong aversion to becoming a burden on the family; entering a nursing home may be a means to avoid the guilt feelings that might develop from living dependently with the family.

Guilt is frequently and sometimes unknowingly instilled at a young age and simmers through adult years, affecting family relations as grown children unconsciously take revenge on parents for damage received in youth. When the family must plan for an aging parent, such guilt can make an already difficult situation even more painful.

In more or less normal circumstances, all other options may be examined before the nursing home is chosen. Occasionally, an elderly couple may choose to enter together. In addition to daily supervision, including nursing and medical care, the nursing home also provides companionship for residents. This is especially important in alleviating the loneliness and isolation common to many of the elderly.

When the need for a nursing home has been established and those concerned have agreed on a choice, the question of cost arises. Nursing home care is expensive, and financing is often a critical factor. Possible sources include Medicare, Medicaid, Blue Cross/Blue Shield, and private resources.

A Federal program for those over 65 and for others who qualify as disabled, Medicare is administered by the Social Security Administration. It reimburses care in a skilled nursing facility when certain criteria are met, covering up to one hundred days for each benefit period. Determining eligibility can sometimes be confusing. The handbook published by the Social Security Administration lists five conditions:

(1)   The applicant must have been hospitalized at least three
      days in succession before transfer to a skilled nursing
      facility.

(2)   Transfer to the nursing facility is desired because care is
      needed for a condition which was treated in the hospital.

(3)   Admission to the facility occurs within a short time—-
       usually fourteen days or less—after discharge from the
       hospital.

(4)   A physician certifies the need for skilled nursing or rehabili-
       tation services on a daily basis.

(5)   The facility's utilization review board does not disapprove
       the admission.

"Skilled nursing facility" is defined as one that is specially qualified
with staff and equipment to provide skilled nursing care or rehabilitation
and related health services. "Skilled nursing care" is defined as care performed by or under the supervision of licensed nursing personnel; rehabilitation by or under supervision of a professional therapist; and all under
the general direction of a physician.

"Skilled" is not easily clarified, although defined more strictly than
formerly. Family and patients often incorrectly assume that 100 days of
care in a nursing home are automatically approved for qualified individuals. However, recent experience suggests that nursing home care will
be granted to fewer Medicare applicants, and it is unlikely that all patients will be entitled to maximum coverage. Checking with a local Social
Security office or nursing facility is advisable to determine the extent of
eligibility in individual cases.

Medicaid programs fall under the jurisdiction of both state and federal governments, so that eligibility and benefits vary in different states.
The program generally pays for "skilled" and what is defined as "intermediate" care in most states for those who meet medical and financial
requirements. The application procedure can be time consuming, so it is
best to start the process well ahead of pressing need, if possible. Detailed
information concerning eligibility and application procedure can be obtained from local Public Assistance offices.

Depending on the terms of the policy held, Blue Cross/Blue Shield
occasionally covers skilled nursing home services. Definitions of skilled
care appear to follow those of Medicare. Local Blue Cross/Blue Shield offices can answer questions concerning eligibility and will also furnish lists
of participating nursing homes in a given area.

Not surprisingly, private resources afford the patient the greatest flexibility in choosing a nursing home. Some nursing homes will not admit applicants unless they can demonstrate financial resources sufficient to cover expenses for a period ranging from six months to two years. If personal funds have been exhausted following the stipulated period, some nursing homes will apply for and accept Medical Assistance to cover patient costs. Since private payments are negotiated between the patient and the nursing home, it is always advisable to make sure what the daily rate includes and excludes.

Choosing a Nursing Home

Locating a home adequate for the patient's needs can take a good deal of time and extensive investigation, but certain guidelines can ease the task a bit and reduce the chances of making a poor selection:

(1) The patient's physician should determine the kind of nursing care needed—skilled, intermediate, or rehabilitative.

(2) The home should be within easy traveling distance of those who will be visiting most frequently.

(3) Visit selected homes unannounced to inspect patients' rooms, kitchen, and recreation facilities, and to assess cleanliness and the attitudes of residents.

(4) Consult the administrator concerning proper licensing for the home and complete charges, including those for laundry and medication.

(5) Secure information about nursing and physician services, physical and occupational therapy, and activities and socialization programs.

(6) Inquire about the quality and variety of the food served and provision for special dietary needs. Are portions adequate for good nutrition and personal preferences?

(7) Are state and local fire safety standards met? Are smoke detectors, sprinklers, alarms, and extinguishers visible?

(8) Safety features should include well-lighted passageways and stairways, and grab-bars next to bathtubs, showers, and toilets.

(9) The ratio of help to the number of patients served should be high enough to assure optimum care and attention.

The Boarding Home

Some states regulate care and services in boarding homes, but the federal government does not because boarding homes are not eligible for direct participation in federal programs. Local offices of licenses and inspections, for example, may regulate for fire, safety, and zoning.

According to HEW's (now HHS for Health and Human Services) "Master Facilities Inventory" of 1973, there were approximately 7000 personal care and domiciliary homes in the U.S. with an average of 32 beds each. An 85-percent occupancy rate accounted for 186,400 residents. Available help equaled 73,000 full-time personnel, or one per two and one-half residents, allowing two and one-half hours of staff time per resident per day.

A boarding home has been defined as "an establishment operated and maintained to provide residential accommodation, personal services, and social care to individuals who are not related to the owner. These individuals, because of impaired capacity for self-care, elect or require protective living accommodations, but do not have an illness, injury, or disability for which regular medical care and twenty-four hour nursing services are required."

Boarding Home Guidelines

Regulations covering boarding homes may range from merely requiring an administrator and certain safety features to provisions for licensed nurses, admission by a physician, and details of building construction. When evaluating a boarding home, it is good practice to make up a checklist including items such as the number and qualifications of personnel, and toilet and bath facilities with handrails, grab-bars, and night lights. It should be determined whether staff is sufficient to perform essential tasks such as bathing residents and assisting the infirm to dress and eat. At least one attendant should be available on a 24 hour basis, and nursing personnel should include a registered nurse and a licensed practical nurse. Bed linen should be changed regularly and nutritious meals served three times daily.

While some boarding homes restrict their clientele to one sex, the majority accept both men and women. Selection of a boarding home close to the patient's former neighborhood, if possible, will help to ease the transition and lessen feelings of isolation from family and friends.

Mrs. G., owner and administrator of a boarding home in a large eastern city, suggests that those referred to homes should be completely ambulatory. Clients with manageable organic brain syndrome (senility) are also admissible, but alcoholics and drifters are excluded because they tend to be disruptive and troublesome to others. Mrs. G. also recommends that the home should not have an institutional appearance and that the administrator should be on call whenever needed, especially in smaller homes. Meals should be easy to change and all boarders should have a spending allowance to encourage independence and self-esteem. Boarders' rooms should have no more than two beds, preferably hospital-type, with firm mattresses. Boarders will appreciate and benefit from regular, periodic visits by a physician, podiatrist, and barber.

Above all, the boarding home administrator must genuinely like older people and be thoroughly competent to fulfill the management role.

THE HOSPITAL

Gary T. Aden, M.Sc.

Vice President, Pennsylvania Hospital

The average American had 16 chances in 100 of being hospitalized in 1975. The odds for people 55 years of age and older almost doubled—-29 in 100. For people over 65, the odds rose to 36 in 100, and at 85, they were 54 in 100. This means that more than half of all individuals over 85 will be hospitalized in any given year. Because the need for hospital care increases rapidly after 55, some knowledge about hospitals can be useful to most of us.

Hospital Discharges per 1000 People, 1975

Age	Discharges
0–14	72
15–24	142
25–34	173
35–44	155
45–54	178
55–64	215
65–74	300
75–84	443
85 +	539

There are approximately 7100 hospitals in the United States, ranging in size from small dispensaries to large corporations.

The low end of the spectrum is represented by over 300 hospitals with fewer than 25 beds, for example, the Kennedy Center Hospital in

HOSPITAL STATISTICS

Size (No. of Beds)	No. of Hospitals	Total Beds	Admissions	Occu-pancy %	Surgical Opera-tions	Outpatient Visits	
						Emergency	Clinic
6-24	363	6,774	215,565	48.0	52,968	578,739	2,455,167
25-49	1,307	47,218	1,505,426	54.7	430,278	3,217,850	7,679,699
50-99	1,672	120,281	3,811,435	63.8	1,412,800	8,224,994	10,138,007
100-199	1,587	223,280	7,362,595	70.2	3,496,330	15,712,015	13,177,620
200-299	811	196,567	6,759,854	76.1	3,693,311	15,218,601	13,667,940
300-399	449	152,307	4,953,291	78.2	2,693,830	10,912,940	10,432,700
400-499	316	141,356	4,287,641	79.6	2,256,025	8,523,644	11,204,339
500 or more	594	519,314	8,163,975	81.3	4,085,912	15,244,857	38,250,939
Total	7,099	1,407,097	37,059,782	75.8	18,121,454	77,633,640	107,066,411

Morgantown, West Virginia, which has 11 beds. At the other end of the scale are hospitals such as Mount Sinai, in New York, with about 1200 beds. A new entity, known as the multi-hospital system, includes corporations which may own or operate many separate hospitals under one corporate structure. An example of this form of hospital organization is the Sisters of Mercy Health Corporation, headquartered in Farmington, Michigan, which operated twenty hospitals with a total of over 5000 beds in 1978. This new movement may well change the corporate status of hospitals over the next decade. It is too soon to tell whether the change will be as vast as predicted or if it will have any real impact upon the patient. However, it is likely that individual patients will never realize that they have been hospitalized in a multi-hospital system.

Types of Hospitals

Ownership

What kinds of hospitals are there and what difference do they make for the individual patient? It is important to note that hospitals are generally classified according to their ownership or the type of patients cared for.

In 1977, 5881 hospitals in the United States were classified as community hospitals. These are defined as hospitals whose facilities and services are available to the public. They may be owned by the community, a religious order, investors, or government.

Hospitals owned by religious groups do not serve only patients of the same religious affiliation. Rather, they reflect the religious organization's desire to carry out its mission of service to God and mankind.

Government-owned hospitals that serve the public are termed public-general. Well-known examples are Bellevue Hospital in New York City, Cook County Hospital in Chicago, and Los Angeles County Hospital in Los Angeles. These large city hospitals have long served the indigent segment of society, but, with the advent of Medicaid, may be changing their role. Other hospitals owned and operated by the federal government serve a specific population for which the Congress has accepted responsibility, e.g., armed forces personnel, veterans of the armed services, American Indians, and so on. These hospitals are not available to the general public.

Patients Served

Hospitals classified according to the type of patient served vary wildly. Individual hospitals may be dedicated solely to children, maternity, eye, cancer, rehabilitation, tuberculosis, respiratory diseases, or other special patients or patients' needs. These are considered specialty hospitals as opposed to general hospitals which serve a wide variety of problems.

Tax Status

Hospitals are also classified by tax status. The religious and many other community hospitals are not-for-profit, and any excess earnings must be returned to the hospital. Another category is investor owned, which included 751 of the 5881 comunity hospitals in 1978. Many were started by physicians who desired to operate their own hospitals, either for convenience or because practicing privileges were not available at existing local hospitals, or because the physicians saw them as good business investments. These hospitals were generally small. Today, however, large corporations have a prominent role in investor-owned hospitals. For example, in 1978, Hospital Affiliates International, Inc. of Nashville, had 135 hospitals with a total of 18,381 beds.

These corporations, as their investor-owned status indicates, bring the profit motive to the health field. Their detractors argue that taking of profit inevitably lessens the quality of service provided. However, investor-owned corporations do thorough market research to find hospitals which provide a good return on investment, and operate the hospitals accordingly. In 1978, the average size hospital operated by the investor-owned chains had 133 beds as compared with 198 for all hospitals. This generally means that investor-owned hospitals provide less extensive services than larger hospitals. Size, however, gives little indication of the quality of health care.

Teaching Hospitals

Another type is the teaching hospital affiliated with a medical school. Physicians do not go from medical school directly into practice, but, must first complete at least one year of postgraduate training in a teaching hospital. To become a specialist, the physician must then advance to a residency program ranging from three to four years, depending upon the specialty. In the year ending June 30, 1978, there were 51,107 physicians in residency programs in about 1200 teaching hospitals.

The hospitals committed to postgraduate medical education often do not limit their programs to physician education, but may also provide clinical experience for nursing students or operate nursing schools. They may offer training programs for such specialties as nurse anesthetists and respiratory therapists. Thus, the patient in the teaching hospital may see or be treated by more professionals than the patient in a non-teaching hospital, and may also receive more technically sophisticated care. Students gravitate to those institutions which have the best teachers, and it is often thought that the best teachers also make the best doctors.

However, the patient in a teaching hospital pays for the medical sophistication. In some teaching hospitals, and in the eyes of some teachers, technical skills become paramount, so that attention to the patient becomes somewhat impersonal and lacks the traditional "bedside manner." Furthermore, the number of people involved in a patient's treatment may be overwhelming. On the other hand, the non-teaching hospital may offer more moderate technical skills but provide more personal service.

In recent years, serious questions have been raised as to the appropriate level of technology in hospitals. How much complex apparatus do we really need? Have we reached the point where still more technology may only slightly, if at all, improve the odds for patients' recovery? It is generally agreed that the nonteaching hospital can satisfactorily treat patients whose medical problems are within its range of expertise. If more sophisticated treatment such as open heart surgery is needed and is availably only at the teaching hospital, most of us will gladly put up with the parade of people poking and probing at us because we believe it is in the best interest of our personal welfare.

Treatment in a teaching hospital is almost always more expensive than in a community hospital. The reason is that the cost of education programs must be passed on to someone and, in most cases, that someone is the patient. While the cost has little direct impact upon most of us because of insurance coverage, a patient who faces unreimbursed, out-of-pocket payments may want to think carefully before having a simple procedure such as a tonsillectomy performed in a highly sophisticated teaching hospital.

Evaluating Hospital Quality

How does a patient evaluate the quality of hospital care? This question is often difficult enough to answer by the patient who is already in the hospital, but is even more difficult for someone who has never been a hospital patient. Even professionals encounter problems in judging the quality of care in a particular hospital. Quality is easier to express by subjective opinion than by objective measurement. For example, in a 1976 report, experts used a complicated system called the Delphi method to assess hospital administration and patient care. However, few of us have access to the kind of data involved in such ranking. Even if we were given information on items such as "the surgical procedures assessment," "the autopsy rate," or "the average length of stay," it is doubtful that we could interpret it usefully to help us make a personal decision about the choice of a hospital. One distinctly influential factor is a patient's personal satisfaction even if it is not an accurate indicator of the quality of medical care, as the following example illustrates (excerpted from an unpublished 1979 thesis by William McCune):

A 76-year-old woman was admitted to the hospital because of a degenerative skin ulcer which was a complication of recent orthopedic surgery. She was initially reluctant to be interviewed, but after the questioning began, proved to be quite articulate in expressing concerns about her hospitalization.

"I must lie on my side all the time and they don't move me enough. I can tell you that they're murdering me slowly in P.T. (Physical Therapy)—it's a bad atmosphere down there—they let you sit up for hours half naked in the cold; it's a torture chamber. When I asked how long I would be in physical therapy, they said, 'Just as long as they could keep me they would.' Very unsociable."

Asked about the food, she stated, "This special diet stinks! I would like to have a sandwich. I'm 76 and I want to eat what I want." When asked if she had spoken to a dietitian, she responded, "Talking with her is like talking to the wall." However, she felt that the attitude of the nursing personnel was acceptable but claimed they sometimes "took their own time" getting to her room when she called.

Asked about bedside assistance, she said that she had no trouble so far with her bedpan, but warned, "When I have to go I can't wait." Once again, she complained that she had to lie on her side and that the nurses did not move her often enough for her satisfaction and comfort. As to her physician keeping her informed about her condition and her contributing to decisions about her own treatment, she stated, "I don't see the doctor enough to know anything." She had no expectations about the hospital or its personnel.

When questioned about financial concerns, she said "If not for Medicare and my son, I would be in trouble." Other worries centered around "heavy expenses" her son was incurring. "My son has a new house and a child in college, and it appears that my daughter-in-law's parents may have to go into an old folks home."

She was asked her feelings about her room. "It's all right. They put a new picture on the wall today. I didn't come for the room." Apart from her financial concerns, she did not believe she had any serious family problems. Away from the hospital, she lived in a nursing home. Of this she said, "I would like to tell my son that those nursing home nurses are for the birds. They watch TV all the time and don't bother with the patients."

When asked her opinion about the outcome of her medical condition and hospitalization, she stated, "I don't know why I should get well so something else can go wrong." After some hesitation, she added, "At least I can look forward to the good dining room where I live."

In this study, McCune found that patients' concerns involved hospital food, attitudes of nursing personnel, adequacy of bedside assistance, and the hospital room. Nevertheless, most limited their demands on the nursing staff who they felt were busy with other patients "worse off" than they. Finances were generally not a concern; patients were inflexible about the lack of toilet and bathing facilities within their rooms.

While these concerns do not directly effect the success, for example, of a hip joint replacement, they are nevertheless important for the patient. Sociologists have described a hospital stay as an experience which strips people of their identities along with their clothes when they step into a hospital gown. It is therefore important that the setting attempt to ameliorate the harsher aspects of the stay. Good food, cleanliness, personal service, and other considerations go a long way to mitigate difficulties and discomfort. The patient can inquire about a hospital's accreditation, local standing, staff members, and similar factors, but the best test may well be personal satisfaction or a friend's reassuring account of a previous experience in a particular hospital.

Choosing a Hospital

Some patients select a particular hospital by choosing a physician who has privileges there. Others are neither so sophisticated nor willing to take the time to investigate various hospitals before choosing a physician. Most of us see a doctor first when we are sick before we even think of a hospital. The average American sees a physician 5 times a year, but enters a hospital only once every six years. For people over 55, physician visits increase to 6 per year and hospitalizations to once every three years.

Table __. Mean Delphi Rankings and Mean Weights of Effectiveness Measures

Measure	Round I	Ranking Round II	Round III	Index[++] Weight (Round III)
PATIENT CARE				
Surgical procedures assessment	1	1	1	17.0
Expert evaluation	4	2	2	15.9
Medical staff qualification	5	3	3	15.3
Medical audit	8	6	4	15.1
Accreditation	3	4	5	9.9
Patient satisfaction	6	7	6	9.6
Autopsy rate	12	10	7	6.6
Average length of stay	9	8	8	5.9
Adjusted death rate	7	9	9	5.0
Patient outcome	2	5	*	—
Hospital-acquired infections reported	11	12	—	—
Hospital-acquired infections treated	10	+	—	—
Professional staff qualifications	§	11	—	—
Special care unit utilization	13	+	—	—
Special care unit availability	14	13	—	—
Malpractice incidence	§	14	—	—
Professional staff training	§	15	—	—
Community involvement	§	16	—	—
ADMINISTRATIVE				
Use of management studies	1	1	1	18.6
Cost per unit of output	2	2	2	14.9
Expert evaluation	4	3	3	11.1
Accreditation	3	5	4	9.7
Personnel per occupied bed	5	7	5	9.5
Employee satisfaction	7	4	6	9.1
Man-hours per patient day	6	6	7	8.5
Administrative staff qualifications	9	8	8	8.1
Use of employee development programs	10	9	9	5.8
Occupancy rate	11	10	10	4.4
Services provided	8	11	—	—
Management planning activities	§	12	—	—
Financial stability	§	13	—	—
Community involvement	§	14	—	—

* Dropped from list because data could not be obtained.
+ Dropped from list on basis of panel suggestions.
§ Not on original list, but added by experts in first round.
+ + Only assigned to Round III.

Adapted from R. M. Grimes and S. K. Mosley, "Approach to an Index of Hospital Performance," *Health Services Research*, Fall, 1976.

Some physicians maintain access to several hospitals, but most limit their practice to one or two. Selection of a doctor then restricts the choice of hospital, which may be further restricted by geographical distances, for example, if only one is nearby. However, some patients may willingly drive 100 miles to a hospital in sparsely populated areas of the country, particularly to see a specialist in a distant city.

People who choose the hospital first will usually find that the administrator or medical director can refer patients to a suitable list of staff physicians upon request. Generally, patients receive several names from which they can choose a physician whom they then contact themselves.

Patient's Rights

The concept of rights for a hospitalized patient is often thought to be new and controversial. It is not new. Patients have always had rights, although they may not always have exercised them because the anxieties of hospitalization and the attitude of some hospital personnel may have been intimidating. What is new is the codification of these rights, and they are controversial because they developed during the conflicts of the socially turbulent sixties.

The American Hospital Association's Patient's Rights are as follows:

1. The patient has the right to considerate and respectful care.

2. The patient has the right to obtain from his physician complete current information concerning his diagnosis, treatment, and prognosis in terms the patient can be reasonably expected to understand. When it is not medically advisable to give such information to the patient, the information should be made available to an appropriate person in his behalf. He has the right to know, by name, the physician responsible for coordinating his care.

3. The patient has the right to receive from his physician information necessary to give informed consent prior to the start of any procedure and/or treatment. Except in emergencies, such information for informed consent should include but not necessarily be limited to the specific procedure and/or treatment, the medically significant risks involved, and the

probable duration of incapacitation. Where medically significant alternatives for care or treatment exist, or when the patient requests information concerning medical alternatives, the patient has the right to such information. The patient also has the right to know the name of the person responsible for the procedures and/or treatment.

4. The patient has the right to refuse treatment to the extent permitted by law and to be informed of the medical consequences of his action.

5. The patient has the right to every consideration of his privacy concerning his own medical care program. Case discussion, consultation, examination, and treatment are confidential and should be conducted discreetly. Those not directly involved in his care must have the permission of the patient to be present.

6. The patient has the right to expect that all communications and records pertaining to his care should be treated as confidential.

7. The patient has the right to expect that within its capacity a hospital must make reasonable response to the request of a patient for services. The hospital must provide evaluation, service, and/or referral as indicated by the urgency of the case. When medically permissible, a patient may be transferred to another facility only after he has received complete information and explanation concerning the needs for and alternatives to such a transfer. The institution to which the patient is to be transferred must first have accepted the patient for transfer.

8. The patient has the right to obtain information as to any relationship of his hospital to other health care and educational institutions insofar as his care is concerned. The patient has the right to obtain information as to the existence of any professional relationships among individuals, by name, who are treating him.

9. The patient has the right to be advised if the hospital proposes to engage in or perform human experimentation affecting his care or treatment. The patient has the right to refuse to participate in such research projects.

10. The patient has the right to expect reasonable continuity of care. He has the right to know in advance what appointment times and physicians are available and where. The patient has the right to expect that the hospital will provide a mechanism whereby he is informed by his physician or a delegate of the physician of the patient's continuing health care requirements following discharge.

11. The patient has the right to examine and receive an explanation of his bill regardless of source of payment.

12. The patient has the right to know what hospital rules and regulations apply to his conduct as a patient.

While the attraction of giving everything in our society a legalistic tone is obvious in these Patients' Rights, they are really just good common sense. These rights may serve as guidelines for what to expect from a general hospital. Except for patients in mental hospitals, the rights should not be invoked legalistically. The medical patient is not a prisoner and is not limited to these precepts alone.

The best way of insuring your rights as a patient is to use common sense and expect it of those who treat you. It is their task to serve your medical and personal needs within reason, but they are not your servants. The patient who understands what to expect of hospital service will have no trouble obtaining proper rights. If a personality clash develops between you and a staff member, ask to discuss the matter with the employee's superior. This will generally lead to a resolution of the problem.

Some hospitals have ombudsmen whose specific task is to respond to patient complaints. It should not be assumed that a hospital that lacks a special patient's rights representative is ignoring the patient's well being or attempting to deprive patients of their rights. There are two schools of thought on patient ombudsmen. The first sees them as beneficial to patient care because they free nurses and others to concentrate on medical tasks. The second holds that they openly invite other staff to forget about the patient as a person because the ombudsman takes care of that. If your hospital has patient representatives, use them. If not, don't be afraid to ask hospital employees for what you need.

Medicare Payments of Hospital Costs

How you pay for your hospital stay is obviously important. If you are over 65, you probably have Medicare coverage which is composed of two parts: A, which pays for hospital expenses, and B, which pays for the doctor.

In 1977, the average Medicare beneficiary had $1,745 in health expenses, of which $769 was for hospital care. Medicare paid 74 percent ($569) of this. The $200 to be paid by the patient included a deductible approximately equal to the cost of one day's hospitalization. (This deductible can change and increased every year since 1968.) After the deductible amount, Medicare pays in full for up to 60 days of hospital care for the duration of each illness. At 61 days, co-insurance takes effect. All Part A co-insurance is based on the inpatient deductible. From the 61st through 91st day of hospitalization, the patient must pay as co-insurance one-fourth the hospital daily deductible. When the 90 days are exhausted, the patient can dip into a lifetime reserve of 60 days, which pays one-half the inpatient daily deductible. Each day of coverage used from the lifetime reserve is never again available. However, a patient who has used the 90 days but who, after discharge, stays out of the hospital for 60 days restores eligibility for 60 days of paid-in-full hospitalization (with the deductible in force) per spell of illness, plus an additional 30 days subject to co-insurance, plus whatever remains in the lifetime reserve subject to co-insurance.

In 1979, a spell of illness requiring 150 days of hospitalization would exhaust the patient's Medicare benefits and cost an additional $6,160. Many people purchase private insurance to cover this gap. Careful examination of such extra coverage is essential to make sure it fills only the gaps. Purchase of several policies should be avoided to prevent wasting money for unnecessary, overlapping coverage.

MEDICARE/PART A COST-SHARING

Year	Inpatient Deductible	Co-Pay 61-90 days	Co-Pay 60-Day Lifetime Reserve	Skilled Nursing Facility Co-Pay 21-100 days	Home Health Agency Co-Pay—up to 100 visits a benefit period
1966	$40	$10	$20	$5	None
1967	$40	$10	$20	$5	
1968	$40	$10	$20	$5	
1969	$44	$11	$22	$5.50	
1970	$52	$13	$26	$6.50	
1971	$60	$15	$30	$7.50	
1972	$68	$17	$34	$8.50	
1973	$72	$18	$36	$9	
1974	$84	$21	$42	$10.50	
1975	$92	$23	$46	$11.50	
1976	$104	$26	$52	$13	
1977	$124	$31	$62	$15.50	
1978	$144	$36	$72	$18	
1979	$160	$40	$80	$20	

Appropriate Use of the Hospital

The appropriate use of health-care resources is currently in debate, and hospital care is one of the central topics. It is not yet clear how or if the results of the debate will affect individual patients. If the present situation is left unchanged, it is doubtful that either the patient or the physician will be penalized for inappropriate use of hospital facilities. Under the current system, the hospital loses reimbursement from Medicare, Medicaid, and some Blue Cross programs if the physician orders inappropriate hospital care for the patient.

What is inappropriate health service? Assume that a patient is scheduled for admission on Monday for surgery on Tuesday, but because the hospital is full, a bed is not available. The surgeon reschedules the operation for the next Tuesday and then, to beat the system, schedules admission on Saturday. Sunday admission is out of the question because the hospital is already booked for Monday surgery. Saturday and Sunday spent in the hospital would be disallowed as inappropriate because they were unnecessary for the surgical work-up, and none of the three healthcare programs will allow payment for these two days. The hospital must take the loss.

Do patients have a responsibility to minimize unnecessary stays? The answer has to be yes, at least in a moral sense. Will patients take this responsibility seriously? The answer probably is no. The patient will be too anxious about surgery, pain, and other concerns to worry about a financial loss someone else will sustain.

Nevertheless, the public can help conserve resources by using alternatives to inpatient hospital care whenever possible, for example, when outpatient services such as ambulatory surgery are appropriate. If transfer to a nursing home is likely to be necessary after a hospital stay, make plans early so that you don't unnecessarily occupy a hospital bed while awaiting a nursing home vacancy. If your medical coverage does not pay for alternatives to hospitalization, for example, home care, press your employer to include such benefits. Employers may erroneously consider this coverage an extra cost, but it is logical to assume that alternative care is less expensive than hospitalization and should result in lower insurance premiums. Last, but not least, ask your physician about alternatives to hospitalization. If the doctor knows that you are open minded to other approaches to treatment, other choices may become available to you. Do your best to learn about all facets of the health care system and use them wisely.

Hospital Jargon

If you must be hospitalized, you can make your stay more comfortable and minimize anxiety by learning the special language of the territory so that you can keep abreast of events. The following definitions are from a pamphlet prepared by a foresighted hospital staff for their own patients. Abbreviations vary somewhat from hospital to hospital and may also change as advancing technology introduces new terms.

Abdomen: Area between your belly button and hip bones.
Ambulate: To walk.
Anesthesia: A way to remove sensations, including pain during surgery. General anesthesia puts you to sleep; local or spinal anesthesia stops pain in a specific part of your body.

Attending Physician: The doctor in charge of a patient's care.

Barium enema (B.E.): Injection of liquid into the intestine by way of the anus so that the lower bowel can be X-rayed.

B.M.: Bowel movement.

Boarding schedule: Schedule of surgical procedures to be done on a particular day.

B.P.: Blood pressure.

BRP: Bathroom privileges; permission to get out of bed to visit the bathroom.

CAT: Computerized axial tomography; a specialized type of X ray that provides much more information than general X rays.

Catheterize (Cath): Remove urine from the bladder through a tube.

CCU: Cardiac Care Unit; special part of the hospital where people with heart problems are cared for.

Critical Care Units: Intensive Care or Cardiac Care Units which provide extra nursing care and continuous electronic monitoring of each patient's condition.

Dermatology: Specialty that diagnoses and treats skin problems.

Discharge planning: Plans made before leaving the hospital for continued care at home.

Echocardiography: An examination of the heart using sound waves.

Electrocardiogram (ECG or EKG): A recording of the heart's action.

Electroencephalogram (EEG): A recording of brain impulses.

Electromyography (EMG): An examination of the muscles.

Electronystagmography (ENG): Electronic recording of eye movement.

Emesis basin: Container used to collect vomit.

Enema: Method by which bowels may be cleaned out or medicine given.

ENT: Medical service dealing with ear, nose and throat. Another term for otolaryngology.

E.R.: Emergency room.

Fasting: No food after a certain time.

Fasting blood sugar (FBS): Blood sample drawn before eating.

Fellow: Physician on a fellowship to obtain specialized advanced education.

Foley: Tube (catheter) inserted for urine drainage.

Force fluids: Encouraged to drink extra fluids.

Fractional: Testing for the amount of sugar and/or acetone in the urine.

G.I.: Gastrointestinal; the digestive system.

Head Nurse: Nurse in charge of a unit. Also see PCC, patient care coordinator.

Home Care Coordinator: Nurse who arranges for a patient's care after discharge from the hospital.

House Officer (H.O.) or House Staff: An intern or resident physician; a doctor who has graduated from medical school and is obtaining advanced training in a hospital.

H.S.: Hour of sleep.

Ice chips only: No liquids or food, only ice.

ICU: Intensive Care Unit.

Injection: Puncture of the skin with a needle, usually called a "shot".

Intake and output (I. & O.): Measure of fluid taken in and urine put out.

Intravenous pyelogram (IVP): X ray of kidneys and urinary tract.

Isolation: Procedure used to prevent spread of disease or infection to other patients.

I.V.: Putting fluid into a vein (intravenous).

IVPB: Intravenous piggyback; injecting a second fluid into a vein by putting it into another intravenous fluid (I.V.) first.

L. & D.: Labor and delivery area of the hospital; the maternity section.

LPN: Licensed practical nurse.

Meds: Medications, medicine.

M.D.: Medical doctor.

N.A.: Nurse assistant, nurse aide.

Neurology: Specialty dealing with the nerves and brain.

Neurosurgery: Operations on the brain or nerves.

Non-invasive: Refers to examinations of the heart or other internal organs using methods, such as sound waves, that do not pierce the skin.

NPO: Nothing by mouth.

Nuclear medicine: Examinations somewhat similar to X rays that use tiny amounts of radioactivity.

OB: Obstetrics, dealing with childbirth.

Ombudsman: Member of patient relations staff who solves patient's problems or complaints.

Oncology: Specialty related to the diagnosis and treatment of cancer.

Oncology Intensive Care Unit: A hospital unit where special measures are taken to protect patients from germs; sometimes used for leukemia patients.

Ophthalmology: Specialty related to the eyes.

O.R.: Operating room, where surgery is performed.

Orientee: A new employee being oriented to the hospital.

O.R. only: Patient who comes to the hospital for minor surgery, and does not need to remain overnight.

Orthopedics: Specialty that treats bones.

Otolaryngology: Specialty dealing with the ears, nose and throat. Same as ENT.

Pathology: Hospital department that provides many types of tests, especially on blood, urine, and body tissue.

PAR: Post anesthesia recovery room where patients are taken immediately after an operation.

PCC: Patient Care Coordinator; nurse in charge of a unit. Also see Head Nurse.

PEU: Protected Environment Unit; another name for Oncology Intensive Care Unit.

Physical therapy (P.T.): Heat and exercise treatment.

Post Op: After surgery.

Pre Op: Before surgery.

Prep: Preparations for surgery; may include shaving the skin.

prn: As needed; medicine is sometimes prescribed to be given *prn*, or as the patient needs it, with a certain time interval between doses instead of on a rigid schedule.

Psychiatry: Specialty that deals with mental illness.

q.: Every; often used in conjunction with other Latin abbreviations in prescribing when medicine is to be taken. *q*4h means every four hours.

Radiation therapy: X-ray treatments.

Radiology: Use of X rays for diagnosis or treatment.

Restrict fluids: Limit the amount of fluid that is drunk.

Reverse isolation: Procedure used to protect a patient from infection. Called reverse because it protects that patient from others, just the opposite of regular isolation.

R.N.: Registered nurse.

Specimen: Sample of urine, blood, saliva, or tissue for laboratory analysis

Stat: Immediately.

Stool: Bowel movement.

Suture: Stitches used to close a wound or incision.

Temp.: Temperature.

T.A.: Trained aide.

TPR: Temperature, pulse, and respiration (breathing).

Upper Gastrointestinal Series (Upper G.I.): X ray of upper bowel.

Urine testing: Testing of urine for sugar.

Urology: Specialty that treats the organs that form and discharge urine.

Venipuncture: Insertion of a needle into a vein, usually to get a blood sample.

Vital signs (V.S.): Blood pressure, temperature, pulse, and breathing.

VNA: Visiting Nurse Association; organization that provides nursing care in patients homes.

Void: Urinate.

Summary

The modern hospital is a complex organization. However, if as a patient, you take the time to learn, you will find that you can master its intricacies. This is more important than you may think. Anxieties about your illness are sufficient challenges for you to cope with. If you gain an understanding of the hospital and do not allow it to overwhelm you, you put yourself in a position to concentrate on the most important matter, your recovery.

THE U.S. HOSPICE MOVEMENT

Edward D. Viner, M.D.

Head Associate Clinical Professor of Hematology
Pennsylvania Hospital

D. Jeffrey Hartzell, M.D.

Assistant Professor of Hematology
Pennsylvania Hospital

The word hospice means a place of refuge for travelers. Like the words hospitality and hospital, it stems from the Latin word *hospes,* which can mean host or guest. Until recently in our society, the term, if familiar at all, conjured up an image of an Alpine hut and brown-robed monks with St. Bernard dogs rescuing snow-bound travelers, or a rescue mission clothing and feeding human derelicts in a city slum. Both images are historically accurate.

Today, the word hospice has a new meaning that remains true to its origins. It now refers to a way of caring for people nearing the end of their journey through life, who are faced with dying and in need of refuge. Also, the modern notion of hospice is comprehensive. It may refer to a special place, a literal refuge, where the dying are sheltered and cared for. St. Christopher's Hospice in England is perhaps the best known model of such a specifically dedicated inpatient facility. Hospice also connotes a team of individuals working together to provide comprehensive care. Such a team is recruited from many disciplines, including the clergy, nursing, social work, medicine, the allied health professions, and, very importantly, lay volunteers.

Hospice may be a place; it is people, and it is a philosophy. The hospice philosophy is a system of care that seeks to restore dignity and a sense of personal fulfillment to the dying. The hospice philosophy and hospice team together provide palliative and supportive care to meet the special physical, emotional, spiritual, and social needs that arise for both the patient and family during the final stages of illness and in bereavement. Hospice care implies a continuum of appropriate institutional and home care, available twenty-four hours a day, seven days a week. The focus is on the patient and the family rather than the disease. The aim is not to extend life but to improve the quality of the life that remains.

Traditionally, the patient has a chronic disease, most often cancer. Recently, however, hospice service has sometimes expanded to provide care in certain crisis situations. Eligible recipients might include the cancer patient dying at home, the end-stage cardiac patient dying in an intensive care unit, the bereaved couple in the labor room who have just lost a newborn, and the spouse of an accident victim who has just died in an emergency room.

Introduction of the modern hospice concept implies the question, "Why is it necessary?" Who among health professionals would not want the dying to benefit from unhurried and compassionate sharing of time? Who would willingly deprive the dying patient of dignity or peace of mind? Who is not moved by the words of the Psalmist: "Cast me not off in the time of old age; forsake me not when my strength faileth?" The answer to these questions is, of course, no one.

The truth is, however, that many people die in loneliness and despair, their dignity stripped away and their infirmities laid bare. With technological marvels protruding from body orifices and needles piercing their flesh, they die in physical, mental, and spiritual pain. Their wretched condition has many causes and implications. To understand some of them, consider the reaction to impending death, first from the point of view of the patient and the family, and second from that of the health establishment.

In most cases, death seems to come too soon or too late. "He was only . . ." is the common lament, citing an age considered too young for death. Someone dying young may be filled with resentment and frustration at being denied dearly held dreams of the future. At the other end of the spectrum is the dreary and distressingly common spectacle of one who has lived far too long—past reason and sentience. Infantile, combative, incontinent, the superannuated patient lives on, exhausting resources of love and money until death finally arrives too late to be dignified. Anger, futility, resentment, fear, loneliness—these are powerful feelings that afflict both the dying and their families.

Now consider the impact of the dying patient on members of the health establishment. Doctors and other medical professionals are equipped with a vast armamentarium of drugs and devices to fight the battle for life. The word armamentarium is deliberately chosen to describe the forces at the command of the health profession. The image of a war against death is intentional. When it occurs, death is tantamount to defeat, and the medical staff feels the humiliation of failure. Before yielding to defeat, therefore, the health professional finds it difficult to resist bringing to bear the incredible array of esoteric diagnostic tools, exotic drugs, and electronic and mechanical devices available for extending life. As the limits of survival approach, the medical team is so personally committed to the success of their efforts that even more is done to try to help the patient. The patient too often becomes a dehumanized biomedical object. Ultimately, the accomplished feat is postponing death rather than prolonging life. Indeed, the distinction between life and death is now so nebulous that an acceptable definition of death is still debated in medical-legal circles. Gone are the days when a patient was dead simply because breathing stopped.

Still another factor contributes to this dismal picture. As the physician does more to keep the patient alive, less tends to be done to control symptoms, especially pain. When the hold on life is especially fragile, the physician tends to avoid doing anything that might weaken that hold. Narcotics relieve pain but may also depress respiration and cause other problems. The physician may thus use analgesics too conservatively for adequate pain relief.

We cannot blame the health profession alone for this situation. As Elisabeth Kubler-Ross pointed out a number of years ago, we had become a death-denying society. Not only physicians and nurses, but lay persons, too, felt compelled to fight death at all costs. Often, even when the physician was ready to stop aggressive therapy, the patient's family pressed for one last "goal-line stand."

In the past decade, however, both physicians and laymen began to recognize the risk that the patient might become the victim rather than the beneficiary of applied technology. This led to a proliferation of articles and books in both the medical and lay press about death and dying. The subject became a popular one for television programs, public debates, and church group discussions. Importantly, but belatedly, these issues have also been included in the medical school curriculum. Quite suddenly, it seems, we have realized a need collectively to examine whether we have been using our tools properly or whether we were departing from the best interests of the patient. We have begun to question our practices, not only medically and scientifically, but also from the economic, legal, moral, and human points of view.

By 1979, attitudes changed to the point where it is no longer absolutely necessary for a physician to use every weapon in the medical armamentarium. We have progressed to the point where it is ethically appropriate to withhold chemotherapy that may do more harm than good to the end-stage patient, and to abstain from the use of antibiotics when pneumonia would provide a peaceful and welcome end to a prolonged battle with cancer.

Certainly, this re-evaluation of death and dying in the United States was a prerequisite for the implementation of the hospice philosophy. It is important to reiterate that the hospice concept does not imply cessation of care, but rather the substitution of proper care of the terminally ill patient. In short, it means appropriate sensitivity and personal support instead of machines, chemotherapy, and antibiotics.

A Personal Example

One of the present authors has had a unique opportunity to confront these issues directly. The story is told in the hope that it will underscore some of the philosophical bases of the hospice concept.

I was an apparently healthy 36-year-old hematologist-oncologist when I went for a routine physical examination at the urging of my then pregnant wife. My physician unexpectedly found my liver to be enlarged, and studies revealed an apparently malignant *hepatoma* (liver tumor). Fortunately, surgery disclosed only a benign blood vessel tumor. There were, however, myriad postoperative complications. After I suffered a month of shaking chills, 104-degree fevers, hundreds of miserable hours on an ice blanket, and a second operation, an abscess was found in the remaining liver. A postoperative bloodstream infection with circulatory collapse then culminated in a severe complication called shock lung. This led to a *tracheotomy* (incision through the neck) and 31 days on a respirator receiving pressurized oxygen. The oxygen pressure produced a series of *pneumothoraxes* (lung ruptures), each requiring insertion of a tube through the chest wall. Following many other lesser but nonetheless difficult problems and a prolonged period of pulmonary and general rehabilitation, including four months in the hospital and another three months recuperating at home, I was able to return to work.

Obviously, I am very glad that my doctors did not give up. I have to admit, however, to times of significant ambivalence when I yearned to quit and just die unmolested. Ambivalence, born of exhaustion, is one of the arguments some doctors offer to oppose a patient's having the choice to discontinue aggressive therapy.

I was privileged to learn indelible lessons which I had once thought were self-evident. First of all, despite our self-image of empathetic, caring people, we doctors really do not appreciate what we ask our patients to endure physically and emotionally. Patients would benefit immeasurably if all care providers could experience the preoperative terror that comes from imagining an end-stage malignancy, the nostalgia inherent in believing that they will not see their children grow up, and the preterminal mourning over the thought of leaving loved ones and friends.

A question frequently asked of me afterwards, and pertinent to the hospice issue, is whether I thought of dying as I lay there critically ill. Indeed, I thought of little else. Doctors frequently worry that talking about death with the patient will prompt a morbid dwelling on the subject or make the patient think that the doctor feels the situation is hopeless. What physicians do not realize is that the critically ill patient is totally preoccupied by thoughts of death, and yet unable to relieve anxieties through words because death is a taboo subject. I frequently wanted to communicate my anxieties but didn't dare. When I finally gave in to the overwhelming need one morning, I remember feeling empathy for the retinue of house officers and nurses at the bedside when they reacted with a subtle but nonetheless obvious, physical withdrawal from the side of the bed. After all, in the years of my own arduous training, when had I been taught to handle that kind of situation?

As noted, I had great ambivalence about death, at times being afraid that I would die, and at other times being afraid that I would not. The depth of this emotional interaction with death is best reflected in the incessant dream of being autopsied, which seemed to recur whenever I shut may eyes. I believe, therefore, that it is not only right but imperative to overcome the longstanding conspiracy of silence and avoidance with respect to death, and to bring these aspects up for discussion with patients who are obviously seriously ill. Patients need the opportunity to talk about their perceptions of the situation and their anxieties. Such discussions need not imply that there is no hope, but where there really is none, clearly it is preferable to discuss the issue than to evade it.

There were many other lessons to learn. The patient lies in a narrowly circumscribed world so that those who enter it assume a disproportionately important status. It is unfortunate that the janitor mopping the floor, the ward clerk, the respiratory therapist, the aides who make the beds, and the orderlies who transport patients to the X-ray department are not ready for this responsibility. They simply do not recognize the implications of being the patient's only link to the outside world. I found that a remarkable degree of nonverbal communication goes on between the patient and the staff, and that it quickly becomes apparent whether or not the health professional really cares about the patient. I experienced firsthand the personal degradation that stems from a total lack of privacy, the noise and resulting sleep deprivation, and the periodic offensive nonprofessional behavior of the staff. I learned what it is really like to have tubes coming out of every natural and a few man-made orifices. I learned about the difficulty of communicating when unable to talk with a tracheotomy in place for many weeks. I learned about the sense of futility at being completely dependent, and how frustrating it is when the doctors and nurses do not listen to the patient. I came to realize that being miserable is a more difficult symptom to alleviate than focal pain, and that after a time, comfort rather than survival becomes the paramount desire.

It is really too bad that every doctor and nurse has not experienced an ICU psychosis and the state of complete emotional and physical exhaustion that can ultimately reduce even the strongest patient to a lip-quivering, eye-watering mass of protoplasm. Most pertinently, I lay there thinking frequently of how inappropriate all that I was being subjected to would have been if indeed I had had an incurable terminal illness. Actually, only at this point did I really believe that my doctors had told me the truth about my tumor being benign for I knew my senior surgeon was too wise and mature to have put me through all this if I really could not have gotten well. I became angry at the neurosurgeons caring for the patient next to me. It was apparent to me that they were knowingly and inappropriately administering the same kind of heroic care that I was getting to an unfortunate man with an inoperable, highly malignant brain tumor.

In the end, my experience taught me that death is not always an enemy and that, indeed, it may well be preferable to a life of pain without dignity and without hope. Coincidentally, it was after my personal experience that the hospice philosophy of care began to be espoused in the United States. Clearly, the concepts inherent in the hospice approach were in concert with my own reflections while attached to that respirator for so many weeks. Accordingly, I determined to learn more about hospice care and to do what I could to advance its implementation at Pennsylvania Hospital.

The Hospice Program at Pennsylvania Hospital

In exploring the form that our hospice at Pennsylvania Hospital might take, we found a number of models available for study. Partly because hospice care means different things to different people, and partly because of funding problems, the hospice movement in the United States has grown somewhat haphazardly. Certainly the best known hospice in the world is St. Christopher's Hospice outside London, founded and directed by Dr. Cecily Saunders. This is a free-standing institution to which only preterminal patients are admitted. It is the prototype for several similar institutions in the United States—Hillhaven Hospice in Tucson, Arizona, is one example. This facility, owned by a nursing home chain, provides the full range of continuous care necessary for dying patients and their families. Another pioneering American hospice activity is Hospice, Inc., in New Haven, founded in 1974, which at first provided only home care. In November 1977, it broke ground for a 44-bed inpatient facility not to supplant, but to supplement the home care program.

There are pros and cons in having a separate hospice facility. One of the major cons is the possibly negative emotional effect in which admission seems to the patient to be entrance to a "death house." Such a misconception is quickly dispelled upon the patient's arrival. In fact, the atmosphere is one of serenity, informality, and peace. There is no sense of despair. Visitors, including young children and pets, come and go freely, unrestricted by established visiting hours. Music is playing, poetry is read, the patient's own rocking chair may be brought to the bedside, and favorite foods may be brought from home. Even if the connotation of a "death house" is overcome, however, economic considerations prevent the construction and staffing of enough free-standing hospices to satisfy the estimated need in the United States.

The Royal Victoria Hospital in Montreal has incorporated hospice care into the general hospital setting. There, a hospice team sees patients on a consultative basis throughout the hospital, and also tends patients in a separate area in the hospital designated the Palliative Care Unit. St. Luke's Hospital in New York City was the first major American medical center to offer a similar in-patient hospice program.

This concept of integrating hospice activities into the hospital has several important advantages. Hospice care is really good medicine in the fullest sense of the term. A hospice team functioning in the general hospital environment can start a ripple effect, radiating the philosophy, idealism, and sensitivity of the hospice approach to general care throughout the hospital.

Ultimately, the Pennsylvania Hospital program was patterned to a large extent on the Royal Victoria approach. Because hospice care has been classified as custodial by insurance carriers, however, they do not cover its costs. Consequently, like others in the United States, we have had to "hide" these patients, and have not been able to establish a distinct, designated hospice area.

We have tried to make the program as flexible as possible. Hospice care has been traditionally offered to patients expected to die within three months and whose physicians have abandoned aggressive therapy. We believe, however, that the criteria for admission to hospice care should not be rigid, and that acceptance of the patient should depend on the individual situation. For example, discontinuation of chemotherapy and other significant therapeutic measures is not a requirement for admission to our program. We believe some cancer patients need the supporting embrace of the hospice team to help them get through the period of rigorous treatment before there is any medical decision or patient awareness that death is impending. While it can be argued that support at this stage might be provided by other hospital personnel, the interdisciplinary approach of the hospice team and the relative facility of experienced team members in talking with such patients make it advantageous to involve these specially trained people sooner rather than later. As noted above, we feel that crisis situations that may arise in the labor room, the open heart surgical theater, and the emergency room, may also benefit significantly from the expertise of the hospice team.

It is also our goal to emphasize the importance of home care. The research of Hospice, New Haven, has demonstrated that patients who can possibly remain at home during their last days experience less anxiety towards death, and their families suffer less guilt. We are working cooperatively with an already established community nursing service to provide home care. Basically, the home care program offers the same type of comprehensive support implied by the hospice concept. The visiting counselor assesses the physical situation in the home and the available family resources. She maintains communication between family members and teaches them basic nursing skills. We anticipate that the security of knowing that help is continuously available will decrease the number of readmissions to in-patient care precipitated by understandable patient and family panic over such symptoms as coughing, vomiting, unremitting pain, and emotional decompensation. In this way, many patients may be able to stay at home longer. It is ultimately hoped that as family and community confidence grows, more and more patients will be permitted to die peacefully at home.

Comfort

Providing comfort is perhaps the single most important goal of hospice care and deserves special consideration. The specter of the dying cancer patient, suffering great physical and emotional pain, is terrifying to us all. Why then do physicians seem unable to use available analgesics adequately to relieve pain? The answer is multifaceted. Unfortunately, doctors have been so preoccupied with lifesaving that many fail to become sufficiently adept at pain control. Furthermore, physicians tend to dwell inordinately on the theoretical risks of addiction, excessive sedation, and interference with natural breathing. Also, regrettably, doctors sometimes compete with patients over who is in charge of the situation. If the physician is relatively enlightened, the nurse may become an obstacle, since the nurse really controls what the patient gets, especially when medication is ordered on an "as needed" basis. Nurses, albeit well-meaning, are often afraid to administer adequate doses of narcotics because they fear they will push the patient "over the edge." They, too, get into contests of will with patients and worry unnecessarily about addiction and other theoretical risks. The basic problem is recognizing the proper therapeutic goal and accepting the fact that all we can realistically do for the terminal patient is to afford comfort. This really should not be so difficult since, after all, helping one's patient die more easily is the ultimate responsibility of every health professional.

Doctors also often fail to understand the difference between acute pain, which is usually short-lived, reversible, and psychologically tolerable, and the chronic pain of the cancer patient. Cancer pain is compounded by anxiety, depression, insomnia, and financial and family concerns. The terminal patient cannot escape dreaded thoughts and preoccupation with death. Frequently, suffering is due less to focal pain than to general misery from such problems as mouth sores, the discomfort of lying immobile, the presence of multiple tubes, nausea, lack of appetite, heartburn, abdominal distension, constipation, incontinence, itching, difficulty with secretions, shortness of breath, and last, but certainly not least, pervasive fear.

Obviously the answer is not just pumping in more painkillers. The need to achieve comfort in a broader sense makes hospice team care most helpful. Implied in the hospice concept is acceptance that, medically speaking, pain relief is not *a* goal but *the* goal. Following hospice precepts, the physician should feel secure in giving narcotics in dosages and at intervals necessary to achieve the purpose. This also requires becoming skillful in the supplementary use of non-narcotic drugs such as tranquilizers, sedatives, and antidepressants, to reinforce the narcotics with the hope that pain relief can be achieved without clouding the patient's mind and senses. Morphine, given by mouth in easily swallowed liquid form, is perhaps the drug of choice. A second drug may be added to relieve nausea or anxiety. Pain medications are most effective when given on a routine schedule so we must try to anticipate pain and use the various drugs before severe pain becomes entrenched. The usual approach is to wait, but this is often ineffective and frequently then requires a higher total dosage of narcotics.

The entire hospice team is concerned with the alleviation of fear and anxiety, and with helping the patient and family deal with often overwhelming psychologial, social, and economic problems inherent in the circumstances. A study at the Royal Victoria Hospital corroborated the value of the hospice approach and the long known fact that less anxious patients require smaller doses of analgesics. The pain study at the Royal Victoria Hospital is of interest. There, it was clearly demonstrated that patients in the hospice unit obtained significantly more pain relief from the same doses of medicine than did patients in general medical wards and private rooms.

Illustrative Case Histories

The following case histories illustrate well both the hospice approach and the type of patients it can help.

Case 1   Anthony D., a 57-year-old man, is dying of lung cancer. He has been in the hospital for two weeks for evaluation of a persistent cough, weight loss, and severe back pain. He has received many blood tests, a variety of X rays and scans of his chest, liver, and bones, a bronchoscopy, and a lung biopsy.

While these investigations were in progress, Anthony's son called the doctor. Their conversation went like this:

Son: Is it cancer, Doctor?

Doctor: Yes.

Son: Please, you mustn't tell my father he has
          cancer; he wouldn't be able to take that.
          His own father died of cancer, and he
          would just give up if he knew he had it.

Anthony's wife, Mary, also spoke with the doctor. She had guessed the truth and suspected Anthony knew it also, even though he had said nothing about his condition and asked no questions. Mary's immediate concern is how she will care for her husband if and when he comes home from the hospital. She has been afraid that the physical and emotional strain would be too much for her to bear.

To add to their worries, Anthony and Mary's daughter gave birth recently to a child with a congenital heart defect and the baby has not been doing well. Also, their son had left home in anger at age 17. Although he and his parents have begun to speak to one another again, the relationship is still uneasy.

Anthony's case is a typical one which might be expected to progress along the following lines. Anthony will have cobalt treatments. His doctor will use the word "tumor," but the words "cancer" and "malignant" will not be spoken by either the patient or his physician. Mary will visit Anthony faithfully, but the strain will begin to tell on her. They will talk about trivial matters, and will often bicker about little things. They have not attended religious services for many years, but in their private thoughts, both have become eager to reopen this part of their lives. They will not share these thoughts, however, because of their need to deny Anthony's cancer. In time, Anthony will suffer more and more pain and grow weaker by the day. When the pain is very severe, the nurse will inject an analgesic which provides some relief but seems to wear off quickly, long before he is scheduled for another shot. By now, Anthony and Mary are aware that the doctors and nurses visit Anthony less often than before, and do not linger at his bedside.

This is the stuff of soap operas, but also the substance of real life and death in our society. Fortunately, hospice care can relieve some of the stress and dreariness of this case.

A hospice counselor, usually a nurse or social worker, could arrange a conference with all members of the family and explore their patterns of interaction, specific fears, resentments, and feelings of guilt. Anthony's needs—physical, emotional, and spiritual—would be assessed. The hospice counselor could then meet with the other members of the hospice team, including physicians, nurses, social workers, clergymen, and volunteers, to review the case and develop a plan of hospice care. The plan might include specific ways to minimize the patient's and family's physical, social, spiritual, and financial suffering. For example, the team physician might suggest more effective measures to relieve and possibly even eliminate pain. The team psychiatrist might help to open communications between parents and son and devise strategies to help the daughter share Anthony's dying experience. A volunteer could be assigned to help Mary with her continuing responsibilities at home, and give her the necessary "time off" from her long daily visits with Anthony. The hospice counselor could work with the family on a regular basis to help them exchange their thoughts and feelings honestly, and help the couple obtain religious counseling. The plan might also include guidance in obtaining insurance benefits and preplanning funeral arrangements.

In a case like Anthony's, it is often possible for the dying patient to spend the last weeks of life at home. Although Mary has realistic doubts about her ability to cope with the situation, the important home care programs being provided by hospices could lend enough support to the family to allow Anthony and his family the benefit of having him die peacefully at home, surrounded by the persons and things dearest to him.

If Anthony died in the hospital, the hospice team members would try to foster an atmosphere of calm serenity and reduce the intense anxiety and depression. Grandchildren would be allowed to visit. The hospice counselor could help relieve the family and support them during the terminal vigil at the bedside. She could make sure that the wife was notified when death was actually impending so that she could be present at the critical moment. The counselor would also try to be present.

Anthony's situation is a common one, and most hospice programs would approach his problems in a fashion similar to that described. A joint effort by team members would focus on the patient and family as a unit and emphasize the quality rather than the mere quantity of the remaining life.

Often, quite remarkably, family members are later able to speak of the dying process as a positive experience. If the patient has died peacefully, and unfinished emotional difficulties between the patient and his loved ones have been resolved, the family may be left with fond memories and a sense of peace, rather than guilt and anxiety. Of course, there is grief, but this is a healthy emotion to be expressed openly during bereavement. It will eventually dissipate, aided by the hospice team, and, one would hope, by positive future family interaction.

A few hospice programs extend their services to other kinds of life and death situations, a goal which we at Pennsylvania Hospital believe appropriate. The following cases illustrate other types of crisis intervention where the special sensitivity to life and death issues provided by hospice care is greatly needed.

Case 2   Paula K. is a 34-year-old housewife admitted to the maternity floor of a hospital. She and her husband, Steve, married when both were 30 years old. At 32, Paula had a difficult pregnancy and delivered a stillborn 28-week-old male. Paula and Steve never saw their child, but were told that he could not have lived even if born alive. They were afraid to imagine his appearance.

Eventually, Paula and Steve decided to try again. The second pregnancy has not been easy either. Paula has gained an excessive amount of weight, and her blood pressure has been difficult to control. Recently her doctor had transferred her care to a specialist in high-risk pregnancy who arranged for the present admission when signs of fetal distress became apparent.

In the hospital, Paula has had a number of blood and urine tests, a special scan of her abdomen, and even an amniocentesis. In this test, a fluid sample is drawn through a needle inserted through the abdominal wall into the uterine cavity. Analysis of amniotic fluid provides essential information about the condition of the baby. Two nights ago, the doctor had to tell Paula that her baby was dead. She and Steve are now in the labor and delivery suite, and her labor pains have begun. Both are still too numb from the shock of the news to think clearly. When they recover, they will be confronted by troubling questions: What should they do about funeral arrangements? Was the baby a boy or a girl? Why did it die? Did the amniocentesis harm the baby? Was the baby normally formed?

If Paula and Steve had been fortunate enough to have a hospice program at their hospital, the following steps might have been taken. When the obstetrician first realized they would lose the baby, the hospice counselor would have been asked to meet with the couple to explore the strengths and weaknesses of their relationship, and find the best way to offer maximum support. When Paula went into labor, the counselor would come into the hospital to be with her and help her through the labor by explaining procedures, giving backrubs, aiding proper breath control, and, importantly, by being a caring person close at hand. During the labor, the counselor would explore the couple's feelings about the loss of this baby and the death of the first one.

After the still delivery, the counselor would arrange to have the baby washed, wrapped in a blanket, and taken to the parents so they could see and even hold their baby. She would point out features of the infant that resemble the parents and might encourage the parents to give their baby a name. This process emphasizes that the baby, though dead, was real, their own flesh and blood, and existed as a part of their lives.

After this intimate time, the counselor would help the parents to cope with such difficult matters as autopsy and burial arrangements. In the days that followed, she would arrange the appropriate religious service.

Finally, during the bereavement period, the counselor would help alleviate the anguish of grieving. Guilt feelings would be examined and put in perspective. For example, having authorized the amniocentesis, the parents might blame themselves for their child's death. The skillful counselor could help the couple work through such feelings and so ward off a possible source of marital stress.

Ideally, the hospice activities would permit the bereaved couple to bring to an emotionally satisfactory end the series of events that started with the first awareness of Paula's pregnancy. The pregnancies might otherwise linger unhappily and inconclusively in the emotional lives of the parents. With hospice care, Paula and Steve could be freed to move on from this pregnancy, turn their energies toward each other and the future, and look forward to the time when Paula can carry and bear a healthy baby.

Case 3   Walter B., a healthy, happy, and successful 42-year-old attorney, has been celebrating with his wife Susan and some close friends by dining at a nearby restaurant. Without warning, Walter gasped for breath, his face became blue, and he slumped over the table. He was rushed to the emergency room of a city hospital.

In Susan's mind, the events were a blur of frantic, nightmarish sounds and motions. Now she is aware of commotion in the tiled room where her husband lies. At the core of her being, she knows her husband is dead, and the doctor will soon come to confirm her certainty. The doctor will also mumble, in an awkward and apparently insensitive way, about an autopsy being necessary to determine the cause of her husband's death.

A hospice program can provide much needed help in this kind of situation. A counselor would stay with Susan in the emergency room, not only giving moral support as a caring person, but also explaining the activities going on around them and assisting with such necessary tasks as autopsy arrangements, calling a funeral director, and notifying family and friends who can come to Susan's aid in the crisis.

Hospice care does not stop at this point. During the bereavement period, the counselor would contact Susan as often as necessary, knowing that she may be haunted by feelings of guilt, for example, at not having pressed her husband harder to have a physical examination when he complained of indigestion some weeks earlier. Susan may also be suppressing anger that Walter left her in such a predicament, an emotion she feels is too shameful to express. These are powerful emotions which Susan must learn to manage, a task in which the hospice counselor can be of great help.

Economic and Regulatory Problems of Hospice Care

Unfortunately, while the idealistic goals of hospice care are eminently worthy, serious problems confront the movement in this country. Not the least of these is how to pay for hospice care. Five major sources of funds have been tapped, including private donations, membership fees, hospital revenues, private and government grants, and federal, state and local contracts. Several hospices have received federal funding from the National Cancer Institute and the Comprehensive Employment and Training Act (CETA) program. However, donations and special grants are not sufficiently stable and reliable to support the necessary continuing service programs.

Two local Blue Cross organizations in the country are conducting experiments in hospice reimbursement, but Blue Cross and the private insurance companies in general have not become significantly involved in hospice care. Third party reimbursement is essentially nonexistent for care in freestanding hospices and, as noted, patients receiving hospice care in general hospitals often do so secretly by being hidden among the hospital's general population. Furthermore, there is no mechanism to fund the home portion of the terminal patient's care. This is vitally important, since a basic tenet of hospice philosophy is home care for the patient as long as possible.

Considering the emphasis in hospice care on trying to keep the patient at home and the fact that hospice inpatients can be cared for in institutions that are much cheaper to build, equip, and maintain than today's hospitals, one would expect that the hospice movement could significantly reduce medical bills. Indeed, retrospective studies support the premise that hospice care would be less costly than traditional terminal care, potentially saving over two billion dollars per year nationally. Yet, those wise in the economic history of medicine counter with the charge that hospice care is a "systems add-on" rather than a less expensive alternative, and would therefore raise the total cost of medical care.

Facts rather than opinions are needed. Recently, the Comptroller General of the United States tried to get facts for his report to the Congress on hospice care. Unfortunately, the detailed information needed to compare the cost of hospice care with traditional terminal care is not available. The Department of Health, Education and Welfare (now Health and Human Services) is planning to fund experiments that should provide hard data on this basic issue. In the end, though, it is probably not realistic to expect immediate national cost savings from the hospice movement.

The Comptroller General's report also noted that there is no standard definition of hospice care, which is one of the difficulties confronting the government and third party insurers. As of 1979, approximately two hundred organizations in the United States, either operational or in varying degrees of planning, consider themselves to have hospice programs which provide many different combinations of medical and other supportive services to terminally ill patients. Many of these services are potentially coverable under present law by Medicare, Medicaid, Social Security, and the Older Americans Act. Other services probably cannot be covered without a change in the law. For example, while Medicare and Medicaid both cover home health care services, under present regulations these must fit the definition of skilled nursing care. Also, the patient must be totally homebound after first having been hospitalized for at least three days. Medicare and Medicaid provide some coverage for emotional support services, pain control, physical and occupational therapy, and homemaker services, but coverage is not uniform, and current rules may be too stringent for a successful hospice program. Neither death education nor bereavement followup is covered by present law, and many potential hospice patients are not eligible for any coverage under any of the four programs. Ultimately, the Department of Health and Human Services and the individual states will determine the specific services covered under existing programs. To a degree, old laws may have to be waived and new ones created.

Establishment of hospice care standards, licensing procedures, and some degree of regulation are other problem areas facing the hospice movement. These are ripe opportunities to milk the public. There is much more to establishing a hospice program than simply changing the sign over the door of what was once a proprietary nursing home, or is now an underused section of a general hospital in an overbedded community. While many of the individual components of hospice care may already be covered by existing standards and licensing procedures, it is advisable to formulate standards applying to hospice care as a whole. This may seem unduly restrictive, but patients must be assured that they will receive full services from any institution calling itself a hospice.

Legal Aspects

If both doctor and patient agree on a proper time to cease aggressive therapy, what are the legal implications? For the most part, we are not dealing with dramatic situations like the Karen Quinlan case, or with determination of the moment of death so that an organ may be removed from a potential donor for transplantation. On the other hand, some physicians hold that similar principles should be applied in deciding when and if to end treatment of a patient with an incurable disease.

While the raising of legal issues by doctors may often be smoke screens to cover unresolved personal feelings, there is a legitimate basis for questioning the legality of various actions. Clearly, legislation cannot prevent controversy, since the innumerable individual patient situations each have their own special nuances. Fortunately, legal responsibilities in this nebulous area are being clarified, and doctors are becoming less afraid to withhold treatment. In large part, this salutary change results from changes in societal attitudes towards death in the last decade.

The doctor is also not alone in the decision-making role. The legal doctrine of "informed consent," under which no medical procedure may be performed without a patient's knowledgable permission, also applies to the terminal patient. Legally, the terminal patient must be fully informed about the nature of the fatal affliction and the alternatives of accepting or rejecting heroic medical efforts to prolong life. Thus, the doctor has the same duty to discuss the prognosis and treatment alternatives with the dying patient as with the non-terminal patient. Both patients have the same right to accept or reject treatment, and the physician is liable for failure to make proper disclosure. If the patient expressly forbids a lifesaving procedure, the decision cannot legally be ignored, and the physician is not liable to malpractice charges for abiding by the limitations imposed by the patient. If concern for the patient's physical and mental condition dictates the disclosure of certain information that would unnecessarily harm the patient, the physician need not tell the patient that he or she is dying. However, if the legal issue is raised, expert medical testimony is required to establish that the decision to withhold information was appropriate. If the patient is incompetent and lacks the legal capacity to decide, the doctor must turn to the closest family member or, if necessary, to a court-appointed guardian.

The concept of a living will is relevant here. This is a written document which attests to both the patient's competence and the absence of duress, and which directs the physicians concerning the patient's desired treatment when later faced with imminent death. The document usually states that the signatory does not wish to be kept alive by artificial or heroic measures if there is no reasonable expectation of recovery from physical or mental disability. While it is only an expression of attitude, with no binding legal effect at present except in California, a living will does advise the physician of the patient's philosophy.

The question of euthanasia is also appropriate to a discussion of the hospice movement. There is a good deal of confusion over this term and its derivatives, and much debate over whether it is really a euphemism for criminal homicide. The word *euthanasia* comes from the Greek for good death. The present connotation is usually a well-intentioned killing to relieve the victim of a painful or handicapped existence. It is plainly against the law. Death by an act of omission rather than commission is described as negative or passive euthanasia. A key question is whether the physician who intentionally omits positive steps to prolong the life of a dying patient is criminally liable if such inaction either causes or fails to delay death. The law is vague, imposing on the physician only "a duty to act reasonably towards the patient." Practically speaking, the doctor should not withdraw or withhold treatment that might significantly lengthen meaningful life. With a hopeless cancer patient, however, it is generally safe for the physician to hold back after appropriate discussion with and approval by the patient and family.

Debates over the right to life versus the right to death will continue, and the medical and legal professions will continue to make necessary decisions which affect life and death. The physician cannot evade responsibility by hiding behind theoretical legal concerns. It is to be hoped that legal confrontations will be avoided by open discussion among the physician, the patient, and the family.

Conclusion

It seems safe to say that the hospice movement is not a fad, but a valid and worthy idea whose time has come. With approximately 400,000 Americans dying each year from cancer alone, and many more from other chronic diseases, the need for hospice care is clear. Since death ultimately comes to all of us, the nature of its coming is of obvious interest. Institutional death in the United States today has many repellent aspects which are causing increasing numbers of people to seek an alternative.

There are many unanswered questions. At the national level, these concern funding, definition of what constitutes proper hospice care, establishment of criteria for patient selection, and determination of the best model or models for our country. At the local level, establishing a good hospice requires months or years of painstaking planning to define specific goals, set up operational guidelines, achieve funding, educate the local medical community, and assemble a staff. A hospice can only be as good as its foundation, its planning, and its people. Design short cuts are likely to lead to program shortcomings.

Now is the time for innovation and experimentation with diverse hospice forms. Integration of the hospice concept into the U.S. health system depends on the development of stable patterns of funding, staffing, and regulation.   Now is the time, also, for each of us to identify and redefine attitudes and feelings about critical illness, dying, and death.

INSURANCE

Frederick A. Tucker, C.L.U.

President, Biddle, Bishop & Smith, Inc., Philadelphia

We are all aware that health care costs have risen and continue to rise at an alarming rate in recent years. While the Consumer Price Index rose 150 percent in the period 1950–1977, health care costs increased 280 percent. In 1962, the daily rate for room and board in a good city hospital ranged between $20 and $25; today's rate for the same semi-private room exceeds $250 per day, not including charges for such services as nursing, surgery, drugs, or intensive care. The rise in costs has been offset to some extent by better services, more sophisticated equipment, and shorter hospital stays, but the increase has nonetheless been extraordinary, making it the subject of numerous governmental studies and reports and the focus of heated debate over the need for national health insurance. It is no wonder that many aging men and women fear the loss of lifetime savings because of major illness and a need for protracted medical care.

Commercial Hospitalization Insurance Prior to Age 65

While most group health insurance plans offered through employers provide satisfactory coverage, the base plan—hospital and physician services—and the major medical program should be carefully studied to determine whether full protection is assured.

The following items in the basic hospitalization plan should be checked:

(1) Does the plan provide a semi-private rate for room and board? Many older plans offer only a fixed rate, such as $75 or $100 per day, making no allowance for inflation. An employee in such a plan may discover that he or she is liable for a much larger share of the charges than expected. A plan that pays standard semi-private room and board rates is preferable.

(2) Does the plan provide additional benefits to cover intensive care?

(3) Is the surgical schedule satisfactory for most procedures? This should be reviewed with a health insurance specialist or surgeon.

(4) How long is the period covered by room and board rate? Most plans range from a period of 30 to a maximum of 120 days, with the better plans covering the longer period. In some plans, the 30-day benefit is extended by the major medical supplement.

(5) Are emergency accident procedures covered? Any limitations?

(6) Diagnostic X-ray and laboratory services are often treated as separate benefits with a fixed limit for each incident. The amount should be checked to determine its adequacy for your area.

(7) Is there a provision for blood transfusions and plasma? Some plans exclude blood, which can be an expensive item.

Suggested Benefit Schedule
for the
Basic Hospital Benefit Program

Service	Benefit Schedule
Room and Board	Hospital's basic semi-private room charge with maximum duration 120 days
Intensive Care Unit	100 percent of all charges
Ancillary Charges	Unlimited during confinement
Other Services	Usually limited per confinement
Physicians' fees	$10 per visit
Surgical Schedule	Fees as defined, including anesthesiologist
Emergency Outpatient	$300 per accident
Diagnostic X-ray and Laboratory Services	$100 per accident or incident
Radiation Therapy	As defined by schedule

The standard contract will usually have certain exclusions, as follows:

(1)   Cosmetic or elective surgery is rarely covered.

(2)   Special duty nursing may be covered in the major medical plan, but is often excluded from the basic plan.

(3)   Coverage for convalescent and custodial care is usually limited, with a lower rate for room and board than is allowed for the hospital. Such care must follow a period of hospital confinement.

(4)   Charges for mental and nervous disorders for patients in a regular hospital are usually fully covered. However, payment of outpatient charges and institutional confinement are greatly reduced.

(5)   Dental procedures are excluded unless they are disease or accident related.

Major Medical Coverage

Major medical coverage differs from basic hospitalization in that it is catastrophe insurance designed to protect the insured from extraordinary financial loss. It can be written alone or as a supplement to basic hospitalization. When written alone it usually has a deductible of $300 to $500, and co-insurance (80% coverage) for the first $1,000 to $2,000 of expenses. When co-insurance ends, the program pays 100 percent of the excess.

Supplemental major medical coverage is a very important part of any complete hospitalization plan. It should be designed to provide benefits not specifically covered under basic hospitalization, with an upper limit of coverage when the plan is in effect. This should not be less than $50,000. Today, $250,000 is quite common , and many insurance companies now offer a $1,000,000 or an unlimited program.

With very few exceptions, major medical plans have a deductible, usually $100 in group health plans. In most plans, expenses incurred in October, November and December can be applied to satisfy the deductible for the following year. When major medical coverage supplements a basic hospital plan, the deductible is an out-of-pocket expense; benefits under major medical are paid when hospitalization coverage is exhausted and the insured has paid the $100 deductible amount. Often there is a family deductible of $300, and no matter how many illnesses may occur within a given year, the amount paid by the insured family will not exceed this figure.

Co-insurance plans, in which the company pays 80 percent and the insured pays 20 percent of the amount of claims, are common today. In one popular plan, the co-insurance clause applies only to the first $2,000 of expenses, with the company paying 100 percent of each claim in excess of $2,000. Another plan offers full payment of allowable expenses after a deductible amount, the latter based on the calendar year. Thus, if an illness continues for more than a year, the deductible is applied a second time.

Limits in major medical coverage tend to parallel those in basic hospitalization plans. Thus, room and board is covered only on a semi-private basis and nursing home or extended care will be limited, usually to periods ranging from 30 to 45 days. However, most plans will offer broad coverage for intensive care and surgical procedures.

Comprehensive Major Medical Plans

Available as individual or group contracts, comprehensive major medical plans feature simplicity, covering basic hospitalization and major medical in a single plan which operates like the supplemental major medical plan. In this arrangement, co-insurance or deductible contracts may be selected, with limits and benefits similar to those described above.

Group and Non-Group Plans

Generally, group plans of ten or more participants will accept any new applicant regardless of pre-existing health problems. Smaller group and individual plans require medical certification of health for all members of the family, and insurers retain the right to exclude or limit coverage for those with pre-existing health problems or illnesses.

As increasing numbers of business firms and institutions acquire group insurance plans for employes, and the number of people who must take individual contracts dwindles, fewer commercial insurance carriers offer individual health insurance. The individual contract has also been subjected to increased rates resulting from the narrowing market as Blue Cross/Blue Shield acquires more and more of the individual and family contracts.

For those who are not enrolled as members of employee groups, or who are unable to obtain coverage through trade, professional, or fraternal organizations, Blue Cross/Blue Shield is the most practical option. While sometimes costly, it has individual health insurance plans that provide satisfactory benefits. Preexisting conditions may be excluded for a period of time.

Blue Cross/Blue Shield Plans

Blue Cross/Blue Shield plans were originally developed in conjunction with local hospitals in the United States to assure collection of hospital fees. Hospitals were willing to accept reduced rates in return for the guarantee that fees would be paid.

Blue Cross/Blue Shield is not one plan, but over 60 plans throughout the country, with differing rates and varying quality of service. Many plans have hospital discount arrangements that are available only to subscribers and save money for plan operators. Because of increasing hospital cost, however, more plans are paying fees in full.

Blue Cross payments for hospital services normally cover charges for room and board, emergency services, operating room charges, intensive care, drugs, and some miscellaneous expenses. Hospitals that accept such payment as full reimbursement for services are classed as member hospitals whose affiliation with Blue Cross is covered by an agreement. In a similar arrangement, Blue Shield contracts for the services of participating physicians. However, many physicians balk at accepting Blue Shield payments, requiring the patient to pay fees directly and to apply to Blue Shield for reimbursement.

Major Medical After Age 65

At age 65, major medical plans usually become supplemental to Medicare, and some group programs drop such coverage at this time. As a result of amendments to the Age Discrimination in Employment Act in 1978, changes in retirement practices will encourage more people to continue working after 65, leaving them enrolled in group health plans. This will probably stimulate corporate interest in major medical coverage for the aging and bring attention to a much needed benefit.

The Health Maintenance Organization (HMO)

HMO's began under the auspices of a government supported test program in the early 70's, following the success of similar programs on the West Coast, and are not yet widely available. The HMO combines in a single organization the financing of health care and treatment services. Participating physicians are contracted by salary or fee, but specialists who are not under direct contract may also be included in the plan. Hospital services may be provided under direct contract with the HMO, or such services may be purchased through Blue Cross or other commercial sources.

Monthly premiums for HMO coverage usually are higher than those for standard hospitalization plans, reflecting broader coverage of diagnostic services, lower deductibles, and co-payments. Designed for regional health care, an HMO works best with local, non-transient groups.

The future success of HMO's is uncertain. Much will depend on continuing support by the federal government.

Medicare

The Medicare Act, known officially as "Social Security Amendments of 1965," was a significant development in the U.S. health care program. Statistics for 1976 show 25,662,921 persons enrolled and disbursements of $17,551,290,952. These figures will of course continue to grow as the U.S. population ages and the cost of health care increases.

Medicare is a two-part program in which Part A provides basic protection against hospital and related health care costs, and Part B, a voluntary supplementary program, covers the cost of physicians' services. Part A is known officially as "Hospital Insurance Benefits for the Aged and Disabled," and is funded by the federal government through the Social Security Administration. Part B is financed by a monthly premium paid by those enrolled, supplemented by matching contributions from the federal government.

Eligibility for Medicare benefits is established in one of four ways:

(1)   The great majority automatically qualify on reaching age 65 as retirees or as others entitled to survivors' benefits.

(2)   A special transitional provision permits benefits for those who reached age 65 before 1967 or 1968 and who can show a minimum number of eligible quarters of social security coverage.

(3)   For those unqualified under the above rules, enrollment may be accomplished by payment of a monthly premium.

(4)   The age requirement of 65 is removed for those who are
       qualified for benefits by reason of disability. In this cate-
       gory, individuals with chronic kidney disease are qualified
       for Parts A and B if disability is established.

The following information with respect to Medicare coverage is accurate as of July, 1980. Because of probable changes in benefits in future
years, it is advisable to check with your local Social Security office to determine the current status of services and benefits.

Part A benefits cover hospital, nursing home, and home care services. A deductible of $204 is payable for each hospitalization. The first
60 days of hospital care are fully covered, and a co-payment of $51 per
day is required for the next 30 days. A lifetime reserve of 60 additional
days requires co-payment of $102 per day. Provided that it follows a three
day stay in a full service hospital, convalescent care is covered for a maximum of 100 days, with co-payment of $25.50 per day after the 20th day.

Home care benefits can be expected to expand with steadily increasing costs of hospital care and mounting pressures to avoid needless expense. Currently, one hundred visits by nurses and technicians within a
twelve-month period are fully covered as long as the patient is confined
to home and unable to travel for treatment.

Part B benefits are available on enrollment and payment of a
monthly fee of $8.80 per person. This Medicare plan includes services of
physicians and surgeons, supplementary services and supplies such as
diagnostic tests, laboratory fees, and physical therapy, and outpatient
hospital benefits. The plan has a deductible of $60 per calendar year,
with benefits limited to 80 percent of the charges after the deductible.
Home health services, outpatient surgery, and pre-admission diagnostic
services are 100 percent covered without a deductible requirement. The
plan also reimburses psychiatric services on a limited basis.

Blue Cross and a number of insurance companies have been designated by the federal government to administer Plan B. The general enrollment period runs from January through March 31 of each year, with
coverage commencing in July for those enrolling in this term. Otherwise,
applicants should enroll three months before their 65th birthday for
coverage beginning three months after the birthday. Monthly premiums

can be deducted from the Social Security check, or for those who are not eligible for Social Security, paid quarterly to the federal government.

If the retiree is physically unable to come to an office to enroll, a close relative may complete the arrangements and, if necessary, pay monthly premiums. The choice of a physician is up to the patient or family, and payments for treatment by the physician or a hospital are limited to reasonable charges.

Supplementary health insurance to provide protection in areas not covered by Medicare may be desirable. It is offered in such a variety of forms that the potential applicant is well advised to study them carefully or to seek guidance before purchasing such coverage. It should be kept in mind that since Medicare coverage is quite broad, additional coverage is necessarily limited. Some plans offer to pay Medicare deductibles and co-insurance expenses. However, the purchaser of supplemental health insurance must be wary. Policy wording often excludes payment for any illness covered by another plan, so that premiums paid would simply be money wasted. A few elementary precautions can prevent such payment for non-existent benefits.

When purchasing insurance supplements to Medicare, the purchaser should first be sure to understand limitations, especially a waiting period or exclusion for pre-existing illness. Specified illness policies, such as those for cancer, should be avoided as the odds do not favor the insured. It is important to note whether the policy covers Medicare deductibles, hospital stays beyond the 150-day period covered by Medicare, and 20 percent of those charges not covered by Medicare Part B. In general, any worthwhile supplemental policy should focus on major health costs rather than the more affordable expense of minor illness or injury.

Many older people buy hospital income policies as a form of supplementary coverage on the theory that a modest added income while hospitalized will help to offset expenses not covered by other insurance. However, these policies normally restrict payment to daily stays in "regular" hospitals, thus excluding payment for confinement in nursing or rehabilitation institutions where the elderly often go after a surgical procedure or other treatment. Purchase of such a policy is best avoided unless nursing home benefits are included.

Life Insurance after 55

Isn't the purchase of life insurance after age 55 inappropriate? Not necessarily. Those who do so have much the same objectives as younger individuals: to provide continuing income for replacing economic value lost with the death of a spouse; to reduce debt, for example, by relieving surviving family members of a heavy mortgage; to finance childrens' education; to cover the final expenses of illness and death; or to cover taxes and estate costs. Life insurance may be used for many other purposes, but the aim in any plan is to guarantee that sufficient insurance remains in force throughout life.

The years just ahead seem to promise continuing inflation and constantly rising values of home, business, and real estate forcing greater attention to be given to estate taxes, which may also rise. The tendency of the aging to continue working beyond 65 to avoid living on fixed incomes is another factor which tends to make an adequate life insurance program important to the economic survival of the family unit. However, for most individuals, planning must begin well ahead of the later years if the desired benefits are to be realized.

Three main types of life insurance are available. *Term insurance* provides relatively low cost protection for a specific number of years. However, when the term ends, the insurance must be renewed at a higher rate or be discontinued. Rates are especially high for individuals in their fifties or sixties, who may find the insurance too expensive when it is most needed. Payment is made only on death.

Group term coverage is a common fringe benefit given by employers. In most cases, benefits cease or are sharply reduced at retirement to avoid high costs to the employer.

Whole Life, or *Ordinary Life Insurance* normally requires that premiums be paid throughout the lifetime of the insured. The policy may be maintained beyond age 60 at no change in rate if it is a non-dividend policy, or at a lower rate than prior to age 60 if it is a dividend policy. However, because most individuals change their policies at various times, for example, surrendering a larger one for a paid-up policy of a smaller face amount, or surrendering it for an annuity at retirement, only a small proportion of policies now in force remain as they were originally written.

Because of the pace of economic change today, it is recommended that the needs of the insured and family be reviewed every two years to determine whether changes or additions are in order. Such review should include the individual's will, the current value of owned property, the insurance program in relation to both, and the cash needs that might arise in the event of death.

Lastly, *Disability Income* coverage provides short-or long-term benefits during inability to work because of illness or injury. Short-term coverage normally commences after a brief waiting period in the case of sickness, or immediately in the case of accident, and continues for a limited number of weeks. Long-term coverage may continue from 60 months to age 65, depending on the plan, following a waiting period ranging from 90 to 180 days. Both forms of insurance are usually offered under group plans sponsored by employers.

RETIREMENT INCOME:
SOCIAL SECURITY AND
SUPPLEMENTAL SECURITY

Jeffrey P. Korn, Esq.

Former Associate Director, Mayor's Committee on Aging
City of Philadelphia

Social Security

Insured Status

The Social Security system provides both retirement and survivors benefits, which may be payable to the worker, spouse, dependents and survivors. The range of these benefits are determined by the worker's insured status, which, in turn, depends on the amount of work credit the worker has accumulated under Social Security. The exact amount of work credit required depends on the worker's age.

Work credit is measured in quarters of coverage that a worker has accumulated in jobs covered under Social Security. In 1982, employees and the self-employed receive one quarter of coverage for each $340 of covered annual earnings. (In 1981, the figure was $310; in 1980—$290.) No more than four quarters of coverage can be credited for any one year. The amount of earnings needed to get a quarter of coverage will increase automatically in future years to keep pace with average wages.

For work performed before 1978, credit was given for each calendar quarter in which $50 or more in wages was earned, up to a maximum of four quarters of coverage per year. The self-employed, prior to 1978, received four quarters of coverage if they had self-employment net profit of $400 or more in any year.

A worker who retires in 1982 needs a total work credit of 31 quarters to achieve fully insured status. For 1983, the number is 32, and it rises one quarter each year until it reaches the maximum of 40 quarters (10 cumulative years in a covered job or jobs) in 1991. The required number of quarters merely establishes the worker's eligibility for retirement and survivors benefits. It does not determine the dollar amount of benefit checks (which is based on average earnings during working years), nor does it entitle the worker to maximum allowable monthly benefits.

Monthly retirement benefits are payable to the following:

1. The retired worker, who may elect to receive checks as early at age 62.

2. The wife or divorced wife of the worker, age 62 or older.

3. Where the woman has been the primary worker, the husband or divorced husband, age 62 or older.

4. The wife—at any age—when she is caring for a child who is under 18 or disabled, and the child is receiving benefits based on the retired worker's earnings.

5. The worker's unmarried children—or grandchildren under certain conditions—if either (a) under age 18 (b) age 18–22 if a full-time student (c) age 18 or older if disabled before 22 with the disability continuing indefinitely.

Survivors' benefits are payable to all of the following if the worker dies fully insured (if the worker was not fully insured, benefits will be paid only to the widow and to unmarried children under the conditions indicated in the fourth and fifth categories below):

1. The worker's widow, surviving divorced wife, or widowed husband age 60 or older.

2. The worker's widow, surviving divorced wife, or widowed husband age 50–59, if disabled and under certain conditions.

3. The worker's dependent parents age 62 or older.

4. The worker's unmarried children—or grandchildren under certain conditions—if either (a) under age 18 (b) age 18–22 if a full-time student (c) age 18 or older if disabled before 22 with the disability continuing indefinitely.

5. The worker's widow, surviving divorced wife, or widowed husband, if caring for a child under 18 or disabled, and the child is receiving survivor's benefits.

Computing the Amount of Benefits

It is important to keep in mind that *fully insured* means only that the worker and family are eligible for benefits when the worker retires, and that the family is eligible for benefits following the worker's death. The dollar amounts of benefit checks payable to the worker and benefits payable to dependents or survivors are based exclusively on the average earnings during working years.

Social Security contributions withheld from wages throughout the period of employment are credited to the worker's earnings account. Thus, the account becomes, in effect, a history of annual earnings. It is from this record that Social Security will calculate the worker's covered average earnings. Up to a limit that is likely to change from year to year because of inflation or other factors, higher benefits will be payable to those with the highest average earnings. It should be noted, however, that regardless of the amount earned in the working years, the worker is credited only up to the maximum *covered* earnings. The following table indicates the amount of earnings covered under law by Social Security.

In any year in which the worker earns less than the amount indicated by the following table, the credit will not exceed the actual amount earned.

An accurate estimate of individual benefits is best obtained by asking the Social Security office to make the calculation, which will be based on the work record in their file. For those who reached 62 or died before 1979, benefits are based on actual average earnings. For those who reach

Year	Maximum Amount of "Covered Earnings"
1937–1950	$ 3,000
1951–1954	3,600
1955–1958	4,200
1959–1965	4,800
1966–1967	6,600
1968–1971	7,800
1972	9,000
1973	10,800
1974	13,200
1975	14,100
1976	15,300
1977	16,500
1978	17,700
1979	22,900
1980	25,900
1981	29,700

62 or die after 1978, actual earnings for past years will first be adjusted, then averaged before final calculation is made by application of a formula. A transitional method, which computes benefits both the old and new ways and then takes the higher figure, assures that those who reach 62 after 1978 and before 1984 will not be disadvantaged. Pamphlets are available through Social Security for those who wish to estimate the amount of benefits due them, but it should be kept in mind that only the figure given by Social Security is valid.

By filling out and mailing a post card—Form 7004—supplied by any Social Security office, individuals can obtain a printout of their earnings record on file at Social Security headquarters in Baltimore, Maryland. Any discrepancy between personal records of earnings and those on file in Baltimore should be reported immediately to Social Security. Especially for those who change jobs often or who have more than one employer in any year, it is advisable to verify earnings records every three years.

Retirement Benefits

While most individuals elect to retire at 65 when they can be eligible for full retirement benefits, others accept reduced benefits by retiring as early as age 62. Such a reduction is not a penalty, but rather an adjustment that takes into account the longer time, on the average, that benefits will be payable. The following table indicates the amount of benefits payable on early retirement:

Retirement Age	Percent of Benefits Payable
62	80%
63	86 ⅔%
64	93 ⅓%
65	100%

It may or may not be an advantage for particular individuals to retire early. The factors that determine such a decision normally involve job satisfaction, financial circumstances, and health. Generally, however, those who retire at 62 and live beyond age 77 will collect *less* from Social Security than those who retire at 65 with full benefits.

Delaying retirement beyond age 65 entitles the recipient to a special credit which increases benefits at the rate of one percent per year for every year of postponement, up to a maximum of seven percent at age 72. This credit has been increased to three percent for workers reaching age 65 after 1981, up to a maximum credit increase of 21 percent.

Family members of fully insured workers receiving retirement benefits may also be eligible for benefits. These are normally calculated as a percentage of the retiree's primary benefit which is defined as the maximum amount payable to the retiree if benefits are started at age 65. However, the total amount of any family may receive is limited to a maximum based on the retired worker's earnings record and calculated from special tables. The following table shows the percentages of primary benefits payable to family members—subject always to the maximum family limit:

Family Member	Percent of Worker's Primary Benefit (%)
Spouse or divorced spouse at age 65	50 (37½% @ age 62)
Unmarried children under 18, 18-22 if students, over 18 if disabled	50
Wife, at any age, if caring for a child who is under 18 or disabled	50

Survivors' Benefits

Benefits payable to family members of a deceased worker are also figured as a percentage of the worker's primary benefit, subject to a maximum family limit on the total payable.

Automatic Cost of Living Increase

Social Security benefits are geared to the Consumer Price Index (CPI), which measures increases in the cost of living. The law provides that whenever inflation rises over 3 percent in any 12-month period, benefits will automatically be increased by the same percentage. Thus, checks mailed in July, 1981 contained an increase of 11.2 percent, reflecting the degree of inflation shown by the CPI. Similarly, checks mailed in July 1982 will contain an increase to adjust for continuing inflation.

Divorce and Remarriage Rules

A divorced wife who has not remarried is eligible to collect retirement benefits if her former husband has filed for his benefits and if their marriage lasted at least ten years. The amount of the benefit is the same as for a wife who is not divorced: 50 percent of the husband's benefit if she is 65, 37½ percent at age 62.

Survivors	Percent of Primary Benefit
Widow, surviving divorced wife, or widower at age 65	100%
Widow, surviving divorced wife, or widower at any age who is caring for a child under 18 or disabled	75%
Widow, surviving divorced wife, or widower at age 60	71½%
Unmarried children under 18, 18-22 if students, over 18 if disabled	75%
Dependent parent—one qualifies —both qualify	82½% 150%
Disabled widow, surviving divorced wife, or widower at age 50	50%

The rules covering survivors benefits and remarriage were liberalized in 1979. Widows or widowers who remarry at age 60 or over, are still eligible with no reduction in their benefits.

Special Minimum Benefit

Individuals who contributed to Social Security for more than 20 years, but had low earnings are entitled to a mimimum benefit which is higher than the amount they would otherwise receive. The amount depends on the number of years of covered work. For 1980, those who retired at age 65 after 30 years or more of coverage received $289 monthly. The benefit will increase automatically as the cost of living rises.

The special minimum should not be confused with Supplemental Security Income (SSI) which is a separate program. It is possible to be entitled to benefits from both under certain conditions.

Lump Sum Funeral Payment

On the death of a worker who was fully or currently insured, a lump sum of $255 is payable to the surviving wife or husband, provided she or he was living with the deceased at the time of death. Where there is no surviving spouse, the benefit may be paid directly to a funeral home or to the person responsible for funeral expenses. It should be noted that this benefit is not payable on the death of a non-working spouse, for example a wife who is neither fully nor currently insured but who was receiving benefits based solely on the work record of her husband.

Work After Retirement

Payment of Social Security retirement benefits will continue provided that earnings do not exceed the annual exempt amount. Earnings above the prescribed limits will reduce benefits by $1 for every $2 in excess earnings. For 1982 the annual exempt amounts are $4440 for those under 65 and $6000 for those 65-72. The lower limit will rise annually as the general wage level increases. The higher limit will rise $500 per year to $6000 in 1982, after which it, too, will rise automatically each year. At age 72, current earnings no longer affect benefits, and in 1982, this provision will apply at age 70.

Only income from a job or self-employment is included in a calculation of retirement earnings. Investment income of any kind is excluded.

A special monthly earnings test is applicable only to the first year of retirement to avoid a financial penalty for those who work and have normal income for part of that year before the date they retire. Under this arrangement, wages or salary earned in that year before the date of retirement do not affect retirement benefits.

It should be noted, however, that the Social Security tax will continue to be deducted from all earnings at any age, even when the worker is receiving Social Security benefits, and no federal income tax is owed. For those who are self-employed, the Social Security tax is payable when net income—total income less expenses—exceeds $400.

Applying for Benefits

It is advisable to contact the nearest Social Security office two or three months before the planned retirement date to apply for benefits. When visiting the office, the insured worker should bring the birth or baptismal certificate, a marriage certificate if applying for a wife's or widow's benefits, and the birth certificates of any children for whom benefits are sought. The office will also require the worker's W-2 tax form for the previous year, or, for the self-employed, a copy of the most recent Federal Income Tax return, so that earnings records can be updated and benefits calculated. If any of these documents are missing, there is no need to delay applying for benefits, since required proof can usually be established by other means.

Receipt of Benefit Checks

Benefit checks normally arrive in the mail on the same day each month, the 3rd, or on the Friday preceding this date if the 3rd is a Saturday, Sunday, or legal holiday. If the check has not arrived by the 6th of any month, the Social Security office should be notified.

Many retirees elect to have their checks sent directly to their banks, to help prevent loss, theft, and forgery. Any bank will provide the authorization form needed for this convenience, and will give any assistance needed to complete the arrangement.

If a check is lost, stolen, or destroyed, it will be replaced. However, this process takes time, so it is essential to notify the nearest Social Security office immediately.

Since a check that arrives at the beginning of a month actually represents the benefit for the previous month, any check received after the death of the recipient must be returned to Social Security. In cases where checks are sent to a bank, the bank should be immediately notified of the death so that checks may be returned. The rule applies regardless of the date of death within the particular month. Where checks are payable jointly to husband and wife, the survivor should inquire at the Social Security office whether the check may be cashed.

Review and Appeal Rights

Those dissatisfied with Social Security or Supplemental Security Income decisions may appeal through a process that advances through several steps. The final decision may be reached by suit in a U.S. District Court if the review at lower levels has proved unsatisfactory. The first step of appeal is for reconsideration by other Social Security personnel who were not involved in the original decision. The second step is a hearing before an Administrative Law Judge, with testimony taken under oath. A lawyer, if desired, may accompany and represent the person making the appeal. The last step before suit in a District court is review, or refusal to review, by the Appeals Council, which meets in Washington, D.C.

Supplemental Security Income (SSI)

SSI is a federal program that provides monthly income to individuals who are 65 or older and in financial need, or who are blind or disabled regardless of age. It is designed to supplement benefits from Social Security or other pensions, although people who have never worked may still be eligible for SSI benefits. Although SSI is administered by the Social Security Administration, it is technically separate in that it is financed from general revenues, not from Social Security contributions.

To qualify for payments under SSI, an individual must meet rather stringent means tests which cover both income and assets such as savings accounts, stocks, jewelry, and other valuables. The value of a home, car, and some household goods are excluded from the test. When assets exceed the limit by a modest amount, the applicant must agree to sell the excess within a specified time—6 months for real property and 3 months for personal property—to be eligible.

SSI benefits may be reduced by one-third if the applicant resides in another person's household, for example, a daughter's or son's, and receives support and maintenance from that person. In addition, the law requires an annual review of the income, resources, marital status, and living arrangements of all individuals receiving benefits under SSI.

Application for SSI benefits may be made at any Social Security office. The procedure is like applying for Social Security benefits, except that there is close scrutiny of personal assets and living arrangements.

BIBLIOGRAPHY

Books

Commerce Clearing House, *1980 Social Security and Medicare Explained,* Commerce Clearing House Inc., Chicago, Illinois, 1980, 436 pp.

Commerce Clearing House, *1981 Social Security Benefits Including Medicare,* Commerce Clearing House, Inc., Chicago, Illinois, 1981 32 pp.

United States Department of Health, Education, and Welfare, *Social Security Handbook,* 6th ed., Social Security Administration, HEW Publication No. (SSA) 77-10135, United States Government Printing Office, Washington, D.C., 1978, 525 pp.

Miscellaneous Publications

The following are concise, informative pamphlets distributed free by the Social Security Administration:

United States Department of Health, Education, and Welfare, *Your Social Security,* SSA Publication No. 05-10035, 1981.

_____, *Social Security Survivors Benefits,* HEW Publication No. (SSA) 05-10084, 1980.

_____, *If You Work After You Retire,* SSA Publication No. 05-10069, 1981.

_____, *How Recent Changes in Social Security Affect You,* HEW Publication No. (SSA) 78-10328, 1978.

_____, *If You're Self-Employed,* HEW Publication No. (SSA) 05-10022, 1981.

_____, *Estimating Your Social Security Retirement Checks for Workers Who Reach 623 in 1979 -83,* HEW Publication No. (SSA) 79-10088, 1979.

_____, *Estimating Your Social Security Retirement Check for Workers Who Reach 62 Before 1979,* HEW Publication No. (SSA) 79-1047, 1979.

_____, *A Woman's Guide to Social Security,* HEW Publication No. (SSA) 78-10127, 1978.

_____, *A Guide to Supplemental Security Income,* HEW Publication No. 78-11015, 1978.

_____, *SSI For the Aged, Blind and Disabled,* HEW Publication No. (SSA) 78-11000, 1978.

RETIREMENT INCOME: PRIVATE

Donald R. Fleischer, F.S.A.

Principal, Towers, Perrin, Forster & Crosby, Inc., Philadelphia

Charles D. Root, Jr.

Member, Board of Managers, Pennsylvania Hospital
Former Vice President and Director, Towers, Perrin, Forster & Crosby, Inc.

Preretirement Planning

One of the most important contributions to a successful retirement is advance planning well ahead of the actual date of retirement. Where you will live, and what your continuing activities will be are questions that should be considered. A location convenient to your children can be a great asset both to them and to you. Many retirees seek a year-round warm climate, while others prefer to remain where their roots are established.

In developing financial plans for retirement, it is helpful to outline personal needs and preferences. Although individual circumstances and goals may differ, the following are general guidelines:

1. An income payable each month of retirement during your lifetime sufficient to enable you to maintain the same standard of living you and your spouse enjoyed before you retired. Because of tax reductions and a different pattern of expenses in retirement, the gross income needed may be

only 80 percent or less of your preretirement income. However, it will be necessary to build protection against the
ravages of inflation that decrease the value of the dollar.

2. Continuing income payable to your spouse after your death
    sufficient to maintain your customary standard of living.

3. Hospital-Medical-Surgical coverage which, combined with
    Medicare, will enable you to meet the major share of medi-
    cal expenses.

4. As large a nest egg as possible for special needs, such as tra-
    vel or unforeseen expenses. The nest egg may include a sav-
    ings account, investments in money-market type mutual
    funds, bonds, or stocks, the equity in your home, and the
    cash values of your life insurance contracts.

Careful advance financial planning can also reduce later retirement
expenses, for example, completing the mortgage payments on your home
before you retire. Plan to enter retirement with a new car or one of recent
vintage in good condition. Consider putting your life insurance on a
paid-up basis at retirement to avoid further payment of premiums. Plan
to purchase desired high-cost items before retirement.

Because it is not possible to predict how long you will live in retirement, you should prepare for a wide range of possibilities: a long life, a
short one, or something in between.

The Teachers Insurance and Annuity Association (TIAA), which
provides pensions to the majority of college professors, reported in 1979
that 778 of its annuitants were over 90 years old and 17 were over 100. Its
oldest pensioner was 107 years old.

Clearly, long life is possible and it is well to avoid outliving your income. Social Security, annuities, and your company pension will continue until your death, and, in some cases, will continue after that in
whole or in part to your named beneficiaries. But if savings are drained
too rapidly, you may outlive them.

The following table shows the number of additional years people
live on the average after reaching a given age. However, these are only,

averages not a basis for firm planning. Many will not live as long as indicated; others will live much longer. As medical knowledge advances, these average expectancies may increase.

Average Additional Years of Life

Age	Male	Female
55	23	28
60	19	23
65	15	19
70	12	16
75	9	12
80	7	10
85	5	7
90	4	6
95	3	4
100	2	3

How Much Retirement Income

Since expenses and taxes should be lower after retirement (for example, Social Security payments are tax-free), less money may be needed from other sources to provide the same spendable income as before retirement. Tables 1 and 2, based on retirement at age 65 on January 1, 1980, illustrate income requirements and calculations for both married and single retirees.

For example, if you are married and your gross income was $20,000 in 1981, only $15,485 remained after federal and state income and Social Security taxes. If you retired on January 1, 1982 and both you and your spouse had reached 65, your combined Social Security checks will equal $12,002; $3483 more after taxes gives you the same $15,485 net income you had before retirement. (Federal income tax would be due on higher non-Social Security income, but at the after-65 rate, and Social Security tax would be due if you continued in part-time employment. Also, your Social Security benefits would be less if you retired before 65).

If you were single, but the circumstances were otherwise the same, only $14,441 remained from your $20,000 1981 income after

Table 1. Example of Retirement Income Needed for Married
Individual to Duplicate Pre-Retirement Net Income after Taxes
(Based on Retirement at Age 65 on January 1, 1982)

Calculation of Pre-Retirement Net Income

Earned 1981 Gross Income	Federal Income Tax*	State Income Tax**	Social Security Tax	Net 1981 Income After Taxes
$ 10,000	$ 702	$ 220	$ 665	$ 8,413
15,000	1,635	330	998	12,037
20,000	2,745	440	1,330	15,485
30,000	5,510	660	1,975	21,855
40,000	8,730	880	1,975	28,415
50,000	12,505	1,100	1,975	34,420
75,000	23,303	1,650	1,975	48,072
100,000	34,278	2,200	1,975	61,547

Calculation of Post-Retirement Required Income

1981 Pre-Retirement Net Income	Age 65 Social Security Benefit Husband & Wife	Needed to Equal Pre-65 Net Income	Gross Needed Before Taxes To Provide Supplement	Gross Needed As % of Pre-65 Gross Income
$ 8,413	$ 7,796	$ 617	$ 617	6%
12,037	10,188	1,849	1,849	12
15,485	12,002	3,483	3,483	17
21,855	12,198	9,657	10,036	33
28,415	12,198	16,217	18,078	45
34,420	12,198	22,222	25,999	52
48,072	12,198	35,874	46,724	62
61,547	12,198	49,349	70,412	70

*Assumes a 10% deduction, married and filing a joint return, no other dependents
**Assumes Pennsylvania State Income Tax Rate of 2.2

payment of taxes. Social Security payments equal $8001, and $6440 more income after taxes will give you the same $14,545 you had before retirement. However, you will need additional gross income of $8621, on which you will pay federal income taxes of $751, to obtain the extra $7906.

These are hypothetical cases. Your own situation will depend on the actual deductions you claim and the level of state and local income taxes

Table 2. Example of Retirement Income Needed for Single Individual
to Duplicate Pre-Retirement Net Income After Taxes
(Based on Retirement at Age 65 on January 1, 1982)

Calculation of Pre-Retirement Net Income

Earned 1981 Gross Income	Federal Income Tax*	State Income Tax**	Social Security Tax	Net 1981 Income After Taxes
$ 10,000	$ 1,177	$ 220	$ 665	$ 7,938
15,000	2,345	330	998	11,327
20,000	3,789	440	1,330	14,441
30,000	6,982	660	1,975	20,383
40,000	10,903	880	1,975	26,242
50,000	15,242	1,100	1,975	31,683
75,000	26,217	1,650	1,975	45,158
100,000	37,192	2,200	1,975	58,633

Calculation of Post-Retirement Required Income

1981 Pre-Retirement Net Income	Age 65 Social Security Benefit Husband & Wife	Needed to Equal Pre-65 Net Income	Gross Needed Before Taxes To Provide Supplement	Gross Needed As % of Pre-65 Gross Income
$ 7,938	$5,197	$ 2,741	$ 2,741	27%
11,327	6,792	4,535	4,573	30
14,441	8,001	6,440	6,832	34
20,383	8,132	12,251	14,124	47
26,242	8,132	18,110	22,435	56
31,683	8,132	23,551	30,616	61
45,158	8,132	37,026	54,215	72
58,633	8,132	50,501	78,714	79

*Assumes a 10% deduction, married and filing a joint return, no other dependents
**Assumes Pennsylvania State Income Tax Rate of 2.2%

were you live. Furthermore, the analysis relates only to income at retirement. Preparation should be made for the impact of inflation, the need for death benefit protection, and other contingencies.

Since living expenses are usually lower following retirement, 100 percent of preretirement income is not needed. The expenses of raising your children are behind you, as is the daily commute to your job. Time may be available to do jobs around the house that were previously hired out. Mortgage payments may be a thing of the past, and life insurance premiums reduced or eliminated. If you have been saving for retirement, either privately or through contributions to a company pension or savings plan, the need for such savings may lessen. A move to a less expensive neighborhood or home, perhaps closer to your children, may be desirable.

Sources of Retirement Income

It has been said about the three sources of retirement income that, like a three-legged milking stool, support is needed from every one: Social Security, company or individual retirement plans (including Keogh and IRA), and personal savings.

Social Security

On retirement at age 65, you are entitled to Social Security benefits but must apply for them. Visit your local Social Security office with your Social Security card in hand at least four months before reaching 65 to get the wheels turning. Your first Social Security check will arrive within the first ten days of the second month after you retire. The amount will be automatically indexed to inflation. Assuming inflation continues, and depending on its severity, you can expect annual increases, probably in July. Also, after your first year of drawing Social Security benefits, you may receive a further increase due to recalculation of your benefits, taking your last calendar year's earnings into account. Your Social Security payment can be automatically deposited in your checking account at your request, for convenience and safety.

Company and Employer Retirement Plans

If you have been employed throughout the years prior to retirement, you probably will have earned retirement income from your employer's retirement or deferred profit-sharing plan. In addition to providing pension benefits at retirement (normally between ages 65 and 70), such plans usually have some provision for early retirement, and may also provide death and disability benefits. Since your company designed its own plan, it may differ from others, and it is important to familiarize yourself with the description of the plan provided by your employer. The plan will be either a ''Defined Benefit'' or ''Defined Contribution'' plan, as those terms are used in the Employee Retirement Income Security Act of 1974 (ERISA).

If the plan is a "Defined Benefit" plan, it will be relatively simple for you to anticipate what your retirement income will be. As the term implies, the benefit you receive under the plan is defined by a formula that applies to all participants. Your employer contributes the amount needed to provide the defined benefit. Here are some examples of retirement benefit formulas:

- A flat benefit, such as $10 per month, for each year of your employment prior to retirement

- A percentage of your average annual salary for the five years preceding your retirement

- A percentage of the salary you receive each year of your employment prior to retirement

  Others are more complex:

- 20 percent of your average annual salary for the five years prior to retirement which was covered by the Social Security Wage Base, plus 45 percent of such average salary which was not covered by the Social Security Wage Base, or

- ¾ percent of the salary you receive each year prior to retirement up to the amount of the Social Security Wage Base, plus 2 percent of the excess of such year's salary over the Social Security Wage Base, or

- 50 percent of your average annual salary for the five years prior to retirement less 50 percent of the Primary Social Security benefit you receive, prorated for services less than 30 years at retirement.

Your employer will, on request, estimate the retirement incomes, at any ages you choose. In making these estimates, the employer will probably assume no change in your salary or in the Social Security law prior to your retirement age. You will have to make reestimates to take account of such changes.

If your company has a Defined Contribution plan, the contribution made to the plan on your behalf is defined by a formula. The formula might be similar to the following:

The company will contribute each year to its retirement plan on your behalf a percentage of your salary for that year (10 percent, for example).

The company will contribute each year to its retirement plan on your behalf a percentage of your salary up to the Social Security Wage Base, plus a percentage of your salary which is in excess of the Social Security Wage Base.

At retirement, you will be entitled to the accumulation of the contributions made on your behalf and all investment income earned by such contributions. In a Defined Contribution plan, it is almost impossible to predict how much the funds will grow, and therefore how much retirement income they will provide. However, the company can make estimates based on various assumed rates of growth, annual changes in the Social Security Wage Base, changes in your salary, and actuarial rates by which lump-sum amounts are converted to annual payment of retirement income

Even though income from the Defined Contribution plan is difficult to predict, it is essential that you obtain an estimate so that you can calculate how much additional savings you should have in reserve at retirement, and the rate at which you may have to withdraw from savings.

In addition to, or in lieu of, retirement plans, your company may have a deferred profit-sharing or a thrift-and-savings plan. A deferred profit-sharing plan is designed to distribute a share of the company's profits to its employees each year. It is similar to a defined contribution pension plan because individual allocations are determined by a formula, but differs in that the amount of profits available for distribution is never known until the year is ended. In a thrift-and-savings plan, the employer matches a proportion of your contribution. For example, for every dollar you save, the employer might contribute $.25 or $.50, or some other amount. Your retirement benefits from such plans will be based upon the amount in your account at retirement from contributions made on your behalf and investment income on those contributions. Once again, it is suggested that you obtain from your employer estimates of the lump-sum or annual income payment available from these plans at your retirement. If the calculations and explanations are not completely understandable, or you have any further questions, do not hesitate to ask for help. Only when this information is complete can you plan the next steps.

Keogh Plans

If you are self-employed, tax law does not permit you to establish the same type of pension and profit-sharing plans available to corporations. Instead, you are limited to the establishment of a Keogh plan, provided your employees, if any, who have been employed for three years or more are also covered.

Under a Keogh plan you may contribute 15 percent of your annual earned income on a tax deductible basis, up to a limit of $7500 annually. Such a plan operates like a defined contribution except that limit is placed on annual contributions. Keogh plans may also operate like a defined benefit pension plan, but again in a more restrictive way than applies to corporations. More information can be provided by the mutual fund, bank, or insurance company which handles your plan.

Individual Retirement Account (IRA)

Beginning January 1, 1982, even if you are covered by a company or Keogh pension plan, you and your spouse can establish an IRA. The limit on the annual contribution was raised to the lesser of 100% of earned income or $2000. Such contributions may be deposited with a mutual fund, insurance company, or bank to be invested according to your instructions and within that organization's guidelines. Basically, such a plan also operates like a defined contribution plan except that the annual contribution is restricted. The funds may be withdrawn on retirement, as early as age 59½, but not later than 70½, and the withdrawns are then fully taxable. Funds withdrawals prior to age 59½ are subject to a penalty for early withdrawal. More information can be obtained from the mutual fund, bank, or insurance company which handles your plan.

Section 403(b) Annuity Plans

Section 403(b) Annuity Plans are special arrangements available to certain educational and tax-exempt organizations which qualify under Section 501(c)(3) of the Internal Revenue Code. Under these arrangements, employees may take a reduction in their salary, with the amount of the reduction being contributed to an annuity contract or to a custodial account investing in mutual fund shares. The employer may also make contributions on the employee's behalf. No tax is paid on the contributions until they are withdrawn, but there are special rules relating to the maximum contribution which may be made in any year; contributions in excess of the maximum are taxable in the year contributed. More information can be obtained from the representative of the mutual fund or insurance company which handles your plan.

Forms of Payment

Your company pension plan, Keogh Plan, or IRA may allow several options for receiving benefits at retirement which you will find in the summary of your plan. Options vary, but the following are typical:

Life Annuity: Benefits are paid monthly as long as you life. However, payments cease entirely at your death, with no payment to your spouse or estate.

Joint and Survivor Annuity: Benefits are paid monthly as long as you live. Following your death, your spouse continues to receive a portion of the income for the rest of his or her life.

Life Annuity with Term Certain: Benefits are paid monthly for as long as you live with the guarantee that they will be paid for a minimum period, for example, five or ten years. If you die before the end of the guaranteed period, benefit payments will continue to your named beneficiary to the end of the period. If you die after the end of the guaranteed period, benefits cease, with no further payment.

Cash Refund Annuity: Benefits are paid monthly for as long as you live. At your death, if the sum of all benefits paid to you does not equal the initial lump-sum value of the annuity, the difference is paid to your named beneficiary as a death benefit.

Installment Payment: You or your named beneficiary receive monthly benefits for a fixed period of time. Payment of the benefits does not depend on how long you live.

Lump Sum: One payment is made for the full value of your benefit. Federal law allows you to defer paying taxes on a lump sum from a pension, profit-sharing, or thrift-and-savings plan if you set up an IRA and transfer the lump sum directly to the IRA. In this way, you can defer receiving such a lump sum until any age from 59½ to 70½. Various other conditions must be met to qualify for these tax exemptions. If you have such lump sums available to you, the advice of a lawyer or a knowledgeable accountant will be helpful. Mutual fund organizations, banks, and insurance companies also provide basic information about IRA's.

Generally, the options have equivalent actuarial value. That is, based on average life expectancies, the benefits payable under the different options are adjusted so they all have the same value at retirement. Because the death benefits differ, the amounts paid can vary considerably. Table 3 shows benefits under different options for a male employee and his wife, both age 65. (Actual amounts will depend on individual plan provisions and your and your spouse's ages at retirement.)

As an example, the 65-year-old man could elect to receive $1,000 per month for life with no benefits payable after death. This might be the best choice for a single man but a married man might wish to provide continuing income to his wife. If he decides that half his benefits should go to his wife after his death, his monthly retirement income would drop to $874, but following his death, his wife would continue to receive $437 (half of $874) for the rest of her life. Alternatively, the couple might take the lump sum of $103,979 and go on the round-the-world trip they always wanted and still have "plenty left over." However "plenty left over" may not be much since taxes must be paid on the whole amount in that year. Furthermore, if the man were to choose the $1000-per-month

Table 3. Life Annuity Terms

Lump Sum	$103,979

Life annuity	Monthly Benefit $1,000
Joint and Survivor:	
100% continuation	776
50% continuation	874
Life annuity with term certain:	
5 years	974
10 years	911
15 years	836
Cash Refund	902
Installment payout:	
5 years	2,036
10 years	1,189
15 years	1,917
	788

life annuity and live exactly 15 years, the average life expectancy of a 65-year-old man, he would receive a total of $180,000, over $76,000 more than the lump sum.

The best option to select depends on each individual's tax situation and the need for death benefit protection for dependents. One word of caution: For plans that offer lump-sum distributions, keep in mind that if you need to withdraw funds from the lump sum in order to live, you may outlive the principal.

Other Employer-Sponsored Plans for Retirees

Most companies continue to provide modest amounts of group term life insurance to their retirees at no cost. Many also provide hospital-medical-surgical coverage designed to supplement Medicare, including dental coverage. ERISA requires companies to inform retired employees of these coverages, their potential value, and the circumstances under which the employeer or beneficiary may receive the benefits. Such plans offer important additional protection during retirement and should be reviewed before you retire.

Private Savings and How They Can Be Use

Other assets at retirement are the third leg of the stool. They might include savings in a savings account or money-market mutual fund, stocks, bonds, real estate or other property, cash values of life insurance contracts, income payable or cash values of annuities, amounts owed to you by others, and the market value of personal property you wish to sell.

It is best to enter retirement with an adequate cash reserve for emergencies and other unexpected expenditures. Most important financially, however, is a satisfactory annual retirement income. You may have to sacrifice some savings or other assets to attain the desired income level.

There is wide range of options for using savings. For example, you might put some or all life insurance contracts on a paid-up basis, thus lowering anticipated expenses rather than drawing from savings to pay the premiums. A reverse mortgage on your home will increase your mortgage and decrease your equity but add periodic payments from the mortgage company to your planned income. You can also liquidate other investments and reinvest the proceeds in a mutual fund which permits periodic withdrawals. The following example illustrates several options:

> James Johnson retires at age 65. He owns his home, which has a market value of $75,000, and has savings accounts worth $15,000, $100,000 of life insurance with a cash value of $40,000, and stocks worth $10,000. His annual income prior to retirement was $25,000. His company retirement plan will pay him $5,500 a year during his lifetime, and then $2,750 to his wife, Vera, for her lifetime, if she survives him. Social Security will pay him $8,000 per year plus an additional $4,000 per year for Vera who is also 65. Their total retirement income for the first year, therefore, is anticipated to be $17,500.

Of his $25,000 gross salary before retirement, $20,000 remained after taxes. According to current tax law, no taxes will be due on any of his income after retirement, including savings account interest and stock dividends.

Therefore, his total retirement income of $17,500 equals about 88 percent of his $20,000 net income after taxes prior to retirement. He wishes to raise his post-retirement income closer to his pre-retirement net earnings without digging too deeply into savings and other assets.

His first decision is to stop paying life insurance premiums of $1000 annually and to use dividends on the policies to purchase paid-up life insurance. This reduces the principal amount of the insurance immediately from $100,000 to $70,000, to which will be added each year such amounts of paid-up insurance as dividends will purchase. By taking this step, he reduces his income needs from $20,000 to $19,000. His $17,500 retirement income is now 92 percent of his post-retirement goal.

Next, he sells stock for $10,000 which he invests in a money-market mutual fund, electing a 10 percent ($1000) annual withdrawal, payable monthly. If the money-market fund earns 10 percent each year, as many did in 1979, the value of the investment will remain at $10,000. If it earns more than 10 percent, the investment will grow. If it earns less, the investment will decrease. With this $1000-per-year withdrawal from the fund, retirement income increases to $18,500. However, about $100 in Federal and State income taxes will be due, so the net income is $18,400, or about 97 percent of the $19,000 goal. Withdrawing interest on savings yields $825, bringing the total spendable income to $19,225, or slightly over 100 percent of the goal.

These steps leave the equity in his home, the cash values of life insurance policies (which increase each year), the money-market fund, and the savings account. In the years ahead, withdrawals from one or more of these assets can provide more income to cover increasing expenditures due to inflation or other causes. Because of a reduction in work-related expenses and a fully paid mortgage, expenditures may be lower than anticipated, possibly freeing surplus funds for investment in savings or a money-market fund.

Income to a Surving Spouse

Proper retirement planning requires provision to maintain your spouse in reasonable comfort if you should die first. Continued Social Security payments to your spouse will generally equal the amount you were receiving prior to your death. In the above example, this was $8,000, not counting adjustments for inflation increases both before and after your death. Your company retirement plan also automatically provides a continuing income to your spouse unless you elect otherwise. In our example, this was spouse unless you elect otherwise. In our example, this was $2,750, bringing your spouse's total annual income to $10,750. In addition, the value of the home, life insurance payments, money-market fund, savings account, and other assets left by you at death will be available.

Part-Time or Partial Employment After Retirement

A successful retirement is usually an active one that may include continued partial employment. Such employment can provide additional inflation protection. Depending on annual earnings, Social Security payments may be reduced or suspended. Check with the local Social Security office to determine the effect of employment. Company retirement and other benefit plans will probably not be affected, but it is well to check on this before accepting employment. Obviously, a part-time job will increase taxes, including continued payment of Social Security tax. The decision whether to continue working after retirement also depends on personal inclination and other factors, but financial considerations such as possible reductions in Social Security or company benefits should be carefully reviewed.

Tax Considerations

Taxes obviously play an important part in planning the financial aspects of retirement. Keeping track of taxes owed and forms to be filed by certain dates is time-consuming. Federal, state, and local income taxes, school and real estate taxes, personal property, wage, and Social Security taxes, to say nothing of estate, inheritance, and gift taxes, must all be considered to insure that only the required minimum amount is paid. Fortunately, Federal and state income taxes on gross income are usually greatly reduced after retirement.

Federal income tax law allows you to double your exemptions after age 65 to $4000 for a married couple. You may also continue to reduce your taxable income by charitable contributions or other deductible expenses such as real estate and other taxes and loan interest. Under certain circumstances, no income taxes are due on the realized gain on the sale of a home up to $100,000.

Currently, all Social Security benefits are free of local, state, and federal income taxes, and probably will be free of most other taxes based on income. Company pensions are usually exempt from local and state income taxes, but are subject to Federal income tax. A company pension may be taxed, depending on the pension plan provisions and the way the money is paid.

Lump-Sum Distributions

If the money from a company or Keogh plan is received as a lump sum, the excess over your total contributions to the plan on an after-tax basis is eligible for favorable tax treatment. Your own contributions are tax free because you have already paid the tax on this money. Basically, taxes on the lump sum are calculated by a special ten-year averaging rule, or, if you qualify and it is to your advantage, by treating that part of the taxable benefits related to employment before 1974 as capital gains, and applying the special ten-year averaging rule for that part related to employment after 1973. Money withdrawn from an IRA is *not* eligible for such favorable tax treatment under current tax laws. If you are to receive or have already received a lump-sum payment, check with your accountant, lawyer, or tax advisor about tax details.

Periodic Payments

If you receive your pension in periodic payments from a company or Keogh plan, or from an IRA, the payments are taxed as ordinary income. However, any contributions you may have made to the plan on an after-tax basis are still received tax-free in one of two ways. If the amount of such contributions equals less than three years of periodic payments, the payments are received tax-free until you have recovered your contributions, then later payments are taxed as ordinary income. If the amount of your contributions represents more than three years of periodic payments, then part of each payment is tax-free and part is traxable as ordinary income. On an overly simplified basis, if you receive a life annuity, that is, benefit payments stop at your death, the part of each year's payment that is tax-free is calculated by dividing the amount of your contribution by your life expectancy at retirement. Other adjustments must be made for different forms of payment.

For example, suppose you are entitled to a monthly pension of $1000 on a life annuity basis from your company's plan, and you determine that over the years you have contributed a total of $30,000 to your plan. Since retirement payments for the first three years ($36,000) exceed your contributions to the plan ($30,000), the first 30 months of payments would be tax-free, and all subsequent payments would be fully taxable. Suppose, however, your contributions amounted to $45,000. Since it will take more than three years to recover your employee contributions, you must determine the part of each payment which is taxable and the part which is tax-free. The part that is tax-free equals your contributions ($45,000) divided by your life expectancy (15 years if you retired at 65), which is $3000 of your *annual* pension or $250 a month. The remaining $750 is fully taxable. Again, check with your accountant, lawyer, or tax advisor for the tax details that apply to your pension.

Death Benefits

Basically, death benefit payments from a company's pension or profit sharing plan are free from federal estate tax, but the beneficiary must pay income tax on them. Exceptions are those amounts attributable to your contributions to the plan, and if the beneficiary is your estate. The income tax rule for the beneficiary is the same as it was for the employee, that is, periodic payments are taxed as ordinary income while lump-sum distributions may be eligible for special tax treatment. Death benefits payable from group term or individual life insurance are generally subject to estate and inheritance taxes, but your named beneficiary will not be subject to income taxes on the proceeds. Professional tax advice is advisable.

Another series of taxes which apply if your assets exceed $150,000, are the federal estate and gift taxes and the state inheritance tax. Like all tax laws and their application, these are complex, and help from attorneys or other experts in these fields is needed to insure that you pass on to your survivors the largest possible part of your estate, and pay the least tax required by state and federal law.

In general, a federal estate tax return must be filed if your gross estate in 1981 or after, as defined by the statutes, exceeds $175,000 (gradually increasing each year to $600,000 in 1987 and later years). You may, during your lifetime, give sums to others (children, for example). Gifts in excess of certain stated annual and total amounts may be subject to federal gift taxes. Finally, state inheritance taxes may also be payable, depending on your state of residence at time of death. The effects of inflation on your estate, particularly that part invested in savings accounts, money market funds, bonds, life insurance, and even real estate and stock, should also be considered.

Effects of Inflation

The declining value of a retiree's dollars over the years of retirement will be a constant concern unless inflation is brought under control—a very unlikely prospect, according to most economists. As indicated earlier, Social Security is indexed for inflation. Many employers also periodically adjust pensions for retired employees. In 1979 studies, Bankers Trust Company of New York reported that 75 percent of surveyed companies had increased pensions to their retirees at least once since 1974, and Towers, Perrin, Forster & Crosby, a Philadelphia actuarial firm, reported that over 90 percent had done so. Thus, some retirees may have less severe inflation problems than others, depending on the actions of former employers, but it is wise to assume that problems regardless of what happens to Social Security or what your former employer may do to increase pensions.

The table shows what has happened to the Consumer Price Index in the United States over the past forty years. As a result the dollar has declined steadily in value:

Comparison of $1 in Previous Years with 1981 Value

$1 in:	1940	1945	1950	1955	1960	1965	1970	1975	1980
Compared with 1981 value	16¢	20¢	27¢	31¢	34¢	36¢	43¢	60¢	90¢

Inflation has averaged 3.5% per year over the last 50 years, ranging from a high of 18.2% in 1946 to a low (drop rather than rise in prices) of −10.1% in 1931. A 1947 dollar bought about four times as much as a dollar in 1981. At 8% inflation, it will take more than $4 to buy as much at the start of year 2000 as $1 did at the start of 1981.

If the future is like the past, a retirement span of 15–20 years will bring more than a doubling of prices. Inflation is thus a serious concern to retirees, but they unfortunately can do little to protect themselves against it. Those who continue to work rather than retire will presumably receive wage or salary increases. Except for increases in Social Security payments indexed to inflation and possible adjustments of pension benefits, retirees may have to meet inflated expenses by drawing on assets such as equity in a home, stocks, bonds, life insurance cash values, and savings. Obviously, a substantial nest egg is desirable when you retire.

ERISA (Employee Retirement Income Security Act)

Since September, 1974, ERISA has protected the rights and benefits of millions of Americans covered by retirement plans established by employers. In effect, it guarantees the funds to support already accrued pension credits up to certain limits if the employer can no longer do so. It also requires the employer to appoint a plan administrator and to inform the employee of the plan benefits, eligibility requirements, and payment amounts. The following is a summary of some ERISA provisions.

SUMMARY OF CERTAIN PROVISIONS OF THE EMPLOYEE RETIREMENT INCOME SECURITY ACT OF 1974

Form of Retirement Benefits

After Retirement

If a participant has been married for at least one year before his retirement date, his retirement benefit must be paid on a 50% "Joint and Survivor Annuity" basis with the spouse as beneficiary. The actuarial cost of this benefit may be charged to the participant by reducing the amount of the pension he would otherwise receive.

Spouse's Benefits if Participant Dies Before Retirement

The plan must also include an option that provides for payment of not less than 50% of a participant's actuarially reduced pension to a surviving spouse if the participant dies after becoming eligible for early retirement. As with post-retirement survivor's benefits, the cost of this option can be covered by adjusting the benefit payable to the employee or his survivor. This option need not be made available until the participant is within 10 years of his normal retirement date.

Maximum Benefit / Contribution Limits

The new law places special maximum limits on:

- employer-provided benefits under fixed-benefit pension plans,

- employer contributions under defined-contribution pension plans or deferred profit-sharing, thrift, and stock bonus plans, and

- the combination of benefits and contributions that may be provided by an employer who maintains both types of plans.

Fiduciary Responsibility

The definition of a "fiduciary" has been broadened considerably and includes, for example, plan administrators as well as plan trustees. Essentially, the "prudent man" rule applies to the investment of plan assets, but investment of pension plan assets in an employer's securities must be limited to 10% of the fund value. Pension plans are to reduce current "excess investments" in employer securities to this 10% maximum level by December 31, 1984 (with 50% of the excess to be eliminated by December 31, 1979). The limit does not apply to profit-sharing or thrift plans that explicitly permit larger investments in employer securities. Nor does it apply to stock bonus plans that typically are invested exclusively in employer securities.

In addition, the list of prohibited transactions for plan fiduciaries has been increased, and the requirement that fiduciaries act solely for the benefit of covered employees is stated explicitly. Greater documentation of plan procedures and policies is required, and exculpatory clauses are void.

Reporting and Disclosure

Reports to Plan Participants

Reporting involves "furnishing" participants with summary plan descriptions, summaries of the annual reports, copies of the latest annual report and plan documents and individual statements of accrued benefits and vested rights. Each of these areas is discussed below.

- A copy of the summary plan description must be furnished to each participant within 90 days after he becomes a participant and to each beneficiary within 90 days after he begins to receive benefits. If the plan is amended substantially, a description of the amendment must be furnished to each participant and beneficiary within 210 days after the end of the plan year in which the amendment is made. All plan participants and beneficiaries must be furnished with a copy of the summary plan description at least once every five years if the plan is updated. If the plan is not changed, a new summary plan description need be furnished only once every ten years.

- A summary of the latest annual report must be furnished by the plan administrator to participants and beneficiaries within 210 days after the close of the plan year. This summary must include at least:

  — a statement of plan assets and liabilities,

  — a statement of plan receipts and disbursements, and

— any other information needed to summarize the annual report

- Copies of the latest annual report and current plan documents must be available to participants at places and times that give them a reasonable opportunity for inspection. If a participant makes the request in writing, he can obtain a copy of the annual report, the plan description and plan documents, but he may be required to pay a reasonable cost for this service. In addition, upon written request (but only once in any 12-month period), the plan administrator may be required to furnish any participant (or beneficiary) with a statement of his total accrued pension benefits, his vested benefits or the earliest date on ehich he will achieve vested rights. If a plan administrator fails to comply with the request within 30 days, he is personally liable to the participant or beneficiary in an amount not to exceed $100 per day.

- A complete statement of deferred vested benefit rights (i.e., the amount payable, date of initial payment, etc.) must be given to each vested terminated employee.

Plan Termination Insurance Provisions

A complex, new insurance program is established to insure the payment of certain pension benefits if a covered plan is terminated with insufficient assets to pay these benefits.

Covered Plans

The insurance program applies to defined benefit pension plans covered by the vesting and funding provisions of the Act.

Insurance Corporation

A pension Benefit Guaranty Corporation is established within the Department of Labor, to be governed by a Board of Directors consisting of the Secretaries of Labor, the Treasury and Commerce. They will be assisted by a seven-member Advisory Committee of nongovernment experts (two representing labor, two representing employers and three representing the general public), appointed by the President of the United States. This Corporation provides that the insured benefits described below will be paid in the event of a termination of a plan with insufficient assets to pay the benefits as promised.

Insured Benefits

Insured monthly pension benefits under the program as limited to the lesser of

- 100% of average monthly pay for the five consecutive years of highest pay (or actual years of plan participation if less the five) or

- $750 increased by the ratio that the Social Security tax base in the year of plan termination bears to the 1974 base of $13,200.

These limits guarantee only the basic pension (on a straight-life basis payable at age 65) provided under a covered plan. The Pension Benefit Guaranty Corporation may also provide insurance for ancillary benefits on conditions it would set forth in regulations.

Recapture and Allocation of Assets

The Pension Benefit Guaranty Corporation may recover from a participant the amount of benefit payments he received in excess of $10,000 (per year) in each of the three years preceding the termination of the plan. The recapture authority does not apply to benefits paid to participants where the first payment occurred more than three years before the plan was terminated. In addition, payments made by reason of death or disability are not subject to recapture.

Asset Allocation

Upon a plan's termination, assets are to be allocated under the following legislated order of priorities:

- voluntary employee contributions,

- mandatory employee contributions (i.e., those required for accrual of employer-provided benefits),

- benefits for employees retired for at least three years before the plan termination (or for employees who were eligible to retire at least three years before the termination date),

- all other insured benefits,

- all other vested benefits, and

- all other benefits.

To the extent an employee's pension is covered by an allocation in a higher priority class, it need not be covered in a later class. If assets allocated to any class are insufficient to provide full benefits, the benefits are to be prorated

Taxation of Lump-Sum Distributions

The Internal Revenue Code accords special tax treatment to certain lump-sum distributions from qualified plans to employees or beneficiaries. The preamendment rules involved a complicated breakdown of a distribution into capital gain and ordinary income components, with the availability of a special seven-year averaging rule to determine the tax on the ordinary income portion. These rules have been simplified and modified substantially. For purposes of special tax treatment, the term "lump-sum distribution" means full payment within one tax year of the value standing in the account under a qualified plan [a plan that meets the requirement of Section 401(a) or 404(a)(2) of the Internal Revenue Code] to or on behalf of an employee who has been a plan participant for at least five years under any of the following conditions:

- upon an employee's death,

- upon an employee's disability,

- after an employee attains age 59½, or

- upon an employee's termination (not applicable to self-employed persons covered under so-called Keogh plans).

Under these rules, all trusts under a single type of plan (i.e., fixed-benefit or defined-contribution plan) and all plans within a given category (pension, profit-sharing or stock bonus) are aggregated and treated as a single plan. Thus, multiple trusts under a profit-sharing or stock bonus are aggregated and treated as a single plan.

The new provisions phase out capital gains treatment for these distributions and introduce a special ten-year averaging rule based on ordinary income treatment. Essentially, the pre-1974 portion of the distribution is taxed as a long-term capital gain and the post-1973 portion as ordinary income.

Individual Retirement Accounts

Individuals not covered by qualified pension or deferred profit-sharing plans or by government plans may make tax deductible contributions to Individual Retirement Accounts established under government regulation. The annual deduction for these contributions, made either by the employee or a sponsoring employer on the employee's behalf, is limited to the lesser of 15% of his annual earnings of $1500.

The new law includes explicit requirements covering how these accounts are to be established and invested, their distribution procedures and their use as a funding vehicle for employer contributions established by a vested terminated employee under a qualified plan "rollover."

Deduction Limits for Self-Employed Persons

The deduction limits for annual contributions on behalf of self-employed persons under Keogh plans (or shareholder-employees under plans for Subchapter S corporations) have been increased to the lesser of 15% of annual pay (but not less than a contribution of $750) or $7500. For determining plan contributions, "covered pay" is limited to $100,000 annually for tax years beginning after 1975.

Alternatively, self-employed persons may establish nonintegrated defined benefit pension plans for tax years beginning after 1975. Under these plans, the annual defined benefit accrual is equal to the appropriate percentage of a covered employee's annual pay for each year up to $50,000.

The new law also establishes specific rules relating to distribution alternatives, excess plan contributions and other plan provisions and procedures and, in general, provides for taxation of benefits under the same rules that apply to other employees.

Section 403(b) Annuity Plans

Section 403(b) annuity plans are special pension plans for teachers and employees of certain tax-exempt organizations [501(c)(3) organizations]. Under these plans, tax deductible contributions [or contributions made under salary reduction arrangements, which, incidentally, do not come under the constructive receipt rules applicable to new non-403(b) salary reduct6ion arrangements] are limited to a 20% "exclusion allowance.'' This 20% limit continues to apply, but it is further restricted by the new 25%/$25,000 annual contribution limit applicable to qualified defined-contribution and profit-sharing plans.

However, certain 403(b) plan participants are permitted additional deductible contributions under special, complicated ''catch-up'' contribution rules.

PROPERTY MANAGEMENT: PROTECTING, GIVING, AND LEAVING IT

Norman H. Brown, Esq.

Ballard, Spahr, Andrews & Ingersoll
Philadelphia, Pennsylvania

This chapter outlines some techniques that are helpful to people who have accumulated a modest estate and now want: 1) to protect it while they live, and 2) to have what is left after they die wisely disposed of for the benefit of their families. Although the problems covered are typical, and the suggested solutions have general applicability, this is not intended to be a do-it-yourself guide to estate planning, tax saving, and investment. People differ, and property matters involve technicalities and subtle differences that may make special solutions more appropriate for particular problems. In many cases, a skilled professional advisor is as necessary for consultation on property management as a physician is on medical care.

Lifetime Management and Gifts

All too often people feel that they have finished their estate planning when they make a will. Wills are fine—anyone who has property should have one—but they do not take effect until death occurs, and even then can apply only to whatever estate is left. To protect your family, it may be equally important to be sure that your property is well managed before you die. For your own protection, it is all important. So let's begin by considering what aids are available to help you manage your property now.

Management

The simplest form of property management is to take care of it yourself. This presents no problem when your background and experience are sufficient to deal with the type of property you hold and you are healthy and available. Even if true now, it may not be so at a later date. Long trips or other absences from home may take you away from your property when decisions have to be made. Illness or accident may reduce your capability. For larger estates, the record keeping necessary to comply with tax laws can become quite burdensome. There are several ways in which you can put another person in a position to help.

Power of Attorney. The commonest, simplest, and in many ways the best means of getting extra help is to give someone you trust a power of attorney to handle all or some designated portion of your affairs. A power of attorney authorizes someone else to act on your behalf within whatever limits you fix when you give the power. You can, for example, appoint someone as your agent or ''attorney'' (the ''attorney'' need not be a lawyer—the word is used in its more ancient sense of ''agent'') with authority limited to a specific act such as selling your house, or to a specific part of your property such as a bank account or your safe deposit box. At the other extreme, you can give unlimited authority under a ''general'' power of attorney to handle any and all aspects of your affairs.

Powers of attorney can be given to spouses, children, parents, friends, or banks or other corporations. There are very few legal limits, although you may find that corporations or persons acting primarily for business reasons are willing to handle only certain types of transactions. You can give the power to two or more people, but if you do so, you should specify whether all must act jointly or whether each can act alone. Powers of attorney can also be given orally, but it is more practical that they be in writing to provide the appointed agent with proof of the authority to act. It is often convenient to provide more than one copy so that if one is left with a bank or mailed to a stock transfer agent, another will be on hand to confirm the authority to perform some other action when the need arises.

For bank accounts or safe deposit boxes, it is desirable to fill out a power-of-attorney form usually available from the bank. Most banks prefer the authority to be given on their own form, and to have the appointed attorney's signature on file.

Power-of-attorney forms are also available from legal stationers, but it may be wiser to ask a lawyer to prepare the form than to do it yourself, to make sure that it contains precisely the authorization for what you have in mind.

Occasionally, the person giving a power desires that it be invoked only in particular circumstances. In theory, this can be handled by making the power depend on a certain event or condition. For example, "I appoint X as my agent to act on my behalf whenever I am outside the United States." In practice, X may have difficulty proving that you are out of the United States, with the result that the power is rendered useless. It may be more appropriate to prepare an unrestricted power and place it with someone who will know where you are, with instructions that it is to be given to X only when you are out of the country (or if any other condition you specify is satisfied). Because the power is not restricted, X will be able to act at the proper time without having to prove to strangers that a particular condition exists.

A serious problem regarding powers of attorney that has now been largely solved arose from the fact that in common law the authority of the agent ceased when the giver died or became legally incapacitated. Probably most powers given in non-business situations were intended to be used only if the giver became seriously ill or otherwise incapable of tending to affairs, just those circumstances in which the powers would lose their validity. Fortunately, banks and individuals dealing with power holders rarely asked too many questions. Nonetheless, the basic rule of law did severely limit the usefulness of the power, especially when substantial sums of money were involved, or the people involved did not personally know the appointed agent.

This problem has recently been eliminated in most states by legislation authorizing so-called "blockbuster" or "durable" powers of attorney, which remain valid regardless of the condition of the giver if the power includes a provision to the effect that "this power shall not be affected by my disability."

Statutes in many states also provide that a power of attorney remains valid, and the agent can exercise the specified authority until the agent receives notice that the person who has given the power has actually died. Most states do not require the inclusion of particular language in the power to take advantage of this provision.

What if you change your mind and want to withdraw a power of attorney? The first step is to tell the person holding the power that you revoke it. This should be done in writing. If there is any question about the power holder's willingness to surrender the power, request written acknowledgment of receipt of the notice of revocation. This can be done by means of a signed and returned copy of the notice, or by giving the power holder the notice in the presence of a reliable witness. If either course is impractical, the notice can be sent by registered mail.

Delivery of notice of revocation makes it improper for the agent to act under the power. However, the danger exists that the agent may show a copy of the power to a third person who is unaware that it has been revoked and may thus exercise control over your assets against your wishes. To guard against this, you should advise any person, bank, or other organization with whom you have filed the power of attorney that it has been revoked, and require the person to whom you gave the power to return all copies of the power to you. If the power has been recorded in a public office, you should also file a revocation in that office. You may need a lawyer's help. Regardless of whether the power has been recorded, if you are seriously concerned about an attempt to use a power that has been revoked, legal advice is advisable.

To avoid becoming involved in such situations, strangers who are asked to accept the authority of an agent acting under a power of attorney—particularly a power that is more than one or two years old—will often check with you, the giver of the power, to make sure that it is still valid. Don't resent such a call. It protects you as well as the other party.

Joint Ownership. Joint ownership is another method of permitting someone else to manage your property, but should be used with great care because of the problems it may cause.

The management aspect of joint property is convenient for things such as bank accounts or safe deposit boxes because you can provide that either of the joint owners can withdraw funds or have access to the box. This convenience may not apply to other property such as stocks or real estate. Before naming joint owners to property, determine whether it will be possible for either joint owner to act alone and, if not, whether it will always be convenient to obtain both signatures for anticipated transactions. It should be kept in mind that all may be well at the outset, but relationships do change. Also, one joint owner may be ill, away on a trip, or otherwise unavailable when needed.

A more serious potential problem with joint property is that it involves ownership as opposed to mere management. An example that arises time and again is the case of the parent who puts money in a joint account with a son or daughter who lives nearby ''to manage my funds if I get sick.'' If the parent dies before the child, the child becomes the owner of at least half the account, and, if it is a survivorship account, the child will own it all. This may not be what the parent intended, especially if there are other children, and if the joint owner refuses to share the account with brothers or sisters—there is probably no legal obligation to do so—the result is likely to be a first-class family row. An alert bank clerk might have suggested to the parent that a power of attorney rather than a joint account was needed in the first place, but usually the joint account is simply established as requested.

Placing property in joint names can also result in gift tax problems. The basic rule is that the original owner of property who puts it in joint names has made a gift to the other person of an undivided interest in the property. If that interest added to any other gifts made to the same person during the year exceeds $10,000, a Federal gift tax return must be filed and tax may be due. (The gift tax is discussed in greater detail below.) There are certain exceptions to this rule. It is not a gift when real property is put in the joint names of husband and wife, and creation of a joint bank account is not a gift to the one who deposits less money than the other (or none at all) until the potential gift receiver actually withdraws more money than he put in. However, there are no exceptions when the joint property is in the form of securities or similar assets, and it is not uncommon for large gift tax deficiencies to be collected upon the death of a joint owner who had unknowingly bestowed gifts.

Joint property can also produce other unfortunate tax results when one of the owners dies. For Federal estate tax, all of the joint property is included in the taxable estate of the joint owner who dies first, except to the extent that it can be shown that the surviving joint owner contributed to the cost of the property, or acquired it by gift or inheritance from some third person. This proof is not always easy to provide, particularly when both joint owners have had income and the property has been purchased from a bank account into which both made deposits. Thus it is quite possible that tax will be imposed on joint property in the estate of a deceased joint owner who actually made little, if any, contribution to its purchase. Revenue agents are frequently, but not always, understanding about these problems. If either joint owner is likely to leave an estate large enough to be subject to Federal estate tax—$175,000 as a rule of thumb—it is important for the joint owners to keep a careful record to show who contributed to the value of the joint property and how much.

State laws with respect to the taxation of joint property on the death of one of the owners vary too widely to be easily summarized in detail. In some states, placing property in joint names, especially of husband and wife, largely or entirely avoids the tax. In other states that follow the Federal rule or some variant of it, the creation of joint ownership gains no tax advantage, and may even create problems if the sources of contributions cannot be proven.

Revocable Trusts. This is a more sophisticated and flexible way to arrange for management of assets. It is particularly apt for the management of security portfolio, but can also be used for real estate, royalty interests, or other investment properties. However, it involves expense and is not likely to be beneficial unless the assets to be placed in trust are at least $50,000–$100,000.

A ''trust'' is created when the owner of property turns it over to one or more other individuals or a corporation (the ''trustee'' or ''trustees'') with instructions to hold and administer the property, and to distribute the income, principal, or both to or for the benefit of a certain person or persons. Although most trusts follow standard patterns, there are few legal limits on the purposes for which a trust can be created. Because of this flexibility, trusts are often ideal for unusual situations.

A common form of trust might be one in which the owner of property (the *Settlor, Trustor, Grantor* or, if the trust is created by a will, the *Testator* or *Decedent*) transfers the property to a Trustee with directions to pay the income to the Settlor for life and to the Settlor's spouse after the Settlor dies, and then after the spouse dies, to divide the principal among the Settlor's living children and the descendants of those who have died. A trust of this kind typically authorizes the Trustee to apply income and principal for the benefit of the Settlor and spouse if they should become incapacitated, and provides for holding the shares of children or grandchildren until they reach some designated age.

The Trustee normally but not always has the responsibility for selecting investments. Some trusts require the Trustee to follow the directions of the Settlor or a designated investment advisor. One arrangement that fits some people's needs is the so-called "standby" trust, under which the Trustee does nothing but hold title to the property, investing and reinvesting as directed by the Settlor, unless the Settlor dies or otherwise becomes incapable of directing investment. Such incompetence might be decided in court, or the family doctor or some trusted relative or friend might certify that the Settlor was no longer well enough to administer the trust.

Trusts created during a person's life time—often called *inter vivos* trusts—can be either revocable or irrevocable. An irrevocable trust cannot be changed. It is usually created for the benefit of persons other than the Settlor and is not likely to be useful as a means of managing an owner's property. A revocable trust remains subject to change by the Settlor, and in many ways is not much more than an elaborate form of agency or custodian account. One difference is that the investment responsibility of the Trustee is more clearly fixed. Another advantage of a trust over an agency is that when the trustee or agent is an individual, it is easier to provide for a successor trustee in the event of death or other incapacity than for a successor agent. Also, you should be aware that a bank named as trustee may use its own common trust funds as a means of investment (frequently the best way to invest relatively small sums of money), but a bank named as agent cannot usually do so.

A further advantage of a trust over an agency or custodian account is that the trust can be used to control the disposition of property after the Settlor's death. In the common form cited above, for example, the terms of the trust may provide that income be paid to the Settlor for life, then to the Settlor's spouse, and after the spouse's death, to children, and so on.

A trust is not a complete substitute for a will because a person seldom puts everything he or she owns in a trust. A will is still necessary to dispose of property remaining outside the trust. However, a common pattern for a Settlor who has put the bulk of assets in a trust is to include provisions in the trust that would normally be found in a will, and then to prepare a simple will that "pours over" the remaining assets into the trust upon the Settlor's death. A collateral advantage of this arrangement that may appeal to those who want to avoid publicity about the disposition of their property is that it is usually possible to keep the trust agreement from becoming a matter of public record at the time of death. Public notice may be required later, but this generally occurs at a time and under conditions that do not attract much attention.

There is no such thing as a "standard" trust agreement, although some banks provide forms designed for simple property management during the Settlor's lifetime and uncomplicated distribution at death, such as payment to the Settlor's estate or distribution among the children. Those interested in a trust should consult an attorney or the trust department of a local bank.

What about costs? Traditionally, trustees have charged annual commissions based on income, often 5 percent, and then, when the trust ends, an amount based on principal, frequently about 3 percent for larger trusts and 5 percent for smaller ones. Many individual trustees still charge this way, but most corporate trustees now prefer pay-as-you-go compensation to waiting for a large principal commission when the trust ends. Bank patterns vary throughout the country, but a typical arrangement with a corporate trustee might be 5 percent of income, plus an annual charge, based on current market value, of $3 or $4 per $1,000 on the first $500,000 of principal and somewhat lower rates on the remainder. There may be a minimum annual charge in the range of $500 to $2,000. Frequently, the minimum is waived or sharply reduced for trusts that are fully invested in one or more of the bank's common trust funds. These charges may be negotiable, but there is an increasing tendency among larger banks to hold to their published rate schedules.

Guardianship, Conservator, Etc. When a person has become unable to manage his own affairs and has made no other arrangements, the legal authorities step in.

Most of us expect to slow down as we become elderly, and less able to look after our business interests. Usually, however, relatives or friends are available to help if needed, making legal steps unnecessary. Unfortunately, demands sometimes arise that are beyond the powers of friends or family to handle satisfactorily, for example, decisions with respect to purchase or sale of securities, and transactions involving real estate, both of which require the personal attention of the owner or someone legally authorized to act on the owner's behalf. If the owner is incapable of acting and has not delegated such authority, the only alternative may be the appointment of someone by the appropriate court.

Details of procedure differ from state to state, but in substance, a court must first find on the basis of credible—usually medical—evidence that the person owning property is unable to administer it. The court may then appoint one or more individuals, or a bank or trust company as *guardian*, *conservator*, or some similar term, to deal with the property on behalf of the owner. Some states permit close members of the family to be appointed. In others, out of concern that family members may act for their own benefit, the court may insist on appointing either someone who is not an immediate relative, or some neutral third person or corporation in addition to a family member.

When appointed, the guardian or conservator generally has the right to take control of all the ward's property. Normally, the guardian would not disturb the ward's living arrangements unless a move is necessary for financial reasons or to provide proper care. However, the guardian would be expected to review the ward's portfolio of securities and other investments to decide which property should be retained, which should be sold, and what costs should be incurred to support the ward and the ward's family. In some states, the guardian, having made these decisions, can put them in effect without further authority. In other states, the guardian must first obtain approval from the court. Court approval may seem safer but tends to increase expenses and makes administration of the ward's estate more cumbersome. Also, if the guardian has been wisely selected, it may be doubtful whether the court can add any useful insight to the guardian's own perception of what needs to be done.

Guardianships provide a reasonably satisfactory solution to the problem of administering property the owner can no longer handle alone. Their drawback is not that they don't work well, but that guardianships are often a last resort, avoided until a situation has gotten more or less out of control. Generally, the subject of a guardianship proceeding is unable to appreciate the need for a guardian by the time the need has become sufficiently clear for a court to be willing to make an appointment. The burden of initiating action falls on family or friends who may hesitate to place family problems on public record or to embarrass their relative or friend. Although judges are sensitive to the problems, and usually manage the proceedings in a way that embarrasses no one, the reluctance is still real. It is not helpful that in recent years, there has been a tendency—springing from what may be an unsound analogy to criminal proceedings—to insist upon greater procedural safeguards, making court procedures more cumbersome and open to unpleasantness.

Prohibitions against the appointment of close relatives also limit the choice and may disqualify the most appropriate appointee. It must also be recognized that some courts regard the appointments of guardians as a form of patronage. In some areas, it was not uncommon at one time for the courts to appoint co-guardians, only one of whom was expected to do the work while both shared the fees.

You cannot appoint your own guardian. If the need arises, you will not then be in a position to make the relevant decisions. However, you may be confronted with this question with respect to a member of your family or a friend. If so, you will need legal advice to determine whether the appointment of a guardian is appropriate and how it can be done. If available, a lawyer who has regularly served the person involved is likely to know the general background of the situation and would be the most logical one to consult.

Although you cannot appoint your own guardian, common sense suggests that you arrange your affairs in a way to minimize the need for such an appointment. This would involve consideration of matters such as the granting of powers of attorney, or perhaps placing your investment securities in a revocable trust.

Lifetime Giving

There are a number of reasons why those fortunate enough to have assets more than adequate to meet their needs during their lifetime should seriously think about giving some away before they die. In any event, those of us who are less fortunate should make plans for the disposal of what is left when we are gone. Decisions about these matters should at first deal with factors that have nothing to do with taxes. However, as soon as we begin to talk about an appreciable amount of money, taxes will enter the conversation. The structure of the gift and estate tax laws was radically changed in 1981. Since the new system is not widely understood, a brief review of it may be the best way to begin a discussion of estate planning.

The "Unified" Gift and Estate Tax. Until January 1, 1977, the Federal Gift and Estate Taxes were separate. Gift tax rates were significantly lower than estate tax rates. Since estate tax rates started at the lowest bracket and applied only to property that was left after all lifetime gifts had been made, wealthy people could realize substantial savings by making large gifts during their lifetimes. This was changed in many important respects by the Tax Reform Act of 1976.

The fundamental change was to unify the gift and estate taxes. A single schedule of rates now grows progressively higher from one bracket to another. It applies first to gifts made during a person's lifetime, and, at death, applies to the remainder of the estate, beginning at the tax level reached by the last lifetime gift.

> *Example:* The unified rate table provides a tax of $153,000 on the first $1,000,000 and a further tax of 41 percent of the next $250,000. If someone has made no previous gifts and dies leaving $1,200,000, the tax will be $235,000 ($153,000) plus 41 percent of $200,000.* If the same person had made taxable lifetime gifts of $1,000,000, a gift tax of $153,000 would have been paid, and if $200,000 is left at death, the tax would be in the 41 percent bracket reached as a result of the lifetime gifts.
>
> *Note: The figures here and in later calculations are simplified by omission of available deductions for debts, funeral expenses, estate administration costs, and other items such as credit against Federal tax for death taxes paid to a state.

Advantages of Lifetime Gifts. This does not mean that there is no longer any advantage to lifetime gifts. On the contrary, some very important advantages remain, as follows:

a. Unless you die within three years of the date of a gift, the gift tax paid is not part of your estate and incurs no tax liability. The example above ignored the fact that the $153,000 tax on the $1,000,000 lifetime gift would necessarily have come out of the remaining $200,000 so that the net taxable amount remaining at death would be $47,000 which at 41 percent would result in a tax of only $19,270. Thus, the combined gift and estate taxes are $62,730 less than if the whole $1,200,000 remained in the estate at death.

b. Unless you die within three years of the date of the gift, any increase in the gift's value between the date of the gift and the date of your death will escape tax in your estate. For unimproved land, or property such as a summer cottage that parents may not be using but are simply holding for the benefit of the family, this can be a very important consideration.

c. Often most important of all is the exclusion from gift tax of $10,000 per year for each recipient. Since this annual exclusion applies to each receiver of the gifts, a large family with many members who have spouses will include many potential recipients and large sums can be given away free of both gift and estate tax by taking advantage each year of the $10,000 exclusion.

What Does the Tax Cover? Gift and estate taxes affect all transfers of property that you may own except to the extent that the transfers are in the nature of sales for which you receive adequate value in return. The tax is not limited to property that is in just your name. It also applies to all jointly held property, unless the other joint owner contributed to the value of the property (when spouses each have income or property of their own, it is obviously important to keep records showing individual contributions to joint holdings), or unless the property was a gift to the joint owners from a third person. You are also considered to own all insurance on your life if you have any of the rights—technically "incidents of ownership"—of an owner, such as the right to change the beneficiary, to surrender the policy for cash, to change to another form of insurance, or to obtain a loan against the policy. You are also considered to be the owner of any property you may have given away during your lifetime if you retain the right to income from it while you live, or the right to change the terms of the gift. You also own your half of any community property.

Employee benefits are difficult to categorize because they take many forms, and the tax status of some of the more common benefits depends on the chosen manner of payment. Pension or profit-sharing benefits are usually paid under "qualified" plans. To the extent that payments under these plans are attributable to employer contributions, and to the extent that similar payments under HR-10, Keogh, or IRA Plans are attributable to contributions that were deductible when made, the benefits are usually free of estate tax. If a death benefit is paid in a lump sum, however, the recipient may have to choose between special, favorable income tax treatment and the estate tax exemption. Other payments under qualified plans, and most payments under non-qualified plans, are subject to estate tax.

You may also be considered the owner of property left in trust for your benefit by someone else if you have certain powers or control over the property, for example, to withdraw the principal for your own benefit to dispose of it or at your death to your creditors or your estate.

Exemptions. In the strict sense of the word, there are no longer any exemptions from gift or estate taxes. Instead, Congress has substituted a "unified credit" of $62,800 against tax that is otherwise due. The amount of property sheltered by this credit diminishes as the top tax rate applicable to a particular estate increases, but in bottom brackets it is equivalent to an exemption of roughly $225,000. The technical inaccuracy isn't significant until an estate is so large that a few thousand dollars one way or another do not make a significant difference anyway.

> **Note:** Until 1977, there were a $30,000 lifetime exemption for gift tax purposes and a $60,000 exemption for Federal estate tax. Although you may still hear references to them, they have been abolished. Some taxpayers, reluctant to forget good news, even refer to the $40,000 exemption of life insurance proceeds that applied until 1942. Since it died almost 40 years ago, you can forget about that one also.

The $10,000 Annual Exclusion. In addition to the unified credit, the gift tax provisions contain a very important exclusion of the first $10,000 of gifts made each year to each of any number of persons. The purpose of this exclusion is to exempt normal Christmas and birthday presents and other relatively small transactions from the gift tax; but when a number of recipients are involved, it is possible through judicious use of the exemption to transfer large sums of money entirely free of tax.

The $10,000 exclusion applies only to gifts of a "present interest." This is a technical term that distinguishes a gift which can be taken and enjoyed at once from gifts that will become available only at a future time. An immediate cash gift is clearly a present interest, and thus qualifies for the annual exclusion. A gift to a trust to use funds for the benefit of grandchildren as a class, with the remainder to be divided among them when the youngest reaches age 25, would be a gift of a future interest and the $10,000 exclusion would not apply.

It is important to note that the exclusion is completely and irretrievably lost for any year in which it is not used. Saving an unused exclusion to be applied against a gift in a future year is not permitted.

In order to take full advantage of the exclusion, it is often necessary to split a gift into a number of smaller parts spread over several years. For example, gifts of a parcel of real estate worth $180,000 to three children and their spouses could be made entirely tax-free if a one-ninth undivided interest is given to each husband-wife combination in each of three years. This would require three separate sets of deeds, but the tax benefit makes the paperwork worthwhile.

Another technique is to take a promissory note, or notes, for part of the gift and forgive the loan obligation in installments as the years pass. For example, suppose a son and daughter-in-law need $70,000 to cover the down payment on a new home. A gift of $20,000 can be combined with a loan of $50,000 covered by a note to prove the existence of the loan. The note can then be forgiven at the rate of $20,000 for each of the next two years, and in the fourth year the remaining balance of $10,000 can be forgiven. If the gift is property instead of cash, you have to be careful about taking back notes because the transaction may amount to a sale on which you will recognize a capital gain for income tax purposes.

Transfers to Spouses: The Marital Deduction. Both the estate and gift taxes contain a special "marital deduction" for property transferred to the owner's spouse. To qualify for the deduction, the transfer must be: (1) an outright gift, or (2) a trust from which the spouse gets all the income and has the right while living or at death (or both) to dispose of the property in any desired way, or (3) a so-called "estate trust" that will pass into the spouse's estate when he or she dies. Gifts with strings attached, such as a gift to a second wife subject to her promise that the property will go to children by the marriage, do not qualify.

There are no limits on the amount that may be claimed for marital deduction. This is a change in the rules. Until 1982 the marital deduction was generally limited to one-half of each lifetime gift to a spouse and one-half of the total estate. (From 1977 through 1981 higher limits were applicable to gifts under $200,000 and estates under $500,000.)

The "unlimited" marital deduction that became available on January 1, 1982 means that married couples can transfer assets freely between themselves, either during their lifetimes or at death, without concern about having their combined wealth depleted by Federal gift or estate taxes.

Bear in mind, however, that unless they have been consumed during the survivor's lifetime, gifts or inheritances qualified for the marital deduction will be taxed when the survivor dies.

From the viewpoint of the children (or whoever else will inherit from the survivor) the effect of the marital deduction is to postpone rather than avoid payment of tax. If we assume that at least one spouse lives until 1987 when the exemption equivalent (the amount sheltered from tax by the unified credit) will have increased to $600,000, this suggests some estate planning guidelines:

a. If your combined assets are not likely to exceed $600,000, there will be no tax when the survivor dies and there is no tax reason not to have as much as you want in joint names and to have "simple" wills in which you each give all you have to the other.

b. Above $600,000 you should probably put an amount equal to the exemption equivalent in trust for the other in order to protect it from tax when he or she dies. This cannot be done with joint property because it passes automatically to the survivor. To make such a trust possible each spouse should hold an amount equal to the exemption equivalent in his or her own name.

c. When the combined assets are relatively large, it may be better not to take full advantage of the "unlimited" marital deduction. Estate tax rates increase with the size of an estate and the tax paid on the survivor's estate if he or she inherited everything in excess of the exemption equivalent may be greater than if part had been taxed in each estate.

Example: If a spouse with $3,000,000 leaves $600,000 in an exemption equivalent trust for the other spouse and gives everything else to the other spouse, there will be no tax when the first spouse dies. When the survivor dies, his or her estate consisting of the $2,400,000 inherited from the first spouse will pay tax of $784,000. If the first spouse left half of his estate in trust for the survivor, there would be a tax of $363,000 when he died and another $363,000 would be paid when the survivor died. The combined taxes on both estates would be $726,000 and $58,000 would be saved by not using the unlimited marital deduction.

Life Estate Trusts. Until 1982 the marital deduction was only available for outright gifts to a spouse or gifts in trust in which the spouse had the right, while living or at death (or both), to dispose of the property in any desired way. This has now been changed. The marital deduction is now available for a trust from which the spouse gets all the income but has no power to control the distribution of principal. The owner of property can now obtain the tax benefits of a marital deduction trust for his or her spouse without any risk that eventual inheritance rights in the property will be diverted from whoever the owner would like to designate, for example children by an earlier marriage.

Gift Splitting. Another tax benefit available to married persons allows one spouse to "join" in gifts given by the other and to have the gift treated for tax purposes as though each contributed half. This means, for example, that if a married person gives someone $20,000, the spouse can join in the gift, and it will then be treated as if each had given $10,000. The entire gift will escape tax because it will be covered by two separate $10,000 annual exclusions available for gifts. Obviously, this doubles the value of the annual exclusion and also the rate at which the exclusion can be used to pass on property free of gift and estate taxes. For purposes of gift splitting, it does not matter whose property was used to make the gift. Even though all of the gift comes from one spouse, the advantages of splitting are still available.

A further advantage of gift splitting is that double use is made of the less expensive tax brackets.

> *Example:* If there have been no prior gifts, a $500,000 gift will generate a gift tax (before the unified credit) of $155,800. If the gift is "split" with a spouse, it will be treated as two gifts, each of $250,000, on each of which the tax (before credit) is $70,800, or a total of $141,600. After allowance for each spouse's credit, a single gift of $500,000 would be taxed at $93,000, as compared with a tax of $8,000 for each of two $250,000 gifts, or a total of $16,000. If the gifts are made in 1983, the unified credit will be $79,300 (more in later years) and if there have been no prior taxable gifts there would be no gift tax at all on a "split" gift of $500,000.

If spouse A joins in a gift made by spouse B, spouse A's own gift and estate tax status may be affected. For purposes of using up the unified credit and computing the rate at which future gifts and spouse A's estate will be taxed, the split portion of the gift is treated as though spouse A made it from his or her own property. This is unlikely to make much difference when both spouses pass their estates on to the same people, such as their common children and grandchildren. However, it may become important in second marriages. If spouse A joins spouse B in gifts to step-children from B's previous marriage, a much higher tax must be paid on subsequent lifetime or testamentary gifts made by A to A's own children.

A spouse can "join" in a gift made by the other spouse by signing the appropriate portions of a gift tax return. This means that gift tax return must be filed to prove the joinder, even though as a result of the joinder no tax will be due. The gift tax return is normally due April 15 of the year following the year of gift.

Deductions. In addition to the marital deduction, estate and gift tax deductions are allowed for property that is given directly to charity, or to a charitable trust that does not have any noncharitable beneficiaries. Deductions are also available for gifts made to charity from a trust that includes noncharitable interest if the trust is the special type known as a "charitable lead trust," "charitable remainder unitrust" or "charitable remainder annuity trust." As discussed later, those who plan to make large charitable gifts in their wills may be able to reduce income taxes by creating a trust of this type during life instead of waiting until death.

For computing your estate tax, deductions are also allowed for funeral expenses, debts, and the cost of administering your estate.

Income Tax Basis of Gifts and Bequests. When you give property to someone during your lifetime, the recipient's (donee's) basis for computing gain upon its later sale is the same as yours with the addition of any gift tax paid at the time of the gift. For purposes of computing loss, the donee's basis is your basis plus gift tax, or the value of the property at the time of gift, whichever is lower.

The rule for inherited property is different. Property included in the estate of someone who dies gets a "stepped-up" basis for income tax purposes equal to its taxable value in the estate of the deceased.

Lifetime Gifts: Other considerations

There are a number of reasons why a well-planned program of lifetime giving can make a lot of sense. Often, the advantages are overlooked because a potential donor doesn't think of them, and those who might benefit hesitate to point out the advantages for fear that they may seem greedy.

Why Make the donee Wait Until You Die? Gifts to your children will often be most advantageous to them when they are young adults and can use the money to meet the expenses of starting a family, purchase a home, establish a business, educate their children, and so on. Most of us hope to live long enough to see our children and perhaps even our grandchildren do these things. If funds can be made available for these purposes, all concerned may enjoy seeing them accomplished during the lifetime of the giver. Also, if the recipient of the gift is to be a charity or other organization, a gift made before you die will enable you to see the effect of the gift and permit the recipient to express gratitude.

Teaching Responsibility. Gifts to your children and grandchildren may also serve as part of their education. Most of us can recall, either by firsthand experience or hearsay, instances of the sometimes disastrous effect of large inheritances upon people who have not been trained to handle money. If you are fortunate enough to have a substantial estate that will eventually pass on to your children, it is virtually a parental obligation to see that they receive some experience in handling money while they are young so that they may be able to deal with larger sums later on. In somewhat the same vein, if you are uncertain about whether some of your prospective heirs can manage your estate themselves or need the protection of a trust, you may find it helpful in reaching a decision to give them a relatively small gift during their lifetimes and observe how they use it.

Spreading Taxable Income. Another occasionally important advantage of lifetime giving is the transfer of income to a member of the family in a lower tax bracket. If, for example, you are paying allowances to some of your children, you must take income taxes into account in determining how much is actually available. If you are in the top income tax bracket of 50 percent, only $500 will be left to give out of a $1,000 dividend check. If your children are in the 25 percent tax bracket, and you can give them stock that produces a $1,000 dividend, they will be liable for the tax. Then, $750 will remain after the tax is paid, thus doubling the yield of the stock.

Gifts to Minors. These present special problems because a minor is not legally qualified to buy or sell the property, to enter into contracts for its management, or otherwise deal with it. When a fond grandparent gives a minor 100 shares of stock, problems can arise if it becomes desirable to sell the stock before the minor grows up. Similarly, if real estate is in a minor's name, the minor cannot contract for repairs, make leases with tenants, and so on.

The classic method of dealing with these problems is to ask a court to appoint a guardian with authority to take possession of the property and administer it until the minor reaches the age of majority, traditionally 21 but now changed to 18 in most states. This accomplishes the intended purpose, but a certain amount of formality, delay, and expense is connected with the appointment of a guardian. Also, the administration of the guardianship may be relatively cumbersome, depending on state laws. In many states, the courts are unwilling to appoint parents or other close relatives because of concern that they will misapply the minor's money, for example, to support the general household.

One way to avoid these problems is to give the gift to a trust created for the minor's benefit. Some states permit the donor to accomplish much the same result by naming a guardian who lacks the broad authority of a court-appointed guardian to deal with all of the minor's property, but who can act with respect to the specified gifts. It is necessary to consult a lawyer to have the instruments drawn to create a trust or appoint a guardian, but the cost should be relatively modest and much less than a court-appointed guardian.

An even simpler method of providing for management of property given to minors is to take advantage of the Uniform Gifts to Minors Acts now in effect in all the states. Gifts of securities or money can be made to minors by registering the security or depositing the money in an account in the name of a individual designated as "Custodian for (name of minor) under the (name of State) Uniform Gifts to Minors Act." The Custodian has broad powers of management similar to those of a trustee, including the power to change the form of the investment, expend funds for the minor's benefit, and otherwise administer the property until the minor comes of age. Even though the age of majority is 18, many states provide that property held under one of these acts is not distributable to the minor until age 21.

Custodianships under the Uniform Acts do not require a special trust agreement or any other paperwork except registration of the donated property in the form provided by the Act. They are intended to be simple to use, and are often the best way for arranging for the management of relatively small gifts to minors.

Before appointing a trustee, custodian, or guardian for a minor, always first consult the person you have in mind to make sure there are no complications and that the arrangement is acceptable. For example, if you appoint someone who is legally obligated to support the minor (traditionally this would be the father, but may be both parents under more modern law) and who dies before the minor comes of age, the property being held for the minor may be included in the appointee's estate and be subject to tax. Generally speaking, property held in trust or custodianship would be so included. On the other hand, the chance is usually small that the parent will die before the minor is of age to receive the property so that, unless large amounts of money are involved, the convenience and economy of appointing a parent to hold the funds may outweigh tax risks.

Can You Afford It? This is probably the first question you should ask yourself when considering a program of lifetime gifts. It is gratifying to consider what you can do for your children by giving them money now, and the prospect of reducing death taxes is pleasing. Also, the children sincerely believe that "if Mom and Dad ever need this money, we will certainly give it back to them." However, while death-tax savings look fine on paper, if you unexpectedly need the money you have given away before your death, the savings may be largely illusory. Also, when your need arises, your children may have unforeseen problems of their own and be unable to give back the money, however good their intentions.

Just as it was suggested earlier that many people should give more gifts while they live but fail to do so because they are unaware of the advantages, so do many people sometimes give gifts they later regret. Gift giving should be considered carefully to avoid both pitfalls.

Charitable Gifts We are all familiar with tax deductions for gifts to charity. Their effect is to reduce the net cost of the gifts to you by the amount of income tax you save. Thus, if your top tax bracket is 55 percent, a $100 gift to charity reduces your income tax by $45 and the actual cost of the gift to you is $55.

There is an additional tax advantage for larger gifts of securities or certain other kinds of property which have increased in value and which are suitable for giving to a charity.

Example: Suppose you wish to make a cash gift of $10,000 to charity. You also have securities worth $10,000 which cost you only $3,000, but which you have been hesitating to sell because of the tax payable on the capital gain. If you make your charitable gift in the form of securities instead of cash, you will receive the same $10,000 income tax deduction, but you will not realize a gain on the transaction and no capital gains tax will be due. The charity, because it is exempt, can sell the securities for cash and also have no tax to pay. Of course, you no longer have the securities but you have retained an equivalent amount of cash. **Caution:** The tax advantages for gifts of appreciated property to charity are best with securities. The Internal Revenue Code restricts the type of property other than securities or cash that can be given with a full deduction for the value of the gift. If you are considering giving any form of property except cash or securities, consult a tax advisor.

Lifetime gifts to charity can also produce deductions that can shelter some of your other income. If you are planning a large charitable gift in your will, consider the advantages of several arrangements by which you can make the gift sooner and receive income from the donated property as long as you live. This can be done in ways that yield an immediate tax deduction for the value of the interest the charity will receive on your death without reducing the income to you during your lifetime. Gifts of this sort can be made through "pooled income funds" which a number of larger charities, particularly educational institutions, maintain, or by creation of a "charitable remainder unitrust," or "charitable remainder annuity trust." These types of gifts are required by law to meet some rather specific requirements, so qualified professional advice is necessary. They can produce welcome income tax benefits during your lifetime *but* (this point is not always sufficiently emphasized by people advocating these arrangements) they are not advisable unless you are definitely interested in making an equivalent gift to charity when you die.

Should You Have a Will?

What the Law Requires—Intestate Laws

To enable orderly disposition of the affairs of someone who dies, the law provides machinery for payment of debts, death taxes, and expenses of administration, and for distribution of remaining assets to those entitled to the estate under the terms of the will or, if there is no will, under the applicable intestate laws. This is done by appointment of a personal representative, generally called an "executor," if named in the will or an "administrator" if not named in the will. The personal representative has the right and obligation to take possession of the property and to apply it to the payment of funeral expenses, debts, and the costs of administering the estate. Costs of administration usually incude compensation to the personal representative and a fee to counsel for the estate. The remainder is distributed to the individuals named in the will.

If there is no will, the person is said to have died "intestate," and the estate is distributed according to the intestate laws of the state where the deceased lived (if the estate includes land located in another state, the intestate laws of the second state apply to the land). The intestate laws in most of the United States derive from English common law. The surviving spouse, if there is one, gets a share of the estate, usually one-third or one-half (the fraction varies depending on the number of children), and the rest of the estate goes in equal shares to surviving children and descendants of children who have died. The descendants divide the equal share the deceased child would have received if living. If there are no children or descendants of children, the property that does not go to the surviving spouse will typically go to parents and, if there are no parents, to brothers and sisters. Many states limit inheritance by remote relatives; if there are no next of kin closer than some designated degree such as first cousin or children of first cousins, the property that does not pass to the surviving spouse will go to the state.

The intestate pattern is frequently unsatisfactory to a married person who primarily wants to make sure that his or her spouse will be adequately taken care of and wishes to provide for children or others only out of funds not likely to be needed for the spouse. Intestate laws may also fail to take care of the special cases of adopted children or stepchildren and, of course, make no provision for non-relatives or favored charities.

In the absence of a will, the probate court must select an administrator to settle the estate. Preference is usually given to those who will inherit under the intestate laws or to their nominees. Depending upon the family situation, these may or may not be persons the deceased would have considered qualified.

If minors are among the next of kin of someone who dies without leaving a will, it will usually be necessary, unless the amount involved is small, to have a guardian appointed by the court to receive their shares of the estate. In many states, the court will not appoint a surviving parent or other close relative who might be the very person the deceased would have chosen.

The expense of settling an intestate estate usually is higher than for an estate administered under a will. The extra costs can arise in various ways. In Pennsylvania, for example, the administrator may be required to post a bond, an expense which is charged to the estate, while executors appointed by a will are normally excused from filing a bond. In other states, such as Texas, estate administration can be greatly simplified by appropriate provisions in a will which permit the executor greater freedom of action than is given to an administrator. An administrator must often incur filing fees, legal costs, etc., by going to court to obtain authority to perform the same duties that the executor performs under the terms of the will.

The point is not that the interstate laws are bad or poorly drafted, but that they necessarily provide only an ''average'' solution to a problem that the owner of property failed to prepare for.

Who Should Draw Your Will?

After five or six centuries of experience since the early days of the English Wills Acts upon which our law is patterned, this question should no longer arise. The homemade will has done almost as much as the automobile accident to foster litigation and enrich lawyers at the expense of bereaved families. Nonetheless, the idea persists that a will is a simple document anyone can write or, if extra care is necessary, create by filling in blanks on a printed form. Part of the problem may be that, like a graceful sculpture or a Picasso line drawing, a well-drawn will can have an economy of style that makes it deceptively simple so that the casual reader does not appreciate the skill and professional knowledge required to discriminate between what can be and what must not be omitted. The purpose of technical provisions may also not be readily apparent.

Too many people still write their own wills, probably expecting to save time or expense. Although they are generally ill-advised to do so, their efforts usually work out better than the following, which came before various lower courts and then twice before the Supreme Court of Texas:

''this letter is written with the idea that Some thing might happen to me. that I would be wiped out suddenly if this Should Happen my business would be in awful shape no relatives, nobody to do a thing So, this is written to try to have my affairs wound up in a reasonable way in case of my Sudden Death. would Like to have all of my affairs, Cash all assets including any Bank Balance turned over to Parties named below with out any Bond or any court action that can be avoided.

They to wind up affairs in any way they See fit.

U.S. Boyles Refrigeration Supply Co.
Charlie Hill superior Ice Co

Should these Gentleman need a third man would suggest Walker.

National Bank of Commerce Each of these Gentleman to receive $500.00 for his Services

I have tried to make my wishes plain. Of course these Crooked Lawyers Would want a Lot of Whereas and Wherefores included in this.

not much in favor of the organized Charities they are too Cold blooded also not much in Favor of any persons over 21—- Benefitting by my Kick off unless there is a good reason am inclined to play the children they are not Responsible for being here and cant help themselves.

                                        Terrell-Feb.7-1950

''have Let this Letter get cold and read it again to See if it Seemed about Right

Dont See much wrong except no wheres and wherefores–excuse me''

                                                Lon Gresham

Although most homemade wills are considerably better than this one, problems are frequent, and the relatively small cost of having a will prepared by a lawyer is likely to be more than recovered by the proper administration of your estate.

How much does a proper will cost? Traditionally, the writing of wills has been a "loss leader" with the legal profession, and 50 years ago very few wills cost more than $100. The lawyer who drew the will was happy to have the business, anticipating later settlement of the estate at a larger fee. To some extent, this remains true, but fees for settling an estate now tend to be more closely related to the time spent and difficulties encountered, rather than a flat percentage. To counterbalance this, lawyers are more likely to charge somewhat higher fees for estate planning and drafting of wills that more nearly reflect the time required for these separate services.

In metropolitan centers, lawyers' hourly charges range from about $50 an hour to perhaps $300 or more for senior members of large firms. Frequently, these charges are heavily discounted for estate planning and wills, so that a consultation followed by preparation of simple, non-trust wills for husband and wife might lead to a fee of $100 to $200. More complicated planning involving such things as transfer of life insurance, treatment of tax shelters, creation of intervivos trusts, and preparation of a more elaborate will can increase the fee to thousands of dollars. Such fees are far from wasted. There are very few million dollar estates for which even a modest amount of planning will not reduce taxes by much more than the fees.

How Should Your Estate Be Planned?

Where Do You Get Advice?

Clearly, professional advice is needed to plan an estate. Traditionally, lawyers, accountants, trust departments of banks, and life insurance agents have been sources of competent help. It is well, however, to bear in mind that the life insurance agent and the banker may be somewhat influenced by the fact that they receive no compensation for their services unless you buy life insurance or use the bank. Accountants are generally knowledgeable about taxes. One whom you may have been using for income tax work can probably also help with your estate planning, and will undoubtedly be able to recommend a lawyer to assist with legal matters.

Inevitably, you will need to consult a lawyer for the preparation of documents and legal advice. The legal advice will probably be as unbiased as any you can find since the lawyer is unlikely to care which bank you use or whether you buy life insurance. However, all lawyers are not equally skilled in estate planning. In less populated regions where lawyers do not specialize, most will have done some probate work and should be able to plan small-to-medium estates (under $500,000). A few will probably have represented wealthier clients and have the experience required to plan an estate of any size. In more densely populated cities where specialization is more prevalent, be sure to choose a lawyer with estate experience. Recommendations from friends are helpful if they have used lawyers for similarly complicated matters.

What Should Your Plan Contain?

The answer largely depends on you. However, consideration of some typical arrangements from the viewpoint of your attorney/advisor may be helpful.

Your advisor will first need to know something about your family and to have an estimate of the assets that comprise your estate and, if you are married, the estate of your spouse.

Avoiding Double Taxes. The next question is likely to be "what would you like to do with your estate?" A typical response is "Use everything to take care of my spouse (or other relatives), and when we are both gone, pass it on to the children (or other relatives.)" At this point, your advisor must decide whether to recommend a simple will in which everything goes to your primary beneficiary and to other designated heirs if the primary beneficiary dies before you do. This arrangement has the merits of simplicity but raises two problems:

a. The property given outright on your death to the first beneficiary will be subject to a second round of death taxes when that beneficiary dies.

b. If the primary beneficiary is old or disabled, auxiliary management may be needed for the property.

Both these problems can be solved if the property is left in trust for the primary beneficiary—usually on terms that provide for payment of income to the beneficiary and give the trustee power to use principal as necessary for the beneficiary's support, medical expenses, etc. In a properly drawn trust, the property will not be subject to tax when the beneficiary dies, and the trustee can be given a full range of powers to use income and principal for direct payment to the beneficiary or for payment to the beneficiary's creditors (medical expenses, bills, etc.) if the beneficiary is unable to manage alone.

Marital Deduction. A related consideration arises when married persons wish to make each other the primary beneficiaries of their estates. This brings into play the "marital deduction" discussed above, and in larger estates this can become a vital element in minimizing taxes.

Obtaining the marital deduction is not difficult. A simple will that gives everything to your spouse will do so while keeping taxes on your death to a minimum. The problem is that your spouse then has everything that you have, plus everything that he or she may own separately, and will leave a larger estate subject to even heavier taxes before it passes on to the children or next beneficiaries. When the sums of money are larger, significant tax savings can be achieved by giving your spouse *only as much as needed* to eliminate the federal estate tax in your estate, while leaving the rest in a trust that will provide benefits for your spouse, but will not be taxed as part of his or her estate.

> *Example:* Suppose you have $750,000 and your spouse has $100,000. There will be no tax when you die if you give your entire estate to your spouse because of the unlimited marital deduction. However, your spouse will leave an estate of $850,000 on which the tax will be $224,500 if your spouse dies in 1982. A marital deduction gift of $350,000 to your spouse is sufficient to eliminate all taxes in your estate, permitting you to leave the remaining $400,000 in trust. When your spouse dies, his or her estate will consist only of the $350,000 marital gift plus $100,000 of separate property, with a Federal estate tax of $17,000. Your children (or other next beneficiaries) will be grateful for the tax saving.

Such savings look fine on paper and may be realistic, but will not be realized until *both* you and your spouse have died. Moreover, the savings are premised on the assumption that your spouse will not use up any of the estate before passing it on. When there are young children or other dependents who may present a large cash drain, a large part of the estate may have to be spent by the survivor. Whatever is used up will not remain to be taxed.

Spouse's Forced Share: Elections Against the Will. In most states, married persons are not entirely free to dispose of their estates as they please. There may be minimum requirements for a share to be given to a surviving spouse. Patterns vary widely, but it is not uncommon that the spouse's share must be at least one-third, and may sometimes be as much as one-half, if there are no children. In certain states, the spouse's share applies only to real estate and does not include personal property such as cash, stocks, bonds and so on.

There is also little uniformity among the states as to the type of property to which the designated fraction is applied. Some states include only the property passed on under the will. Thus, a spouse might get a large amount of property, such as life insurance and joint property, which is outside the will, and could also claim a fraction of other property that passes under the will. In other states, the spouse's claim must be reduced by whatever is received outside the will. If these limits are likely to affect your plans, you should discuss the rules of your state with a qualified professional advisor.

Waiver of Spouse's Rights: Antenuptial Agreements. A will that does not give your spouse all that local law allows may nonetheless be fully effective. In many cases, surviving spouses do not assert their rights, perhaps for personal reasons such as a reluctance to go against the deceased spouses' directions or perhaps because they recognize that good family planning requires that certain assets go directly to children or others without passing through the estate of the surviving spouse.

Spouses may also agree to give up their forced shares in each other's estates. This is common when remarried individuals have children by an earlier marriage. Frequently, both parties want to pass their estates on to their own children, with no need or desire for any additional inheritance from the new spouse should he or she be the first to die. In these cases, it is usually desirable to record the understanding by written agreement. Such agreements are normally made before marriage and are called "antenuptial" agreements but may also be made after marriage, in which case they are "postnuptial" agreements. Generally speaking, the agreements are valid if the parties understand the implications of their action, which normally means that they are aware of the size of each other's estates and the interest they are relinquishing with the waiver of rights. Agreements of this sort should not be "homemade." Since there may be technical requirements under state law, the agreements should be prepared with the help of an attorney. In some cases, a different attorney for each spouse might be desirable.

Antenuptial agreements do not necessarily involve the complete waiver of a party's rights. For example, if one spouse, say the wife, has a significantly larger estate than the other, she might agree that if she is the survivor, she will make no claim against the estate of her husband, but might also agree that if she dies first, a minimum provision will be made for her husband. Nor does the existence of such an agreement prevent a spouse from making a will that is more generous than required. In many cases, even though the parties have waived all rights in each other's estates, one or both may wish to make some provision for the other, and a will that makes such a provision will be effective.

Business Interests. If you have a business of your own, or are a partner in a small business, another matter to be worked out with your advisor is the disposition of your business or partnership interests. This will normally involve such matters as consideration of a "buy-sell" agreement with employees, other stockholders, or partners, whether such an agreement should be funded with life insurance owned either by the company or the other partners, and the formula or other basis on which the price or value of your interest is to be determined. You should also consider making adequate arrangements to provide for managing the business after you have died or otherwise become incapable of managing it yourself. Solutions to these problems may not only require special agreements with other stockholders, partners, or employees, but also provisions in your will directing your executors or trustees with respect to the management of your business and the choice of persons you select as executors and trustees.

Lifetime Gifts. These will almost automatically come into consideration for people with larger estates—say $1,000,000 or more—in the form of a suggestion that advantage be taken of the $10,000 annual exclusion. Quite typically, this might be done by transferring funds both to children and to grandchildren, if any, or to a guardian or custodian for the grandchildren's benefit. This can be an excellent way of helping your children indirectly by providing funds for the college education of their children.

Even though your estate may be far short of $1,000,000, the subject of lifetime gifts may arise in connection with assets such as a summer cottage that you no longer use. It may make sense to give it to your children now to keep it from being taxed when you die. Another excellent choice for a gift is life insurance. Unless you are planning to convert the insurance to an annuity or otherwise use it yourself, it will never be of direct benefit to you and it may be helpful to get it out of your estate by making a gift of it. Gifts of life insurance are valued for gift tax purposes on the basis of the "interpolated terminal reserve," which, for practical purposes, is usually quite close to the cash surrender value. When the policies are group or term insurance, the gift tax value is usually very low or non-existent, so the transfer can be made without any tax implications except for the savings that will result on your death if you survive the transfer by three years.

It should be kept in mind that if you give away your life insurance, the proceeds will be part of the beneficiary's estate when he or she dies. This probably won't present any tax planning problems if you are making a gift to your children, but if you are making the gift to your spouse, you will be building up your spouse's taxable estate, possibly increasing the combined death taxes that will be paid on both estates before the property passes on to children or other beneficiaries. Often, a good way to get around this problem is to give the insurance to an irrevocable insurance trust for the benefit of your spouse. Trusts of this sort present a number of highly technical problems, but if properly drawn, can provide complete protection for your spouse while protecting the insurance proceeds from taxation in either estate.

Minors and Other Incapacitated Beneficiaries. If some of your beneficiaries are minors, very old, or otherwise unable to manage their property, your lawyer will undoubtedly want to discuss what should be done to handle their shares of your estate. All states will permit you to appoint either a trustee or a guardian to look after the property that passes to beneficiaries under your will, and you will have flexibility in specifying the terms on which the property should be held. Thus, it is not necessary to give property to minors when they reach the age of legal majority and you can select any greater age you think would be more appropriate. Similarly, if a beneficiary has emotional problems, or you fear a beneficiary might give the inheritance to an organization whose aims you do not approve of, your lawyer may be able to draw up a trust that will give the trustee discretion in the timing of payments and the payment of only as much as the trustee thinks the beneficiary will use for personal support or for other purposes of which you approve.

Choice of Executors and Trustees. Generally speaking, any adult or trust company can be selected as your executor or trustee. However, some states, such as Florida, impose restrictions on the right to appoint non-residents other than family members and there may also be restrictions on the ability of out-of-state banks to act as executors. Usually, few, if any, restrictions are placed on your selection of a trustee.

For a simple will that gives everything outright to a surviving spouse or children, it may make sense to name the person or persons who will receive the estate as executors. They will be looking after their own money and as long as they are reasonably capable of attending to business and are generally available, they can obtain all the technical advice they need from the attorney for the estate. Do, however, give some thought to geographical availability. Also, it is usually better to avoid appointing so many people as executors (for example, all the children), that there is no pinpointing of responsibility.

For larger estates, particularly when property is passing in trust, it may be advisable to appoint an executor with experience in the administration of estates. Often, there will be some person such as a son or daughter, family accountant, or family attorney who is a logical choice. In metropolitan areas, there are trust companies which are highly experienced in this field and can provide excellent guidance. Frequently, a good combination is a trust company plus an individual such as the surviving spouse, child, attorney, or other family advisor who is appointed to serve with the bank and who maintains contact between the beneficiaries and the bank.

The points to be considered in selection of a trustee are similar to those already described for selection of an executor. In addition, because the principal function of a trustee is to hold and invest funds, it is particularly important to make sure that there is at least one trustee who is experienced in financial matters, or to be sure that the trustees will be sensible about obtaining advice. The fact that most trusts will last for long periods also makes it necessary to consider the effect of advancing age upon individuals who might otherwise make good trustees. It is not uncommon for a businessman to have a number of friends about his own age who seem to be natural choices for trustees. However, they may retire and drift away from business matters, or may not remain sufficiently vigorous to make good trustees for very long after the death of the person who appoints them. It is often better to select younger people.

FRAUD

Michael Mustakoff, Esq.[*]

It is a fact of life that many, perhaps most, of us are sometimes tempted by propositions that seem to offer either something for nothing or something for very little. This makes us prey for unscrupulous persons dedicated to separating us from our money. It is natural to seek bargains, and it is not necessary to be greedy or stupid to fall victim to fraud.

Although fraud is often aimed at anybody who has liquid assets and is also feeling an economic pinch, the elderly are particularly attractive targets for the con artist. Their incomes are more likely to be fixed and more severely affected by inflated living costs. However, there are ways the elderly can protect themselves against fraud, and things they can do when they have been defrauded.

First, it's useful to look at some common frauds.

Some Common Frauds

Some confidence schemes, like the *pigeon drop,* are relatively straightforward. Others, such as those involving investment opportunities, home improvements and repairs, and opportunities for self-improvement, are considerably more complicated. They are often directed at elderly widows and widowers who tend to live alone, to have few relatives or friends to consult, and to be unsure of their economic and social status. They also may have large sums of money in savings, insurance benefits, or inheritances from spouses.

[*] *Formerly with the District Attorney's Office of Philadelphia as told to Marian Bellamy, Editorial Consultant*

The Pigeon Drop

One of the commonest frauds, the pigeon drop is also one of the simplest. One of the conspirators, usually a young woman, approaches the victim in a public place. She shows the victim a large roll of cash, which she claims to have just found, and appears puzzled as to what to do with the windfall. Had she found the money in an addressed envelope, she claims, she could return it to its rightful owner. Appealing to the victim's integrity, she wonders aloud whether the victim would hold the money for a "reasonable time." If the owner is not found, of course, the victim may then keep half the money for his or her trouble. So far, everything seems above board—all the victim must do to earn a sizeable sum is hold the roll of money for safekeeping.

The victim agrees. Now the woman becomes worried. Can she trust the victim? The victim wants very much to appear trustworthy. Would the victim be willing to leave a security deposit of his or her own money, simply as a formality? If the victim agrees, the trap is sprung.

Pigeon drop operators usually work in pairs. The young woman with the new-found cash calls in her partner, who may pose as her accountant or attorney or as an innocent stranger passing by. They persuade the victim to withdraw a large sum, always in cash, from savings—to show good faith. Ordinarily, the amount requested is nearly as large as that of the found money, and is to be handed over to one of the partners.

The criminals accept the "deposit" and set a date by which time they'll notify the victim if they've found the money's rightful owner. They make it clear that "finding the rightful owner" is merely a formality not a diligent search, and that when they return, it will be to divide the loot with the victim.

The victim walks away, satisfied with the prospect of gain until the "found money" turns out to be a false bankroll, such as a genuine bill wrapped around a roll of worthless paper. The criminals have disappeared. Any names or addresses they may have left are as phony as their money. The only real cash that changed hands was the victim's "deposit."

This is a crucial moment. The victim's first thoughts are likely to be, "How could I have fallen for something like this?" "I can't let anyone know how I've been taken!'' Caught between losing money and losing face, the fraud victim too often choses to save face and doesn't call the police. Wishful thinking starts. Perhaps it's all a mistake. Perhaps the young woman and her accomplice were honest and also thought the money was real. The victim resolves to wait until the arranged date before complaining.

The criminals rely on the victim's fear of losing face to gain time. They work the same scheme again and again before the first victim finally, too late, seeks to expose the game.

Home Repair and Improvements

Unscrupulous operators in home repair and improvement may operate door-to-door or over the telephone. Someone may appear at the victim's door, claiming that he has been ''doing some work in the neighborhood,'' perhaps sealing a roof or refinishing a driveway, and materials were left over that permit him to do the same work for the victim at an irresistibly low price. The bargain is possible only because the neighbor has already paid for the materials. As in the pigeon drop, the victim is tempted by the prospect of getting ''something for nothing.'' The victim is enticed further by a request not to reveal the price to the neighbor who just paid much more for the same work. Also, because the job would be done ''on the side,'' The con man asks for payment in cash, ''so the boss won't find out.''

Once the criminal has the money, he may proceed in one of two ways. He may do the ''work,'' but with intolerably cheap and shoddy materials. For example, he may ''resurface'' a driveway or ''seal'' a roof with used motor oil, and get away while the victim is waiting for it to dry. Alternatively, he may begin the work then claim that he needs more materials to continue. He may even ask for more money to cover the additional cost. Once he has left the scene, he never returns.

The door-to-door home repair racketeer is a fly-by-night operator who depends on fast talk and a quick getaway. Telephone home-repair schemes take more time but produce more ill-gotten profit. The schemer solicits the victim's business in advance and receives a deposit. Once he has the money, he delays beginning the work, or begins it but needs more money to continue. For example, he may contract to install a new furnace, then demand more money once he has removed the old one. If he is to add a room to a house, he'll plead poverty after he has knocked out a wall. The victim is trapped. Giving up at this point means losing the initial investment and the money to remedy what has already been done.

The best move is to absorb the loss, complain to the authorities, and take the business elsewhere. However, good sense is often overcome by the fact that a legitimate contractor charges much more than the shady operator. The victim may excuse a rash decision by thinking that the police would not help anyway because they are busy chasing "real" criminals, and then make at least a second payment before complaining.

In a variation of the home-repair scheme, one of the conspirators poses as a building or furnace inspector, declares the victim's property to be unsafe or in violation of the building code, and recommends a contractor, his partner, to do the work. The intimidated victim then hires the contractor with the usual disastrous result.

The elderly are especially vulnerable to a home repair fraud. Their homes are often old and in need of major repair but their fixed incomes cannot stretch to meet the cost of a legitimate contractor. Also, they are more likely to be unable to do their own repair work. They may be lured by a bargain price without being aware of the consequences.

Investment Rackets

Investment racketeers, like shady home repairers, favor older people as victims. The elderly are likely to be seeking a way to invest savings and augment fixed incomes. The easiest prey are those without investment experience and readily accessible sources of sound financial advice.

The simplest investment fraud is solicitation of funds for a nonexistent business. One such scheme, the All-American Hot Dog Company, came to light in Philadelphia in 1976. The company's principals obtained mailing lists from legitimate organizations and approached many Philadelphians, soliciting advance capital for a chain of frankfurter carts that would supposedly operate throughout the city during the summer of the bicentennial celebration. Investors could "buy in" with amounts ranging from $3,000 to $15,000.

By the end of the Bicentennial, no company cart had appeared on the streets, and no investor had received a penny from the company. Yet almost all the victims adopted a "wait-and-see" attitude toward the criminals and did not notify authorities until after the carts failed to appear for the Christmas shopping season.

The "Pyramid" is a more complex and vicious scheme, and, of course, more profitable for the racketeer. This investment fraud hinges upon turning the victim into an agent of the fraud.

The pyramid operator sells franchises. Of course, many legitimate chains of restaurants, cosmetics vendors, auto repair shops, and home service companies operate through franchise. Even some nationwide real estate organizations now franchise local agencies to create a pool of members for better service. The parent company sells the right to use its name, its advertising, and, usually, its supply and supervisory services in return for an initial investment, but retains a share in management and profits and a large degree of control over product or service quality. The franchisees, in turn, sell the product or service to the customer. By contrast, the pyramid is a bogus franchise organization and its specific product or service is irrelevant because it is a fiction. The pyramid operator makes money only from selling franchises not from product sales to ordinary customers.

For example, a potential investor is offered a chance to enter a cosmetics distributorship "at ground level" through the purchase for several thousand dollars of exclusive operating rights in a given area. The pyramid operator shows samples of the company's product, attractive company advertising, and glowing projections of the company's success. After purchasing the franchise, however, the investor discovers that the only way to obtain a return on the investment is by recruiting additional franchisees in the assigned districts. The product or service to be sold never materializes. Before the company can go into production, the pyramid operators take their share, declare the operation a failure, and move on. The operation collapses, and smaller investors are left holding the bag, having to absorb the cost of the company's planned failure and often the legal burden of the fraud.

Operators of pyramid rackets profit by making accomplices of their victims. Those investors who stand to lose most when the scheme collapses are also the most reluctant to call foul when they recognize the fraud.

The pyramid organizers make it clear that the victims will not only lose their shares when the game is exposed, but that the recruiting of additional franchisees has made the victims legally liable partners in crime.

Advertisements offering chances to earn money at home often disguise small-scale pyramid operations. Payment of a small fee brings a brochure on how to set up a mailing business, or stuff envelopes for profit in your spare time. The brochure is long on promises and short on details. It asks for a second, larger fee as an investment in the business. The investor eventually finds that the material to be mailed for profit is a thinly disguised chain letter, offering others the same business opportunity. The investor thus receives little more than a short course in setting up a mail fraud. To continue, the investor must find new "customers." Of course, the victim is at a disadvantage, lacking the professional operator's advertising capital and detailed knowledge of mail fraud statutes.

Loneliness and Loss Rackets

The frauds discussed above take advantage of economic insecurities. Others aim primarily at personal insecurities—loneliness, loss of loved ones, and fear of death and disease—and their victims are almost exclusively elderly.

Crooked "dance studios," "social clubs," and "health spas" prey on loneliness, especially that of widows and widowers and older people whose children have moved away and many of whose friends and acquaintances have died. They advertise an opportunity to meet others, to escape from a depressing daily routine, to become socially active. Minimally, all but the very worst do provide such opportunity. However, the promise is only a front for the real intent which is to lure the victim into paying ever larger sums for extensions of service, private "lessons," and, in extreme cases, personal "loans" to the "instructors" or "counselors."

As always, the initial fee is small to stimulate interest. At the opening session, a deluge of flattering attention urges the victim to sign a longer-term contract. Flattery and attention are the real products, and the purchaser pays dearly for them.

The contracts are first renewed monthly. The victim then comes to depend on the instructor or counselor for compliments, conversation, and friendship, and is encouraged to make this an indispensable source of companionship, perhaps the only one. The relationship may even have sexual overtones without explicit contact. When the victim is irrevocably hooked, the scheme operators offer a very long-term contract at an inflated "bargain" price as the only way the sessions can continue. The victim may then respond very much the way a drug addict does to a "pusher."

Sometimes, after becoming the victim's sole ego support as flatterer, confidant, and confessor, the instructor will let slip a serious personal need for a loan of money. The revelation may be offhand, just after a session, as if unrelated to the business arrangement. A sufficiently softened victim makes the loan without question to help this close friend and thus loses more money. But more than money is lost. Here, the fraud victim's typical reluctance to see through the game and admit to being victimized is most fully exploited. Someone duped into an investment fraud may feel momentarily foolish or guilty of being greedy when the fraud is exposed. But someone deceived into dependence on false emotional support feels utterly worthless when the support collapses.

Frauds aimed at the recently bereaved prey on the confusion that often accompanies the loneliness. A recent widow, especially of an older generation, may know little about her husband's finances. Immediately after his death, she will have had little time to examine or discuss them with relatives or with legal counsel. This is fertile ground for a variation of the pigeon drop.

In this scheme, the conman approaches the recent widow as the "agent" for an alleged insurance firm, claiming that the deceased husband had held a large policy with the company. The policy's benefit belongs to her, but she must first prove that the policyholder was indeed her husband. The victim becomes indignant. Of course he was her husband! She shows the "agent" as much proof as she can muster. But the criminal's request for proof is merely a distraction with a purpose. It increases the widow's desire to claim what is "rightfully hers" and stirs emotions that cloud her thinking during the next phase of the scheme. As in the pigeon drop, the phony agent requests a "security" deposit which the "home office" will return once the identification is confirmed. There is no home office, of course, and the deposit disappears with the "agent" out the door.

Insurance policies figure even more prominently in schemes that prey on fear of illness. So-called "Medi-gap" policies claim to cover the gap between federal Medicare payments and the actual cost of medical care. While such policies can represent real insurance, some are questionable and duplicate rather than broaden coverage or provide little practical protection. According to some estimates, unnecessary multiple coverage makes up three billion of the four billion dollars spent on such policies each year in the United States. In one such case, an 80-year-old woman spent $50,000 on 31 policies in three years. Some salesmen have frightened elderly clients into foregoing necessary living expenses in order to meet payments on unnecessary extra policies.

Miracle Cures and Other Health Frauds

The natural (and sometimes excessive) concern of the elderly with health makes them common victims of this type of fraud. The bogus doctor with a "miracle cure" steals not only money, but also the patient's chance for legitimate care.

The favorite disease for false cures is, of course, cancer. Medical science has made enormous strides against this disease, but treatment still seems painful, expensive, and risky to many, especially older people. They are therefore susceptible to confident promises of a fast, painless, and relatively inexpensive alternative. For the duration of the spurious treatment, the patient shuns accredited doctors, often as a mandatory part of the treatment. If the disease is cancer, it may progress beyond the possibility of effective remedies during this delay.

Some unscrupulous pseudomedical practitioners invent fictitious ailments for which they, of course, have the only "cure," a lengthy course of treatment under their care. Then, after "curing" the patient, they warn of possible "relapses" and recommend continued care under their supervision. They may also invite the same emotional dependence used by crooked dance instructors.

Nursing Home Frauds

Nursing home frauds are the ultimate insult against the elderly. Fraudulent home operators control not only their victims' money and self-respect, but their lives.

Patients in such homes average 80 years of age. Many are widowed. Almost all are chronically ill. In many nursing homes, the patients live virtually at the mercy of the operators. An unscrupulous nursing home proprietor may bill the patient for fictitious services and overcharge drastically for those the home does provide. For a helpless patient without nearby family, or for an elderly "ward of the state," the operator is the only contact with the world. In such a situation, the victim finds it impossible to complain.

Some nursing home frauds can touch their victims even before they have entered the home. For example, a home operator may try to alleviate present financial trouble by fraudulently trading on claims for care not yet given. This is the "Ponzi scheme," in which a business receives funds in trust for future services, but uses them instead to cover present expenses.

This was the basis of the recent scandal in California involving the bankruptcy of Pacific Homes, a nursing community sponsored by the Methodist Church. (Many criminal nursing home operators have fraudulently claimed association with institutions such as churches, charities, hospitals, and schools. Even a genuine church connection such as Pacific Homes is not an absolute guarantee against loss.) According to a November 1979 Wall Street Journal story, Pacific Homes was a 56-year-old nonprofit corporation claiming assets of 40 million dollars. For an advance fee of $54,000, the institution promised lifetime care for residents without additional cost. Many elderly people accepted the offer and made the advance payment, anticipating an increasing need for care and continuing inflation. Pacific Homes seemed eminently trustworthy.

By law, the Homes should have held the received money in trust for future services when the paid-up patients were admitted. Instead, they used the funds to cover current capital and operating expenses and then had to collect more advance payments to stay in business. The situation first came to light when the company declared bankruptcy in 1977. A federal grand jury was impaneled to investigate, and several residents sued both Pacific Homes and the Methodist Church.

A bankruptcy trustee has required that all life-care patients be placed on a monthly-payment plan. However, since their prepayment investments had vanished, many residents were nearly impoverished and sought cheaper care at other nursing homes.

How to Protect Against Fraud

Variations on fraud are numerous and cost elderly Americans billions of dollars each year. Yet it is possible to avoid becoming a victim. First, it must be recognized that anyone can be the target of fraud, not only the greedy or foolish. For example, a self-made Philadelphia millionaire, a financier himself, was recently duped by an investment fraud. When asked what he had learned from the experience, he replied, "Nothing. If someone else who was well placed in the community made me an offer tomorrow, I would ask where to sign...I made a lot of money trusting people." He then added, "Fortunately, I am in a financial position to do it again." Despite his disclaimer, however, even he will be more likely to spot a shady deal in the future.

The following simple precautions can help to avoid becoming the victim of fraud:

Be aware of the possibility. Confidence men and women do not wear funny suits, Panama hats, and sunglasses. They earned their name by gaining their victims' confidence, and this confidence is their stock in trade. Suspect anyone who offers to sell you a product or service you did not previously inquire about. Ask for identification. If the person represents a legitimate company, you should be given any information you request. Ask for details about the company. Where is their headquarters? Who is the person's superior? May you contact recent customers?

Don't be rushed into signing anything. A legitimate business representative will be happy to call again, after you've had time to do some comparison shopping. A good company representative will know the company's advantages over its competition, as well as the competition's good points. You should receive an intelligent discussion of the product's merits. Never rely solely on the salesperson's advice.

Discuss an investment or a franchise with a professional. Consult your family lawyer, a reliable accountant, or an investment counselor. If necessary, ask a trusted friend to recommend someone. A professional adviser will tell you your rights and obligations, if, when, and how you can cancel an agreement, and whether you can get your money back. In some instances, a company is not required by law to return your money, even if you return the product. A knowledgeable advisor can also help you to understand the full cost of a purchase, including hidden interest, insurance, service, and finance charges you may not have been told about. Many business and government agencies will gladly provide reliable advice on products and services. Utility companies will inspect your furnace and electrical system free of charge. Local governments also offer building inspection services. Organizations such as the local Chamber of Commerce or Better Business Bureau can identify known fraud operators.

Never take the first offer. Shop around. If an offer seems too good, find out why. Competitors can be the best guide to a merchant's honesty. Remember, one dishonest business can damage the reputation of a whole community of honest businesses. No matter how good a deal may seem, get competitive bids from established firms.

Never make a down payment in cash. A check has two advantages. First, it gives you a few days to change your mind before the check clears your bank. If you discover misrepresentation, you can stop payment. Second, it provides a legal, traceable record of the transaction. If the business proves fraudulent, the bank record can help the authorities to deal with the perpetrator of the fraud.

As a rule, avoid making a large down payment before receiving the product or service, especially on home repairs or improvements. Above all, never make final payment until you are satisfied with the product or the work. Good businesses build their reputations on satisfied customers.

Report suspected fraud to the police or to the economic crime unit of your local District Attorney's office. They may even be able to identify known confidence artists for you. If you report the crime promptly, the police will be more likely to catch the criminals and return your money. In cases of fraud, time works in the criminals' favor. The longer you delay, the surer their escape. They rely on their victims' reluctance to report the crime. A successful fraud operator can even make the victim feel responsible for the crime and thus afraid to report it.

Local, state, and federal law-enforcement agencies have recognized and are beginning to crack down on fraud against the elderly. The Federal Trade Commission may soon follow the lead of some state agencies in moving against nursing home fraud. Many police departments are initiating special efforts to aid and inform elderly potential victims. In the meantime, awareness and a willingness to report such schemes remain the best protection against fraud.

FUNERALS, BURIAL, AND CREMATION

Charles H. Nichols, Ph.D.

Director and Trustee Emeritus
National Foundation of Funereal Services

Introduction

There is nothing stranger or more morbid about confronting one's own mortality than writing a will, planning an estate, buying life insurance or cemetery property, or in other ways preparing for certain departure from this life. These considerations may not be pleasant, but they are sensible and sometimes necessary. Don't wait until it is too late to discuss your wishes with your next of kin and to make them a matter of accessible record.

The primary facility for taking care of the dead is the funeral home. According to the last published U.S. Census of Business, there are 20,854 funeral establishments in the United States. Excluding cash advances, which are not financially significant to the funeral director, these establishments grossed $2,063,008,770. Cash advances of $155,280,230 were simply accommodation items handled by the funeral home as a convenience for clients. They might include items such as a cemetery's charge for grave space, a newspaper's charge for death notices, a florist's charge for family flowers, or an honorarium for a clergyman. They are not really part of the funeral home's bill.

Total funeral home personnel numbered 83,517, including 13,326 proprietors and partners, plus 70,191 employees. Fifty-seven percent of the funeral homes are organized as private corporations, about 30 percent as proprietorships, and 12 percent as partnerships.

Mortality for 1972 was 1,926,000 deaths, 9.4 per thousand people. As a rough approximation, about one out of every hundred persons dies each year. In recent years, the death rate has been declining slightly due to increasing average length of life and increasing numbers of the elderly. It is expected that this trend will eventually reverse itself as the average length of life approaches biological limits.

From these figures we can see that the average population per funeral establishment was about 10,000; and the average population per worker in funeral service was about 2,500. Average mortality per establishment was about 95 deaths; and average receipts per death were about $1,050, or a per capita death expense of less than $10. It must not be assumed that every death involved a funeral, although a funeral is conducted in the vast preponderance of cases. Some Indian reservations, it is said, handle their own deaths, and a new phenomenon, the immediate disposition organization, about which more will be said later, disposes of a small percentage of bodies without a funeral ceremony.

Half of all funeral homes are relatively small and conduct an average of 61 services annually. Thirty-one percent conduct an average of 138 services, 19 percent an average of 242, and 9 percent an average of 473. Although it varies with the size of the home, the investment is usually substantial. The average for 1977 was $233,534, consisting of $175,155 in facilities, land, and equipment, $45,219 in accounts receivable, and $13,160 in funeral merchandise inventory.

When funerals are discussed, we tend to think primarily of the funeral director and the embalmer—the licensed personnel of the funeral home and their associates. However, others involved may include ministers, priests, or rabbis; florists; musicians; casket, burial vault, and cremation urn manufacturers; cemeterians and cremationists; funeral, cemetery, and crematory equipment manufacturers; livery and transportation services; hairdressers, restaurateurs, and perhaps professional pallbearers. Clearly, the funeral director seldom acts alone, but is usually the primary agent and the one who sees that family wishes are carried out.

Role of the Funeral Director

The funeral director's major role remains what it has always been, even before it emerged from the "undertaker" status of the last century; the care and disposition of the dead and the counseling and comforting of the bereaved. Although the director may be knowledgeable about various physical and theological aspects of death, and such subjects as suicide, euthanasia, and hospices, these are not directly related to the duties of the office.

The dead are beyond pain or feeling, but their treatment must be dignified. Survivors who had loved the deceased and invested a part of themselves in an emotional relationship are in grief and often deeply depressed by feelings of helplessness in the face of an overpowering loss. It has always been a major part of the funeral director's role to soften the blow of death for the grieving. Even though the terms "bereavement counseling" and "funeral counseling" are relatively new, they describe a function that has always been a major responsibility of the funeral director. In fulfilling this role, the funeral director must also be familiar with the normal and abnormal expressions and consequences of grief (see *Coping with Crisis and Psychiatric Problems*).

Most states require the director to have a combined funeral director/embalmer license, while others issue two separate licenses. Normally, the same school and apprenticeship or internship requirements prepare for both, but state boards may give separate examinations. Half the states require one to two years of college, a 12-month curriculum in mortuary science, one to two years of apprenticeship, and successful completion of the examination for license. There are now 35 mortuary schools in 25 states and the District of Columbia, of which 13 are proprietary, 14 are community colleges, and 8 are departments of state universities.

Legal Requirements Following a Death

Legal requirements for the care and disposition of the dead are few but important. They relate to sanitation, public health, and vital statistics.

A *death certificate* is required for every death. It is commonly prepared by the funeral director, but the attending physician must also sign and state the place, date, time, and cause of death. In case of accidental or violent death, or death under suspicious circumstances (often requiring an autopsy), it must be signed by the medical examiner or coroner. In addition to medical, funeral, and disposition data, the certificate records the deceased's name, address, Social Security number, date and place of birth, occupation, U.S. Armed Forces service number (if applicable), name and birthplace of father, maiden name and birthplace of mother, name of person supplying the information, etc. Since this information must usually be supplied by the next of kin, it is wise to have it readily available in personal records.

A permit from the local Board of Health or comparable authority is customarily required for burial, cremation, or transportation (out-of-state funeral or burial). Embalming is a legal requirement in some states if death was caused by certain infectious diseases, or if transportation by common air or rail carrier is planned. Embalming or refrigeration is a practical, even if not always a legal, requirement when a body is to be held for any period of time.

International transportation of the dead is subject to numerous rules and regulations which vary from country to country and generally cover preparation of the body, type of casket and outer shipping case, instructions for sealing, and required documentation. With increased use of air transportation for shipment of bodies, efforts are being made to simplify and standardize requirements, but they remain highly variable. It is wise to consult the closest consular office of the country involved, although your U.S. funeral director knows about such requirements or can obtain the necessary information through national associations.

Burial vaults are not required by law, but many cemeteries require a vault or other outer receptacle to prevent the sinking of graves—a common maintenance problem which extends over long periods of time. Families concerned about maximum protection for the casketed remains will often select a burial vault, even where not required.

Religious Considerations

Funeral service is a complex institution. There is no simple answer to the question, "What is a funeral?" Perhaps the question is best answered functionally. At the lowest level, there is the practical matter of disposing of the dead human body, safely and hygienically. At the next level, there are social considerations: the laws must be observed, customs respected, the bereaved given access to the strength and support of relatives and friends, and the community provided with the opportunity for appropriate leave-taking. At the psychological level, there are the needs of man as an emotional as well as a rational creature. Because we highly value every human life, we want the proper expression of sentiment at the ending of each life. By the practices and rites of the funeral, the bereaved must be led from disorganized shock, guilt, and grief to an acceptance of loss and a wholesome reorganization of life patterns. Finally, at the highest level, there are the spiritual and religious aspects of a funeral. These are reflected in the conscience of each individual, and their direction rests properly in the hands of the clergy. Regardless of denominational differences, faith is the great sustainer for most of us.

In its 1978 Yearbook, the National Council of Churches reported 37 main categories of churches, some containing up to 16 subdivisions. Funeral rituals vary widely among these different faiths, especially when ethnic differences are taken into account. Those in doubt about appropriate procedure should consult their minister, priest, or rabbi, or, if they are unchurched, ask the funeral director to refer them to the desired clergy. The funeral director will be familiar with the procedures normally followed by those in the local service area.

It should be noted that even those who are not members of a church frequently have a religious preference, especially when a funeral is being planned. For those who profess no faith, a Humanist service or no service at all can be held as desired.

Funerals

The Complete Funeral

Based largely upon the concept of a funeral as outlined above—a concept shared by most people to some degree—the standard, or conventional, funeral has evolved in the United States. With some variations, it remains the most common type in the nation.

The "First Call," in funeral service terminology, initiates the procedure. The next of kin, or authorized delegate, telephones the preferred funeral service firm to request its services. The funeral director obtains the initial information needed—the name and location of the deceased and the name, address, and telephone number of the person making the call, in case verification or more information is needed later. The firm then arranges to transfer the deceased from the home or hospital—most frequently the latter today—to the funeral home. The funeral director asks the attending physician to sign the death certificate, if it has not already been signed, and later submits it to the local Board of Health or comparable agency for the burial, cremation, or transportation permit, depending upon desired arrangements. The completed death certificate becomes a permanent record of the Department of Health's Bureau of Vital Statistics.

Preparation of the body is normally begun soon after the deceased is brought to the funeral home. Cleansing, grooming, dressing, and casketing would normally be a minimum requirement. If the body is to be held more than 24 hours—as is the case for most funerals— embalming and, in some instances, refrigeration are necessary for both esthetic and health reasons.

Embalming consists primarily of replacing blood with chemicals that permeate body tissues and is not unlike a surgical procedure. Originally performed by medical practitioners, it was introduced in the United States at the time of the Civil War for the purpose of returning military dead to their homes, a practice that continues today. The funeral director obtains oral or written permission to embalm the body and, in some cases, such as a disfiguring accident or emaciating illness, to perform restorative procedures.

The third part of the complete funeral is the arrangement conference between the funeral director and the family or its authorized representatives. This normally takes place at the funeral home, since selection of funeral merchandise, primarily the casket, is involved. In some smaller communities, this conference may be initiated at the home of the bereaved family and concluded at the funeral home. Its purpose is to arrange the numerous details of the funeral: to secure personal information about the deceased needed for the death certificate, death notices, and obituary; to determine the kind of funeral desired and to set the date and time with the church representative; to establish the place of the funeral—the funeral home, the church, or less frequently today, the family home; to select pallbearers and see that they are notified; to discuss the family's wishes for music; to arrange for family flowers, if any; to find out how many funeral cars will be needed and perhaps prepare car lists for the procession to the cemetery; to learn what final disposition is to be made—burial, mausoleum entombment, or cremation—and to make the necessary arrangements with the cemetery or crematory; to select the casket or suitable container, the burial vault or other outer enclosure if needed or desired, acknowledgment cards, and perhaps a burial garment or a cremation urn. Funerals reflect family differences, and no two are exactly alike.

However, in every case, costs should be freely discussed at the arrangement conference. The family knows its financial limitations, and the ethical funeral director has no desire to exceed them. Because payment for rendered service is necessary to continue operations, the funeral director would be unwise to urge a family to spend more than they can afford to pay, and, in some cases, must tactfully encourage the family to select within their means.

Toward the close of the arrangement conference, the funeral director will complete a memorandum of agreement, or contract, for signature by himself and the financially responsible members of the family. This document lists the service and merchandise selected by the family, clearly states the costs involved, and can be amended only by mutual agreement on items that the family may wish to add later. It protects the family, who will then know what to expect and how much they will pay, and it protects the funeral director with respect to terms of payment.

The fourth part of the complete funeral concerns the period and calling hours of visitation, and this, too, will have been discussed during the arrangement conference. Usually, there are one or two days of visitation, with afternoon and evening hours. Current trends favor one day, but if relatives are coming from a distance, two days are not uncommon. The purpose of the visitation is to provide an opportunity for all who knew the deceased "to pay their respects," and to surround the bereaved with caring, sympathetic people who share the loss and render social support.

If the casket is open, as is most often the choice, the immediate family is customarily given a first opportunity for private viewing before the public viewing begins. This confrontation is a moment of truth, for no one can look upon the casketed remains without realizing that the familiar person is truly dead.

Whether open or closed—a decision made by the family—the casket is surrounded by flowers delivered to the funeral home (except when flowers are not customary). The family flowers are sometimes placed on the foot panel of the casket, or on stands at either end. Those attending the visitation sign a register which is later given to the family, express their condolences, and perhaps, when the actual funeral service is scheduled, participate in the funeral and committal rites. There is no need to worry about what to say to the bereaved family, for the mere act of being present conveys a personal message. Throughout the visitation period, the funeral home staff is in attendance, receiving visitors and making themselves available for any services that may be needed. Preliminary fraternal or Rosary services often will be conducted at a scheduled time during the visitation.

Those unable to attend the visitation or the funeral service may send flowers, write a personal letter of condolence, send a mass card or a sympathy card, make a contribution to a charity favored by the family, or perform other acts of kindness and consideration. It is still commonplace for friends and neighbors to send prepared foods to the family, offer the use of cars, or assist with child care and household chores.

The fifth and most important part is the actual service, the funeral rites. This is most often a public service, but occasionally is private, limited to family, relatives, and a few invited friends. The private service precludes participation by those who may have known the deceased but are not known by the immediate family—occasionally a necessity where a very large attendance might reasonably be expected.

Most often today the funeral service is conducted at the funeral home. For some religious groups, however, such as Roman Catholic or Episcopalian, the religious rites are almost always conducted in the church. Occasionally, the funeral service is in the family home, but less and less frequently.

If a religious service is conducted, the minister, priest, or rabbi is in control, aided in this spiritual role by the funeral director only as appropriate to handle physical details. A church-connected family will invariably have a conference, perhaps several, with clergy prior to the funeral rites.

In a non-religious service, emphasis is placed more upon memorial aspects. Perhaps several of those closest to the deceased will speak of their relationship or of the deceased's achievements and contributions. Selected readings and musical compositions may be included, stressing philosophical and humanitarian rather than religious concepts.

Contemporary variations are sometimes introduced, whatever the type of service. Guitar music may be played; a message previously recorded by the deceased may be delivered; family members may express personal recollections of the deceased; members of an organization to which the deceased had belonged may join in closing the grave. Newspapers have reported motorcycle clubs forming long lines of cyclists in the funeral procession. The funeral may be conducted out-of-doors in a place favored by the deceased, such as a woods, garden, or seashore. Most such variations are designed to emphasize the individuality of the deceased in a special way and can be incorporated into the service with decorum and without loss of funeral values. Such services are sometimes referred to as "life-centered."

The procession is the traditional next part of the funeral. It is literally rooted in tradition, not only in American funerals and their English predecessors, but in those of many foreign lands as well. In today's funeral, the hearse or casket coach leads, followed by the cars of immediate family, pallbearers, relatives in order of kinship, friends, and neighbors. Sometimes, if not actually driving the hearse, the funeral director may be driving a lead car, usually accompanied by the minister, priest, or rabbi. Meanwhile, some or all of the funeral flowers (if any) will either have been hurried to the graveside to be there when the procession arrives, or, if the family has ordered it, be carried in a flower car as a part of the funeral procession, normally following the hearse.

Occasionally, the procession will terminate at a cemetery chapel, if desired by the family, rather than at graveside. For cremations, it will terminate at the crematory, many of which are located in and operated by cemeteries, sometimes with a separate chapel for cremation services.

The final part of the complete funeral is the committal service. This has religious relevance: "Ashes to ashes and dust to dust." It also has important psychological relevance in the sense of imparting a note of finality, not only to the service, but to the physical existence of a human life.

Alternate Forms

In contemporary society, the complete funeral is sometimes modified by what may be called alternate forms. It is possible to classify these in three categories: simplification, curtailment, or complete elimination of the funeral.

Simplification may be best typified by the "memorial society" movement, perhaps not too aptly named, since the funeral is itself, among other things, a memorial to the deceased. Memorial societies have voluntary membership, are manned almost entirely by volunteer workers, and usually charge a one-time individual or family membership fee. Their announced purpose is simplification of the funeral, although economy also seems to be a goal. They keep on file a record of each member's wishes for funeral arrangements. In some cases, they may negotiate an agreement with a funeral service firm to handle one or more basic types of funerals at stipulated fees. It is important to recognize that they act as an intermediary between the family and the funeral director, since only the licensed director can perform the service. A memorial society, a funeral cooperative, a pre-need promoter, a supplier of funeral merchandise, or a cemetery may not provide funeral service unless these agencies actually have state-licensed practitioners on their staffs. The over 100 local memorial societies in the United States and Canada have representation in a parent organization—the Continental Association of Funeral and Burial Societies—although their total membership is only a very small percentage of the total population.

Curtailment, in contrast, is not organized. It is simply a trend toward elimination of one or more parts of the complete funeral as a matter of economy or individual preference. There may be no embalming, either because interment or cremation will occur within a limited time, or because of religious custom, as in an orthodox Jewish service. Viewing may be omitted, usually because, for one reason or another, the casket will be closed. Visitation and calling hours may be curtailed or eliminated. The public funeral may be omitted in favor of a private service for family, relatives, and a few close friends by invitation only. There may be no flowers, signaled by a "please omit" or "in lieu of flowers" phrase in the death notice, indicating curtailment of what friends may freely do in expressing sympathy. There may be no procession to the cemetery, indicating omission of a public committal service. Or there may be a graveside service only, with no services at either church or chapel. Omitting too much risks the loss of funeral values. Rituals and rites of passage have evolved over generations to help and comfort the bereaved and to ease their adjustment to loss. If the old rituals are abandoned, new ones will be needed to replace them.

In the third category, complete elimination of the funeral, there is immediate disposition of the body. Customarily, the body is transferred to a refrigerated collection facility as soon as possible after death, held until disposition permits have been secured and any legally required waiting period is satisfied, then cremated and the ashes either returned to the family or disposed of as prearranged. This is a very recent phenomenon, but several immediate disposition companies now exist. The largest, known as "Telephase," operates primarily in California and Arizona. At least five firms operate in the San Francisco Bay area, one of them, the "Neptune society," featuring a scattering of ashes over the Pacific Ocean, and similar organizations exist in Florida.

Any funeral service firm obviously has the facilities, staff, and equipment to provide immediate disposition, but this should not be confused with funeral service. There simply is no funeral, as the term is recognized. Occasionally, upon return of the ashes (which are really bone fragments sometimes referred to as "cremains"), the family may wish to arrange a memorial service, possibly religious, which at least salvages some of the value of a funeral.

Funeral Merchandise

Although service is paramount in dealing with funerals, funeral merchandise is also involved and the funeral director performs a retail function. He provides a place (funeral home) and an organization. He buys the merchandise, has it shipped to the funeral home, receives and inspects it, pays for it, and perhaps stores it prior to displaying it. He maintains inventory records, eventually sells the merchandise, and perhaps extends credit for the sale, requiring delayed collection, the assumption of risk, and financing.

Caskets are a special type of furniture designed for funerals. They were linked in early American history with the cabinet maker, an association which continued in the formerly commonplace business combination of furniture and funerals. In this context, they do not include what have been called "alternate or suitable containers," most often used for immediate dispositions. These are what the name implies—simple containers constructed of corrugated cardboard, fiberboard, or plywood of sufficient strength and rigidity to hold and transport the body. They are available in many funeral homes for clients desiring immediate disposition, as they also are in immediate disposition organizations, but they are not caskets.

Caskets, as items of funeral furniture, are constructed of wood or metal, or, to a limited extent, of fiberglass polyester resins (loosely termed "plastics"). Wood caskets are either cloth-covered or finished woods; metals may be steel, lead-coated steel, stainless steel, copper, or bronze. Caskets may be protective "sealers," having water-tight rubber gaskets or sealing compounds, or "non-sealers." They vary in many other ways—style, design, color, interior fabrics, type of upholstery, material and design of handles and corners, and so on. Therefore, they also vary in overall quality, depending upon the basic material used, thickness of wood or metal, and other factors. Differences in price, as with any merchandise, are determined by differences in quality.

Outer burial receptacles include wooden boxes, concrete grave liners (separate concrete slabs for bottom, ends, sides, and top), concrete boxes, and burial vaults. The best and most protective is the burial vault, which is designed for strength, durability, and protection from water. These are constructed mainly of concrete or metal, with a few now made of plastic. Most concrete vaults are top-sealed, while metal vaults are air-sealed. The top-sealer is a box-with-separate-lid design, employing a modified tongue and groove principle with a sealing compound. The air-sealer has a flat bottom on which a dome-shaped top rests; air trapped within the dome prevents water from rising inside the vault above a certain point of compression below the casket bottom.

Burial garments are offered by many funeral service firms as an added service, although most families prefer to use the deceased's own clothing. For women in particular, burial garments are somewhat specialized; their high necklines and long sleeves are designed to conceal marks of emaciation, suturing, or transfusion, as well as sagging muscle tone. Garment costs are roughly equal to costs of normal clothing.

Most funeral service firms also offer some selection of cremation urns, including urn vaults if burial of the cremains is preferred by their clientele. Cremation urns (they aren't always urn-shaped) can be very simple and relatively inexpensive, or elaborate and quite costly. The latter are likely to be placed in a columbarium at the cemetery or crematorium. This is a special structure, somewhat like a small mausoleum, with special wall recesses to hold cremation urns. Urns are usually bronze, but occasionally marble, synthetic marble, or a finished wood such as mahogany. Apart from the traditional urn shape, they come in such forms as small caskets, vases, and simulated books. When urns are not used, the cremains may be buried in the container in which they were delivered by the crematory, or, in the absence of restrictions, simply scattered.

Funeral Prices

The average spent for a funeral service in 1978 was $1,402. However, average costs vary in different areas. The following table indicates the range and statistical distribution.

1978 FUNERAL DOLLAR—WHERE IT CAME FROM

Price Category	Percentage of Selections
$ 0– 600	7%
601– 800	4
801–1,000	8
1,001–1,200	11
1,201–1,400	15
1,401–1,600	17
1,601–1,800	16
1,801–2,000	11
2,001–2,200	4
2,201–Over	7

(As Reported by National Selected Morticians, based upon a complete range of prices for a sample of 80,851 funerals.)

These prices cover an adult funeral, including service, facilities, funeral cars, and casket. They do not include such optional items as burial vaults, garments, and urns, or cash advances often made by the funeral director for such items as cemetery expense, death notices, flowers, etc.

A breakdown of funeral costs is shown in the following table, from the same source.

1978 FUNERAL DOLLAR—WHERE IT WENT

Item of Cost	Percentage of Funeral Dollar
Caskets	18%
Salaries	36
Building	12

Autos	5
Advertising	4
Supplies	3
Miscellaneous	18
Profit (Before Taxes)	4

The net profit is a modest 4 percent. This would normally be too small for the funeral director to stay in business, but the selection of optional funeral items by many families raises the return to a more reasonable level of almost 11 percent (as of 1978).

Contrary to some reports, funeral prices have not risen extraordinarily. According to the 1977 Consumer Price Index (the last figures, since the U.S. Labor Department discontinued its separate funeral service index shortly after June, 1977), the price of funerals had increased by 56.2 percent between 1967 and 1977. During the same period, "all items" increased by 81.8 percent, "Services" in general by 93.7 percent, "Legal services" by 114.6 percent, and "Medical care services" by 116 percent.

Paying for the Funeral

Among the sources of funds to ease the burden of funeral costs, the most important may be the personal life insurance of the deceased. (Life insurance was initially called "death insurance," and many people still buy it with coverage for funeral expenses in mind.) There is also explicit "funeral insurance" now available designed to cover funeral expenses, sometimes even coupled with a prearrangement of funeral details.

Another important help in meeting funeral expenses, when the deceased is covered by Social Security, is the lump-sum death benefit, a maximum of $255 in most cases, payable to the surviving spouse or other person responsible for funeral expenses. There may also be survivor benefits for the spouse and/or dependent children who meet age and other Social Security requirements. It is advisable to check with the local Social Security office about potential benefits since they are subject to revision. The funeral director can also give helpful information about these benefits.

For those who die in active military service, funeral benefits are provided by the particular branch of service, and some benefits are also available for veterans of past wars. For qualified veterans, the Veterans Administration will provide an American flag to be placed upon the casket, $250 toward funeral expenses and burial in a national cemetery or up to $150 for burial in a private cemetery (up to $800 for funeral and burial if the death was service-connected), a standard headstone or bronze marker issued by the government, or an "in lieu of" allowance based upon the government's cost. As with Social Security, the amounts and qualifications for these benefits may vary, and the local office of the Veterans Administration or the funeral director should be consulted.

If the deceased held membership in a fraternal organization, union, religious society, or any comparable group, it is well to check with the appropriate headquarters office, as many of these organizations provide a death benefit. Death benefits provided by an employer, either directly or through group insurance should also be investigated. In a few states, chiefly in the South, burial societies still exist; in other states, funeral insurance is more common. Some motor club insurance covers accidental death to car drivers or passengers. Finally, welfare departments, usually at the county level, provide assistance to those without funds who qualify.

Preplanning

Flexibility is desirable when preplanning funerals. However, individuals who are without family nearby, who do not anticipate changes in residential location, and who have firm ideas about preferred funeral arrangements, may plan more definitely. Those who will leave behind close and caring relatives and friends should seek a balance between their own wishes—usually motivated by the desire to lessen the burden for their family—and the risk of depriving the family of involvement in funeral arrangements.

In general, there are three types of preplanning: simple prearrangements, prefinanced funerals, and prepaid funerals. The latter two include prearrangement plans, but also make some provision for meeting funeral expenses.

Prearrangement involves a consultation with the chosen funeral service firm which records your wishes and other needed information. This record is not a contract, no money is exchanged, and normally there is no charge by the funeral director. Such prearrangement may include information for the death certificate, clergy to be called, the desired kind of funeral and casket, pallbearers to be asked, preferences as to Scripture or other readings and music, chosen form of disposition, and so on. Those who do not care to make a prearrangement with a particular firm should consider preparing such a record to be kept with other personal documents.

In prefinanced arrangements, the choice is often establishment of a separate bank account, jointly with next of kin specifically for payment of the funeral bill. Costs may also be covered by a funeral insurance policy payable to the beneficiary responsible for meeting these expenses. Money to cover anticipated funeral expenses may also be specified in a will.

Prepaid funerals take care of all needs but should be arranged with great caution. Who knows when he will die, or where, or under what circumstances? Advance payment in full, or in installments, involves a considerable amount of trust on the part of the payer. However, there are some instances where it may be desirable to arrange a prepaid funeral, usually by entering into a funeral trust agreement. This should not be an irrevocable trust, and it should conform to any pre-need legal requirements, which vary from state to state. Don't lose control of your own funds or your right to change the plans, and take careful note of any penalties for default or cancellation. In short, "pay now, die later" plans require close scrutiny!

Criteria for Selecting a Funeral Firm

A 1976 study by National Selected Morticians, involving responses by 11, 167 families served, shows why a particular service firm is selected, as follows:

Reasons for Selecting Funeral Home

Satisfactory experience on previous service. . . . . 24.79 %
Professional reputation of the firm. 20.41
Observation at times of visitation and funerals 13.12
Convenience of the firm's location. 13.03
Personal acquaintance with a firm member 12.09
Recommendation of friend, clergyman, doctor, etc. 6.53
Favorable opinion of the firm's facilities 5.89
Fair and reasonable pricing policies. 2.98
Other reasons. 1.16

"Other reasons" included factors such as belonging to the same church or lodge as the funeral director, existence of a pre-need arrangement, or, in small communities, the fact that only one firm was available. Advertising was rarely mentioned, though it may exert some influence in conjunction with other reasons.

Since most funeral firms have been in existence for several generations (many are family owned and operated and handed down from father to son), their continuation depends upon public good will. This, in turn, depends upon reliable service, fairly priced. Surveys have repeatedly shown that the most powerful single factor in the selection of a funeral home is previous service: a family has been satisfactorily served in the past and therefore calls the same firm on the occasion of new need.

Final Disposition

Burial preceded by a funeral continues to be the most common method of final disposition. The cemetery provides burial facilities, and many provide mausoleum and cremation facilities as well. There are a number of mortuary-cemetery combinations, especially in the West and Southwest, but they are not common in the nation at large.

Mausoleums may be either public or private. The public mausoleum is usually a substantial granite or marble building containing several levels of crypts built into the walls. These receive the casketed remains and are then sealed, in effect providing above-ground interment. Private mausoleums are smaller buildings constructed by monument companies for individual families. A simpler, above-ground receptacle with one or two crypts may also be available. When many of these are placed in rows to form a kind of low wall in a special section of a cemetery, they are sometimes referred to as "garden crypts."

Disposition by cremation is the reduction of the body by intense heat to a few pounds of bone fragments which may then be pulverized. Modern crematories are usually located in cemeteries, but immediate-disposition companies and some larger funeral homes often possess their own facilities. In some cemeteries, a separate building may be provided for cremations, including a chapel where the committal service can be conducted. In most instances, however, the funeral service is concluded later to be kept in an urn, buried, or scattered.

Anatomical Gifts

Body donation is most commonly arranged with medical schools for the purpose of advancing the education of those preparing to become doctors or surgeons, specifically for dissection classes. Organ or tissue donation is important for the progress of medical science as well as for the continued functioning—perhaps even the life—of the recipient. Neither type of donation precludes the possibility of a funeral, which would either take place prior to the transfer of the entire body to a medical school or follow the removal of the donated organs and tissues.

If body donation is being considered, it is important to make prior arrangement with the medical school involved, as only a limited number of bodies can be accepted at any time, and donations occasionally exceed the need. Transportation expense may or may not be met by the school.

The national *Uniform Anatomical Gift Act* enables willing donors to make gifts of particular parts of the body without legal complications, although the intention should be made clear beforehand to one's immediate family. Uniform donor cards are generally available from the national organizations that endorse and encourage particular kinds of organ transplants. If you are interested in becoming a kidney donor, write the National Kidney Foundation, 116 East 27th Street, New York, NY 10016. If you would like to donate your eyes to someone in need of a corneal transplant, write the Eye Bank Association of America, 3195 Maplewood Avenue, Winston-Salem, NC 27103.

The 1979 *Illinois Rules of the Road* includes the following reference to the organ donor program: "Anatomical gift donors in Illinois may now place an organ donor sticker on the upper right hand corner of the back of their driver's license, to indicate that they are carrying an Anatomical Gift card, which gives specific direction regarding the organs to be donated in case of death. Organ donor stickers and anatomical Gift Cards may be provided by any person, hospital, school, medical group or association interested in assisting the Uniform Anatomical Gift Act." Such associations are usually listed in the classified telephone directory under the heading "Social Service Associations."

Conclusion

"It is the inalienable right of every American to have freedom of choice whether it involves the election of a candidate for political office, the kind of clothes he wants to wear, the kind of schools to which he wants to send his children, the kind of wedding he wants his daughter to have. So it is when it comes to the selection of a funeral. The right remains that of the individual or family to purchase a funeral service of their own choice, at the price they wish to pay, from the funeral director of their choice. No reputable funeral director would presume it should be otherwise.

"Reputable firms urge you to select, in advance of any emergency, the funeral director in whom you can have confidence. Visit his funeral home, observe his facilities, meet his staff, ask questions, inquire about prices, see his selection room. Tell him about the kind of service you desire for yourself or your family. He will respect your wishes and those of your loved ones."

(Excerpt from *Facts about Funeral Service Every Family Should Know*, available without charge from the National Foundation of Funeral Service, 1614 Central Street, Evanston, IL 60201.)

INDEX